GLOBAL
MEDICAL MISSIONS
PREPARATION, PROCEDURE, PRACTICE

EDITED BY
W KUHN · S KUHN · H GROSS · S BENESH

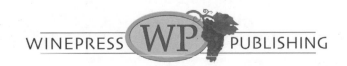

WINEPRESS WP PUBLISHING

This publication is designed to provide accurate and authoritative information in regard to the subject matter covered. It is distributed with the understanding that the publisher is not engaged in rendering legal, accounting, medical or other professional services. If legal advice or other professional assistance is required, the services of a competent professional person in a related field should be sought.

— From a Declaration of Principles jointly adopted by a Committee of the American Bar Association and a Committee of Publishers and Associations.

About the Authors

Susan M. Benesh, RN, MS

Nurse Clinician, community health and academic background, taught nursing at Wayne State University and Oklahoma State University. Now she volunteers with her home church and Mission to the World with Academic Medical Teams. She is married to Bruce and they share their home with three children, two dogs and two cats.

Keith R. Bucklen, MD, FACS

General surgeon practicing in the northwest suburbs of Charlotte, NC. Medicine and surgery are his vocation – family and missions are his passion. Early in his career, he served as a church planter under Mission to the World (Presbyterian Church in America) in West Africa, where he explored new medical missions models. Since his return to the States in 1991, he has been involved in missions at several levels – local church committee, denominational missions committee, various seminars and speaking opportunities, and frequent short-term missionary service. He is often accompanied to the field by his nurse wife, Janet, together with whom he has six children and six grandchildren.

Ann M. Butler, RPh, MD

Assistant Professor - Medical College of Georgia, Augusta, GA. Certified in Family Medicine. Licensed Georgia Pharmacist. Member of Crestview Baptist Church where she volunteers as pianist. She has participated in several mission trips with MTW including Philippines, Myanmar, Peru, and Bangladesh.

Jim Carroll, MD

Professor and Chief, Child Neurology, Medical College of Georgia. Vice-Chairman, Department of Neurology, Medical College of Georgia. Director of Child Neurology Training Program, MCG. Active in basic neuroscience research in the area of adult stem cell transplantation. Leader for numerous short term mission trips, with specific interest in the Middle East. He worked in Middle East for several years.

Shirley Carroll, MSW

She has a background in social work and is currently rearing eight children. She has participated in numerous mission trips in various capacities. Often runs the eyeglass clinic. She is married to Dr. Jim Carroll and served together with him in the Middle East.

David Foster, NCC, LPC, LMFT

National Certified Counselor, Licensed Professional Counselor, Licensed Marriage and Family Therapist. David Foster is Director of Clinical Services for Warren-Yazoo Mental Health Service in Vicksburg, MS. He also is an Adjunct Instructor in marriage and family therapy at Reformed Theological Seminary. He has been extensively involved in training, disaster relief, and medical missions work with Mission to the World. Clinical Member and Approved Supervisor with the American Association for Marriage and Family Therapy. He is married to Vicki. They have three adult children: Kelly, Colin, and Craig.

Hartmut Gross, MD, FACEP

Professor of emergency medicine, pediatrics and neurology at the Medical College of Georgia (MCG). He is co-director of International Medicine at MCG with Walter "Ted" Kuhn. He is director of both MCG's Special Events Medical Team and the Emergency Department Under-graduate Medical Education. Volunteering on Missions to the World (MTW) in developing countries since 1999, he is also faculty at MTW's annual Medical Mission Leadership Training course. He and his family share their home with a growing collection of insects from around the world.

Jamie L. Johnson Kornegay, MPT
Physical therapist at Baptist Princeton Hospital in Birmingham, Alabama. She graduated from the University of Alabama at Birmingham with a Masters in Physical Therapy and is currently working on her doctoral degree in Physical Therapy with an Orthopedic and Manual Therapy Certification. She is on staff with the Medical Campus Outreach and Christian Medical Ministry of Alabama and is intricately involved with medical and physical therapy student discipleship and organization of short term medical mission trips. Her passion is to use physical therapy as an instrument for the Gospel throughout the world. Jamie is married to Dr. Matthew Kornegay and partners with him in leading short-term student medical mission trips and discipleship training of medical and physical therapy students.

W. "Ted" Kuhn, MD, DTMTH
Professor of emergency medicine and associate professor of pediatrics at the Medical College of Georgia where he is co-director of International Medicine with Dr. Hartmut Gross in MCG's Center for Operational Medicine. He sub-specializes in tropical medicine and travel medicine. Dr. Kuhn serves as co-medical director of Mission to the World, Presbyterian Church in America, with his wife Sharon. Both he and his wife were career medical missionaries in South Asia before joining the faculty at MCG and as staff at MTW.

Sharon Kuhn, MD, DTMTH
Associate professor of Family Medicine at the Medical College of Georgia and also specializes in tropical medicine and travel medicine. She served as a career medical missionary in South Asia before joining Mission to the World as co-medical director with her husband, Dr. Ted Kuhn.

Jill Black Lattanzi, PT, EdD
B.S. in physical therapy, an M.S. in exercise physiology, and a doctorate in education. Her doctoral work focused on cultural competency training for physi-cal therapy students. She has presented internationally and is publishing a text on the topic. She has been taking students and physical therapy professionals on physical therapy medical mission trips to Mexico and other parts of Central and South America and the Caribbean since 1990.

Meghan Lee, MPT, ATC
Physical Therapist at the Joseph M Still Burn Unit in Augusta, GA. Meghan became involved with missions as a physical therapy student. Before graduating in 2003, she was involved as a student leader in planning logistical, clinical, and spiritual aspects of trips. Meghan currently works with Medical Campus Outreach at the Medical College of Georgia where she works with students leading bible studies and discipleship on campus. She is also a team leader for MTW and leads short term trips for students.

Doreen Hung Mar, MD, DTMTH
Career non-resident medical missionary with Mission to the World, the mission-sending agency of the PCA. She is based in Northern Virginia. Though trained in internal medicine and most recently in tropical medicine, she works only part-time in emergency medicine. She delights in being able to share her gifts with others, at home and especially abroad on medical mission trips!

Annette Merlino, DMD
General dentist practicing outside of Pittsburgh, PA. She has been involved in mission dentistry since graduating sixteen years ago, averaging three trips each year, working in Africa, Asia, and Central and South America.

Brian D. Riedel, MD
Pediatric gastroenterologist and served with Mission to the World as a medical missionary from 1999 to 2004 chiefly among the Quechuas of the Cuzco area high in the southern Andes mountains.

health ministry among the poor. Dr. Riedel maintains an appointment as Assistant Clinical Professor of Pediatrics at the Vanderbilt University School of Medicine, where he served on the full time academic faculty for six years before going to the mission field.

John Sexton, RN-C, FNP, MSN Community Health

(University of Virginia). Full time missionary with MTW medical department. He has served in Peru, Mexico, and now serve teams throughout the world with MTW.

Brian Stansfield, MD

Currently a pediatric resident at the Medical College of Georgia and plans to pursue a career in neonatology. His interest in international medical missions developed through Medical Campus Outreach which is a nondenominational Christian ministry to the medical community. He has been on multiple short term medical teams and desires to continue participating in medical missions throughout his career. He is married to Mindy who began her residency in Pediatrics in 2006 and she shares his passion for international medicine.

Tom Stewart, MD

Graduated from the University of Florida College of Medicine and completed residency training in pathology at the Medical College of Georgia. He served as a flight surgeon with the Air Force for three years. Tom was in pathology private practice for 15 years before he joined Mission to the World as director of Street Child ministries in 2000.

Bess Tarkington, RN

Upon graduating from the University of Virginia School of Nursing, Bess worked in the clinical setting at the UVA Medical Center for eight years. While working at UVA and volunteering at the local free clinic, Bess developed a growing interest in the care of HIV positive individuals and their families. She served for three years with the medical department of MTW before returning to the University of Virginia in 2006.

Cynthia Urbanowicz, RN, CEN, HP

Has extensive training in emergency medicine, critical care, flight medicine and disaster planning. She has led numerous MTW teams and also served as the assistant medical director for MTW's medical department. Cyndi currently serves as MTW's director of disaster response.

James Wilde, MD

Associate professor of Pediatrics and Emergency Medicine at the Medical College of Georgia. He is fellowship trained in both pediatric infectious diseases and pediatric emergency medicine. He currently serves as Director of Pediatric Emergency Medicine and as co-director of research for the Department of EM. His work in international medicine has taken him to Liberia, the Peruvian Amazon, Haiti, and Thailand.

Dedication

This book is dedicated to Joshua and Lydia, who throughout the years have shared our vision and our many medical mission adventures.

And to our dear friends and colleagues, Wallace and Opal, without whose vision, persistent support, guidance and loving patience, the medical outreach of MTW would never have become a reality.

I thank my God upon every remembrance of you,
always in every prayer of mine
making request for you all with joy,
for your fellowship in the gospel
from the first day until now.
-Philippians 1:3-5

Ted and Sharon Kuhn

I dedicate my efforts on this book to my wonderful wife, Vickie, and our children Michael and Monica, who encourage and support my mission travels.

Hartmut Gross

Dedicated to those who have encouraged and supported me on this journey and to all of those people who have gone before me. Especially to Bruce, John, Connie and Barbara, Mom and Jack.

Susan Benesh

Acknowledgements

Allie Tsavdarides for her generous assistance in photo editing. Thank you for helping us share the vision.

Lydia Kuhn and Bob Bradbury for their provision of photographs. Thank you for sharing your artistry in capturing the visual impact of stories from around the world.

Final layout by Julie Phinney, Books and Periodicals Prepress Services, Bozeman, MT, 406-586-1297.

Table Of Contents

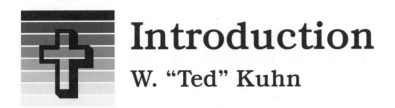

Introduction
W. "Ted" Kuhn

This book was written with you, our fellow health care professional and international sojourner in mind. It was designed to provide the resources and knowledge base needed to effectively minister to the poor and needy around the world often in adverse conditions. Whether your travel includes remote tropical jungles or vast expanses of "concrete jungle," whether it involves the slums of major world cities or the thin air of mountain top villages, or whether it involves the lecture halls of great medical universities, this was written as a vital resource and guide for you from those who have walked before you.

If you have felt God's call to bring healing to diseased ravaged bodies and the message of salvation to a world in need of the touch of the Master's hand, there is something here for you. If your heart is moved by masses dying of AIDS in Africa, or thousands dying of malaria in Asia, or homeless children on the streets of Manila, or if you long to comfort grieving survivors of a major earthquake, read on! If you believe in your heart that there is something more to life than filling out insurance forms and updates on the newest government regulations to US health care and defensive medical practices, you will be refreshed by many of the authors in this text. If you seek to comfort the world's poor, rather than to be in comfort, to give of what you have rather than to receive more financial reimbursement, to extend God's love rather than safely huddle together in our own social circles, to bring joy where there is sadness, hope where there is despair, faith where there is doubt,[1] then come, walk with us as a sojourner and fellow traveler in the most blessed, the most exciting, the most fulfilling path you will ever find this side of eternity.

Some of you, no doubt, are about to embark on a change of direction in your life. If it is true, and I believe it is, that you receive by giving, then you are about to receive much. You have set aside your time and finances, and decided to give to those less fortunate than you. To serve and to sacrifice is always honorable and to be commended.

I have spent many years traveling in underdeveloped countries. I have learned much from my mistakes. I assure you that there is hardly a more uncomfortable feeling than to be sick, even bedridden, in a foreign country with a language barrier and an uncertain medical delivery system. I have vomited in the rice paddies of Southeast Asia and squatted under banana trees in the subcontinent. I have had altitude headaches in the Andes and jet lag in Hong Kong. I have had to drink river water in the Amazon and eat street food in the Middle East. I have had heat exhaustion in Central America and been wet and cold in the Himalayas. The task of this text is to prepare you medically and emotionally for what is to come. While it is not always possible to anticipate every need, and there is never a guarantee that travel in other countries is safe, there is still much to be said for preparedness.

This text was written by my friends and colleagues, all people experienced and interested in protecting you and your team from the hazards of travel in developing countries. The goal of this text is not only to prepare you personally, but to enable you to prepare and lead others into the developoping world. The authors have attempted to give you the latest information, and in the areas where medical information is rapidly changing, they have given you the resources to update current thought. They have also provided contact information for obtaining medicines and supplies for health ministry overseas. While you may not need all the information contained in this text, every traveler will benefit from some of what is included. We wish to speed you safely on your way. God bless and "vaya con Dios."[2]

Blessings,
Ted Kuhn

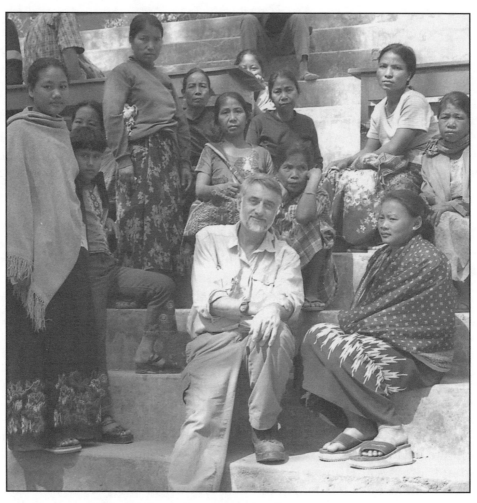

Ted Kuhn/
"Bangladesh"

References
1. Paraphrased from "The Prayer of St. Francis"
2. "Vaya con Dios" translated from Spanish means "Go with God."

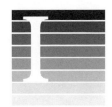

Section I:
Individual Preparation for International Travel

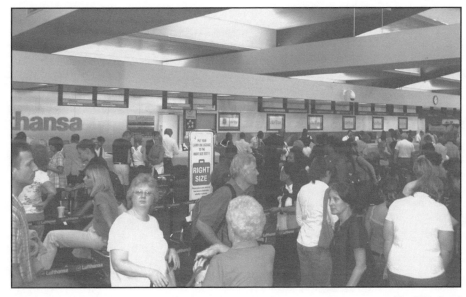

Ted Kuhn/
"One Hour Check-in at Airport"

3

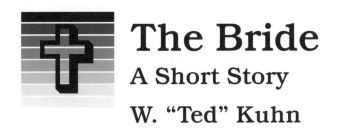

The Bride
A Short Story
W. "Ted" Kuhn

urely the presence of the Lord is in this place, I can feel His mighty power and His grace. I can hear the rush of angels' wings; I see glory on each face. Surely the presence of the Lord is in this place."1 Hands lifted in worship. Eyes gazing toward heaven searching for the glory of God in the face of Jesus. Hearts overflowing with love. Music played softly on a keyboard, words of the praise song projected onto a wall. All brothers and sisters in Christ, for the moment, lost in wonder, love and praise.

Hot, humid, Sunday morning air greeted me through the open window of the small church. I could see the street outside, passersby busy with life and indifferent to the worship inside. A concrete promenade, a mud bank, then the mighty Amazon River. The river, evidently no more anxious than I to rush on this sultry, Sunday morning. Debris and banana leaves floated slowly past. The sprawling slum of Belén just yards from the sanctuary. Fifty thousand people crammed into a watery sewer squeezed between the banks of the Amazon and the promenade of the city of Iquitos. Mid-morning slum-life clearly visible from where I stood. A cesspool of suffering and misery.

I had walked through the Belén market the day before. Climbing ancient stairs, I had entered by a small, dirt path, stepping into the putrefying throat of the immense garbage dump. Men and women, placed there by fate or by providence, a universe away from my world. The smell of rotting fish

and refuse oppressive beyond tolerance. The crowd lightly pushing, shoulder-to-shoulder, a gentle tide of humanity surging between stalls of dried fish, spices, goat heads and fresh meat. Several hundred people rummaged through a table of used clothes, filthy from a thousand muddy hands. Goat entrails hung from a nail above me. A young girl squatted to relieve herself on the path. She pulled her dress above her waist. Her private areas plainly visible to anyone who chose to watch. But curiously, no one watched. No shame, no embarrassment, no alternative. And for a moment, countless eyes diverted, permitting an instant of privacy. Perhaps a shared accommodation, a simple, unexpected gift. Collective decency in a slum offering no respect for human existence.

Mounting the steps, I unexpectedly stood face-to-face with a middle-aged woman blocking the path in front of me. She would have been in her mid-forties. She was

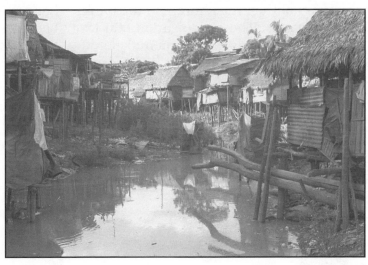

Ted Kuhn/
"Belén"

dressed in a dirty, white, woven, plastic flour sack with holes cut for the arms and neck. The red advertising letters of the flour brand visible around the hem. The sack minimally covered her body exposing her thin legs at the mid-upper-thigh. Her black, tangled and twisted hair, matted on her head. Her face, pockmarked with sores from the bites of a hundred mosquitoes. Her broad, bare, calloused feet, looked excessively large in comparison to her skinny legs, almost like shoes too big. A half-naked, middle-aged harlot, standing on a little mound of fresh garbage in the middle of one of the worst slums in the world. The absolute bottom of the food chain of humanity. Selling her diseased body to any man with a few pesos, not quite the cost of a can of soda.

Thousands of years ago, God commanded one of his prophets to marry just such a woman. An immoral woman, impure, selfish, drunken and full of deceit. Hideous in the flesh. Not surprisingly, she would prove to be an unfaithful wife. For sale to anyone with a few coins. Yet Hosea committed his life to her and redeemed her from her many adulterous affairs. Choosing her, and only her, for his bride from all the daughters of the nations. Giving her what no one else was willing to give, his life and his unconditional love.

On the wings of the hot, humid air, the sweet sound of the praise chorus carried me back, through the window and into the sanctuary of the little church on the banks of the Amazon. The congregation still lost in praise, oblivious to my mental detour through the adjacent slums. Unaware of the beggar woman, whom I had met yesterday only yards from the sanctuary. The church, the beautiful Bride of Christ. Pure and holy, presented without spot or blemish. Greatly loved, redeemed by the blood of the Bridegroom. The Bride, destined before the foundations of the world to be resplendent in her beauty at the marriage feast of the Lamb. Arrangements perfect and complete. And all creation, from eternity past until now waits in anxious anticipation for the revealing of the bride.

The church, the beloved, the betrothed, as filthy and as unfaithful as Hosea's wife and the harlot of Belén. The church, hideous in her sin, standing on the garbage dump of deceit, pride and division. Waiting for the bridegroom, the bride adorned in a white, plastic flour sack. Her hair dirty and matted, feet cracked and muddy, face covered in sores. Fleeing from the unconditional love of the bridegroom. Selling herself to anyone for anything. The church, who could love her? And who would choose her from among all the peoples of the earth to be His bride, His only bride?

Yet this is the beloved bride of the Son. Transformed by the unconditional love of the bridegroom. And that which the Son loves- can we love any less? "Surely the presence of the Lord is in this place, I can feel His mighty power and His grace. I can hear the rush of angels' wings; I see glory on each face. Surely the presence of the Lord is in this place."[1] In Christ, the harlot becomes a virgin again. Your church, your bride awaits. The Spirit and the Bride say "Come." Come swiftly, Lord Jesus.

Reference

1. *Surely the Presence,* Copyright 1977, Lanny Wolfe Music.

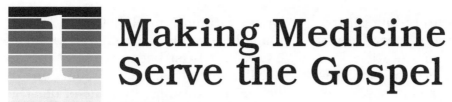

Making Medicine Serve the Gospel

Keith R. Bucklen

If medical missions are to be an effective tool for advancing the Gospel, and not random acts of mercy without a message, it must be strategic. Too often, the demands of health care delivery may be so overwhelming as to consume a disproportionate share of time and resources at the expense of the Gospel ministry. Forethought and planning are necessary for effective Christian medical outreach. This is not a forced fit. On the contrary, medicine and evangelism are fundamentally connected and the Gospel message is imparted quite naturally through medicine. Physical and spiritual man are wrapped up into one being: sickness impacts the whole man, including his mind, emotions and spirit; conversely, habitual sin often leads to physical illness. The very practice of medicine is an opportunity to live out the Gospel. Love, mercy, compassion, sacrifice, and healing are all aspects of Christ's work, effortlessly demonstrated during the course of medical ministries. The health care provider is ideally situated to evangelize rather than to be simply a medical "foot in the door" for clergy.

Regardless of the science brought to bear on a person's illness, the results are at best short-lived (no pun intended) and medical care is not an end in itself. Every patient will become ill again and all will eventually die. Mankind has an inescapably terminal disease, sin, and any health care that does not take this into account is, at best, incomplete. The only remedy offered for sin is the Gospel of Jesus Christ. Only His work in the human heart is able to address both the root cause of sin and its consequences, and is able to alter the natural course of life, both now and for all eternity. So, infinitely more important than the medical care rendered is the impact of the Message of Life communicated in the process by the Christian health care worker.

Given the natural relationship between medicine and the Gospel, are there more effective ways to use medicine as a missions tool to expand the Church around the world? Some traditional medical mission models fail to capitalize on the opportunity health care offers the Gospel ministry in today's environment. With careful planning, flexibility, humility and a servant's heart, the modern medical missionary can move as the Spirit of God moves, providing mercy, healing, compassionate care and effectively communicating the Word of Life. It is incumbent upon us to design Christian medical outreach in such a way that medicine serves the Gospel and not vice versa.

Medical Mission Compounds and the "Traditional" Model

The historically dominant model of medical missions is facility based. Typically, the mission compound is an enclave, or expatriate community, living separately from the local community. There is often a small hospital, support facilities, housing for personnel and a chapel or church. These buildings are usually surrounded by a wall or fence. The expatriate community lives in, but separate from and not quite part of the host community or culture. The mother tongue of the missionaries is the usual default for communication. The culture on the compound is clearly expatriate. Mission compounds produce a sense of separation from the host culture, both for the missionaries and the denizens of the host country.

There were undoubtedly good reasons why this historical model was developed. Principally, the medical missions compound offered control both of medical care and the ministry. The compound provided efficient administration of the work, with all facilities in one place under one administrative structure. The compound also afforded a degree of protection and security in an often hostile culture.

Western mission enterprise has historically benefited from the traditional model. Nevertheless, in the current context of modern missions and the current world milieu, the traditional model has too many shortcomings to be of much contemporary use.

1. "For a church to impact a culture, it must be of that culture."[1] National evangelicals in developing countries have taken an increasing role in ownership for evangelism within their country, often with the assistance of foreign missionaries. But the concept of expatriates assuming total responsibility for this is becoming more and more unwelcome. The most fruitful church planting efforts in the last century are consistent with the culture, and originate *from* the culture of the host country. The success of contemporary evangelical movements in Asia, South America and multiple African nations, sometimes without any outside aid, underscores this point.

2. Western missionaries, living within a western context, supporting a mainly western style of worship is a "colonial" model of church planting which is increasingly unwanted in many developing nations. Not only is this model unwelcome, but it is less successful than nationally motivated and nationally led church planting movements. The Biblical model for missions is an "incarnational" model. Christ "lived, made his dwelling, among us" (John 1: 14, NIV). Christ became one of us, he lived as one of us, he worked as one of us and he worshiped as one of us. The model of a mission compound, a culture within a culture, is not consistent with the biblical model.

3. Common people, who have limited access to health care, may appreciate missionary medicine, even if it is dispensed from a compound. However, at the governmental level, the mission hospital may be an offense to national pride. In many settings, the official health care authority regularly challenges the mission's right to exist with demands for "proof" of compliance with (often unreasonable) regulations, and then it issues only temporary permits to remain in operation and threatens revocation of missionary visas.

4. From a professional perspective, foreign medical institutions, especially ones that are lavishly equipped (by the standards in that country), subsidized with western funds and offering care at discounted fees, pose the threat of competition for national health care providers. Often there is resistance to the mission hospital from this financially and politically powerful group.

5. Western style medicine, as is often practiced in mission hospitals, is too expensive for the local church to longitudinally support and supervise. The frequently stated goal of "turning over" the medical work to the local church is unrealistic and financially unobtainable and is probably poor stewardship of scarce church monetary resources. Without a continuous flow of financial and human assets from the foreign mission agency, the possibility of passing responsibility for the mission hospital to the local church is doomed.

6. The purpose of the missionary compound is advertised at the front gate. There are often labels or signs declaring "Christian" or the name of a sponsoring denomination or affiliated religious organization. But that very same label can become

an obstacle for some. It may become an invitation for manipulation by those who quickly learn that the "price" of a visit is the appearance of receptivity to the message being promoted.

7. When the Spirit of God moves, bricks and mortar find it hard to follow. Putting down roots into a community that God is working in today makes it difficult or impossible for the medical missionary to move when the Spirit of God moves them tomorrow: into a different community, a different village, a different ethnic group or perhaps even different country.

8. The real threat to the survival of the historical medical mission model, however, comes from within. The priority, regardless of stated philosophy, is medicine rather than the Gospel. It has to be. The most common limiting resource is almost always medical personnel and supplies. And since the very witness of the work is based on the delivery of quality health care, inadequate medical staffing (or facilities, equipment, etc.) is self-defeating. So, when resources are scarce, medicine gets center stage.

The need for new models of medical missions seems clear. But what are the alternatives? How do we exercise this ministry of mercy in today's environment? How do we use medicine as a tool for evangelism without creating opposition? What is the best overall stewardship of medical, financial and human resources to achieve our corporate goal of planting churches? In short, how do we make medicine serve the Gospel, and promote local, successful church planting movements?

Blueprints for a New Model

Creative paradigms for medical ministry are derived from sound strategy development. The priority of outreach is most essential. The work must be structured in such a way that nothing threatens the mission of advancing the Gospel of Jesus Christ. Regardless of the excellence of medical care, the model must be judged on the basis of effective evangelism.

First of all, the work must begin and end with the Church. Any medical outreach that is not a well-mitered part of the ecclesiastical whole is only a splinter that has potential to become a foreign body and fester. The medical work must be the answer to a perceived need on the part of the church and not an end in itself. It must be envisioned and developed by the church; and most importantly, it must report to the church. When Christian medical ministries take on a life of their own, apart from the Church, they become self-serving and an eventual drain of resources. Not only must missionary medical projects be a child of the sending church, their ministry and strategy must be ultimately coordinated with the national church, even when that means their termination.

A focus on contacts, rather than on activity, is critical to fruitfulness. In a sense, the medical activity must be incidental, not second-rate, but secondary to the prime directive of reaching people with the true lifesaving Message. Missions must be people-oriented, not chiefly about programs, facilities, plans, etc. The design of a medical outreach must maximize interaction with individuals.

Serving with humility in the host country is a key characteristic. This is demonstrated above all by personal flexibility. An effective medical missionary must not insist on doing what he knows how to do and is comfortable with; but he should exhibit such a passion for the Gospel that he is willing to fill any role that will further the cause of Christ. The work, then, should be adapted to the medical opportunity that God, in his sovereignty, provides, however trivial or obscure. And the workers must be united in both commitment and love; for in this is the power of the Good News visible and the reality of the claims of Christ most convincingly displayed. "Your love for one another will prove to the world that you are my disciples." (John 13:35, NLT) If the Gospel cannot transform the medical team, on both an individual and group level, it has nothing to say to the host culture.

Several years ago, American medical missionaries were sent to assist in disaster relief following a devastating earthquake. Thousands had died and the medical resources of the area were overwhelmed. The first wave of missionary medical personnel arriving in the country were surprised by the local health care workers' reluctance to accept their offers of assistance. In typical western (American) fashion, the "secular" medical teams who had preceded them, took charge. The backlash from the local providers was an attempt to regain some sense of responsibility for their own countrymen and recoup personal dignity. The only request for help came from the lone national pharmacist. The missionary doctors volunteered for the task of sorting through piles of donated medicines and organizing a makeshift tent pharmacy, a job that would take several days. The task was well beneath the capabilities of these missionary physicians. Nevertheless, they lovingly carried out the assignment without complaint, in humility. This humility was a powerful witness and generated harmony between the medical missionaries and indigenous providers. In the end, this simple act of submission and service was a powerful apologetic for the Gospel. It enhanced both the medical care of the disaster victims as well as the Gospel outreach and is remembered and still spoken of years later.

Needless to say, commitment to prayer and personal submission are the spiritual ingredients of humility. These character traits are antithetical to all that we learn in western medicine (and with which our sin-stained personalities fully cooperate): i.e., action and control. Medical missionaries must cultivate these qualities of prayerfulness and personal submission to authority, above all, to God's authority, *before* arriving on the field, since the shock of trying to function in a new culture will only make prayerless activity and the need for man-made structure more attractive.

Beyond the character issues of strategy development, there are certain design aspects that will make new models of medical missions more likely to bear fruit for Christ. Finding (or creating) the right medical niche is paramount. If there is a clear medical need in the host country, filling that vacancy is very likely to yield vast ministry opportunities with minimal competition (or resentment), since there is usually a good reason why host culture medical providers have not filled it. One such work was the lifelong preoccupation of Dr. Paul Brand with lepers, first among the outcasts in India and then in Louisiana.[2] Missionaries have found similar ministry possibilities providing medical care for other disenfranchised groups: disabled, impoverished, orphaned, ethnically marginalized, prostitutes, street children, psychiatrically ill and patients dying of AIDS to name a few.

Minimizing institutional requirements is usually advantageous. As with most material possessions, it often becomes difficult to distinguish between missionaries and their medical facilities. Simplicity is a virtue in cross-cultural medical outreach. Not only do missionary medical institutions require staffing, equipment and maintenance, but all this becomes much more complicated in a foreign environment. What is more, transitioning the church planting work from the mission to the national church is often hindered by the expectation that such medical works should continue.

It may be best to work within the existing health care system, if it is an option. Doing so will place the missionary in the role of learner, something that is sometimes quite foreign (no pun intended). This may be uncomfortable for many American health care workers but is an excellent position from which to offer the Gospel without threat. This is especially true in cultures where the brash, "American" personality is not valued, or is even resented. Supporting the indigenous medical order pays a compliment to the host country and often opens the door to ministry among national health care personnel as well as patients. At the very least, working within the system minimizes the need for investment of missionary resources in facilities and the threat of competition with the country's own providers.

The practice model the medical missionary employs must make sense to both providers and patients in the host country. The medical missionary must be able to explain in an understandable way, why he has left the most prosperous nation in the world to practice medicine abroad. Has he been barred or ostracized from working in his own country? Has his stateside practice failed; or has the drain of American competition propelled him here? Is he hoping to become wealthy from an untapped foreign market? Is he feeling superior with misguided pity for the "poor and ignorant locals?" People must not only understand the reasons, they must find the reasons plausible and acceptable.

One can become just as distracted from a Gospel focus by the demands of medical care as by buildings and personnel; so choosing a health care outreach that has limited (or at least, does not have unlimited) demands is desirable. Avoid a highly-structured medical practice. Flexibility is the key. A missionary health care worker who can regulate his/her own schedule is much more likely to be available for the Gospel enterprise. I have heard career missionary physicians complain, almost without exception, that they are as busy (and often busier) on the field than they were in a stateside practice; and they usually lament the fact that they have almost no time for verbal evangelism, much less for friendship ministry. What a shame (and no accident in the grand scheme of spiritual warfare) that the person so ideally equipped for outreach has so precious little time for it.

Your role in this "new model" of medical missions *could be* exciting, prestigious and high profile, but it is much *more likely* to be enlightening, humbling, discouraging and outside your area of expertise. You can be virtually certain that your part won't be what you expected, it won't be what you are used to; and it won't be what you are comfortable with. That's when we need to be reminded that when our world seems out of control, it is only out of *our* control. As Paul was reassured by the Lord himself: "My grace is sufficient for you, for my power is made perfect in weakness." (2 Cor. 12:9)

Finally, when looking for a place of medical service from which to launch a spiritual outreach, be bold and creative. As William Carey, renowned 18th century missionary

to India is recorded to have said, "Attempt great things for God; expect great things from God." The Old Testament priests did not see the water part until they stepped into it; and neither will we (Joshua 3:15, 16). This attitude is nowhere more crucial to an abundant harvest for the Gospel than in the realm of medical missions. We should adopt the mandate of the Federation Star Fleet from the *Star Trek®* television

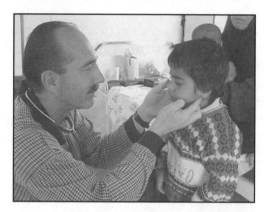

Bob Bradbury/
"Examination of a Patient in the Middle East"

series: "to boldly go where no one has gone before."

Another Residency, Missionary Medicine?

Most of us practicing in a North American health care setting have had as many years of training as we care to have. We consider ourselves ready for medical missions on the basis of our training and experience within the American health care context. But fruitful service in a "new model," the kind described above, will likely require additional preparation. Language acquisition, difficult even for those with an aptitude for it, is essential. On yesteryear's hospital compound, the translated tongue of the missionary was the order of the day. But mastering the heart language of the people is a must for dynamic communication. Consider the Apostle Paul who, on his missionary journeys, spoke at least one of the languages familiar to the people. And how thankful we must be that Christ, known in the Bible as the incarnate "Word," did not come down from Heaven speaking only the tongue of angels!

To be adequately equipped to effectively minister the Gospel, general training in cross-cultural ministry is indispensable. Health care personnel are often "excused" from evangelism and church planting courses (and the cultural *faux pas* the courses help obviate) because of the medical skills and services they offer. But if they are to be more than a springboard for outreach by others, health care workers must have a firm grasp on scripture, basic theology, other belief systems, the contextualized expression of Christian doctrines, etc.

And if medicine is going to truly serve the Church, the adaptability demanded of the Christian health care practitioner may require additional medical (or related) training. As the Lord provides an avenue for outreach, we must be prepared to follow. Whether it is deaf ministry and sign language, community health, or AIDS ministry, the vehicle by which the Good News is offered must be finely tuned. Attempting to make the church planting ministry conform itself around our preferred medical work is contrary to the stated priority of the mission and becomes the proverbial "tail wagging the dog."

Can all this actually be implemented? Innovative and effective Christian medical ministry *is* beginning to take place around the world. It is taking numerous forms; community health, outpatient clinics, academic teaching ministries, and private practice, as many of these principles find expression in the lives of a new generation of medical missionaries.

Short-Term Ministry, Long-Term Gain?

Short-term medical teams are a fresh approach to Christian medical ministry.

Although they can be misused as an excuse for an exciting overseas adventure or a church-subsidized vacation, they can also be used strategically to further the cause of Christ cross-culturally. Short-term teams can provide care to indigent patients, offer academic interaction, administer relief to victims of disaster, help staff a national church medical initiative and so on. As such, they must be part of a larger strategy, a tool for long-term church planters. They suffer from lack of cultural adaptation, and familiarity with the language of the host country, etc.; nonetheless, they are real, proven and valuable tools in world evangelization. In the context of the "new model," where medicine must serve the Gospel, the short-term medical teams "travel light." Since, by definition, such work is not institutionalized, the Church is not generally burdened by heavy demands on its resources. Additionally, short-term medical projects leave no obligation on the part of the national church to pick up the leftovers when the expatriates leave.

Good News at Any Cost

None of the models of medical missions should be considered the ultimate pattern to be reproduced. Cultures and people are dynamic. Missionary teams are as unique as are the individuals who comprise them. The needs and opportunities are ever-changing, and the Spirit of God moves as He wills. Effective Christian medical missions will never be monolithic in design. They will certainly be as varied as the churches themselves. The opportunity to develop a fruitful paradigm for outreach, one in which medicine becomes a "good and faithful servant," is restricted only by the health care worker's submission to the Church, personal and spiritual maturity, imagination and creativity, and determination to promote the Good News at any cost.

References
1. Kooistra P: Toward a Definition of Church-Planting Movements, *Looking Forward*, Winepress, 2003.
2. Brand P: *The Gift of Pain*, Zondervan, 1997.

Preparing Yourself and Your Family for Short Term Missions

David Foster

Potential Benefits of Short-term
     Mission Participation
Preparation Checklist

What if Jonah had been better prepared for his mission trip to Nineveh? How differently would the scriptures have recorded his story? His outright disobedience to God, his cultural bias, deep-set resentment and shortsightedness haunt us through the four chapters of his book. We are left at the end of the account of his ministry in Nineveh with an open-ended question; did he remain bitter or did he get better as a result of having gone to Nineveh? Jonah provides us with a benchmark to check ourselves against as we consider short-term missions work. Like Jonah, we are faced with the potential for success or failure in our short-term missions endeavors. Adequate preparation is critical in heightening the prospects for a positive outcome.

Potential Benefits of Short-term Mission Participation

First, the participant can gain an enlarged view of God and what He is doing in the world. The disciples in John 4 observed Jesus' ministry to the Samaritan woman at the well, likewise, we too can see the power of God at work across cultural and racial divides.

Second, short term mission involvement can yield a broadened view of the Body of Christ. It is no small thing for a "short termer" to return home with the notion firmly fixed in their head that the people they worshipped with in a foreign land are truly brothers and sisters in Christ. (Acts 10:28, 34, 35)

Third, we can gain a heightened sensitivity to the needs of the world. Awareness of issues of injustice, poverty, and illness can pave the way for future mercy ministry and friendship evangelism.

Fourth, increased prayer is often a product of short-term missions participation. Like Paul in Colossians 1:3–14, we may begin to pray for people we know and even those we do not know. We can pray for the missionaries, church members, and particular needs that we are aware of.

There is also a *fifth* benefit. There is the potential for increased giving to the Lord's work at home and abroad. Jesus put it succinctly, "where your treasure is, there will your heart be also." (Mt. 6:21)

Further, it is a well-researched fact that short-term missions involvement results in increased likelihood of long-term mission field involvement. A majority of career missionaries come from the ranks of those who were initially short-term team members. Their hearts were touched and they began to feel the call of God on their lives. All of these benefits and many more are within the reach of those who heed the short-term call.

Of course, there are **negative possibilities** as well. Perhaps you have heard from those who have gone on mission trips and returned home bitter about the money and time expended. Foreign logistics, bureaucracy, and time schedules frustrate some. Others complain about the role they were given on the trip or the lack of response from the nationals. Probably the worst scenario involves those returning traumatized by exposure to violence, illness, injustice, or poverty. Most of these negative experiences can be prevented. Through adequate preparation, even challenging situations can become rewarding opportunities.

Preparation Checklist

There are seven areas of preparation worth highlighting. What follows is a suggestive, though not necessarily comprehensive, list of ways to get ready for short-term missions trips.

1. *Physical preparation*—Are you able to handle the physical demands of the trip? As Paul told Timothy, bodily training is of some value (I Tim. 4:8). You should strive through exercise, nutrition, rest and where needed, medication to insure your full participation on the trip.
2. *Cultural preparation*—Learn as much as you can about the country you are going to: its government, language, customs, taboos, history, and risks associated with traveling there.
3. *Logistical preparation*—Make sure all passports, visas, and immunization records are up to date. Check your packing list. Take clothes appropriate to the climate and setting.
4. *Mental preparation*—Develop a realistic expectation of the trip via learning about schedules, role you will be playing, possible inconveniences, etc.
5. *Spiritual preparation*—This is the most critical aspect of preparation. Pray about all aspects of the trip (logistics, team cohesiveness, opportunities for minis-

try, receptive audiences, etc.). Pray also for the mind-set exemplified by Christ in Philippians 2:3,4: a servant's heart.

6. *Team preparation*—The rebuilding of the wall at Jerusalem by Nehemiah and his cohorts serves as a ready example as to how a team can effectively function. Short-term missions teams work best in the abandonment of a "me" orientation and an adoption of a "we" orientation.
7. *Re-entry preparation*—It is often the case that participants return home to face many difficulties. Sometimes values change regarding material goods. It can be disturbing to return to an opulent US from an impoverished foreign setting. The need to talk about the trip may not always be met with receptive ears. The pace of life sometimes seems accelerated at home. Exposure to extreme injustice, poverty, and illness can be traumatizing. It is absolutely necessary that a debriefing be done following a missions experience. Maintaining connections with team members to process memories is also helpful. It may also be important to talk further with your local pastor or other ministry professional about your experience.

Through adequate preparation, short-term missions trips can be useful to the Body of Christ and personally rewarding. The decision is up to you. If you pursue missions according to Jonah's example, you may return bitter or have missed out on the rich opportunity you have been afforded. If you go with a giving heart and with a receiving heart, you will return a richly blessed individual.

Resources
1. Forward DC: *The Essential Guide to the Short Term Mission Trip*, Moody Press, 1998.
2. Mack J, Stiles L: *Leann's Guide to Short-Term Missions*, Intervarsity Press, 2000.
3. VanCise, M: *Successful Missions Teams*, Birmingham, AL., New Hope Publishers, 2004.

3 The Risk of Travel

W. "Ted" Kuhn

Many Americans travel to under-developed countries each year. Fortunately, only a few will ever experience a life-threatening illness or event. Often much time is spent worrying about terrorist attacks, earthquakes and tornadoes which, while devastating when they occur, are also rare and unlikely to affect most traveling Americans. On the contrary, the chance of developing a mild or a moderately disabling illness or injury during a 1 month stay in an underdeveloped country is actually quite high and a majority of travelers will develop gastrointestinal or respiratory symptoms during their travel. "During a 1 month stay, there is a 65–75% chance that a traveler will have some sort of illness or physical symptom. However, the chance of being hospitalized will be less than 1%."[1]

This figure obviously depends on the country you are visiting, the conditions of your stay and your personal risk-taking behavior, including your compliance with vaccinations, malaria prophylaxis and safe food practices. A stay in a 5 star hotel in a major third world city would put you at a much lower risk than sleeping in a tent in a rural area and working in squalid conditions with a refugee population in that same country, all else being equal.

Death and Disability During Travel

The good news is that most travel-related illnesses and injuries can be prevented or at least anticipated. Mortality while traveling is quite low and usually from only two circumstances: cardiac-related events; and, deaths due to trauma, the majority of which are motor vehicle and motorcycle related.[1] Our greatest fear, fatality from exotic infectious disease, actually accounts for less than 1% of all travel-related deaths. Heart attacks have the greatest overall mortality but usually occur in older individuals (defined here as those over age 55) with preexisting cardiovascular disorders. The individual with a known cardiovascular disorder should consider the possible consequences conferred by the significant stress of travel and seek the advice of his/her personal physician or cardiologist.

Fatality from accidents, mostly motor vehicle and drowning, are the leading cause of death for those under the age of 55. Mortality from motor vehicle accidents is much higher in underdeveloped countries than in the U.S. secondary to limited access to emergency medical systems and hospitals that may not be equipped to handle major (or minor) trauma. Also, vehicles often are not fitted with seat belts, air bags or child restraints. Likewise, Americans may often be driving on unfamiliar roads, in an unfamiliar vehicle with unfamiliar traffic signs and even on the "wrong" side of the road. For example, in the United States, there are 1.1 vehicle related deaths for every 100 million kilometers driven compared to 44.1 deaths over the same distance in Egypt.[1] Nearly three-fourths of the deaths in the world resulting from motor vehicle crashes occur in developing countries and that number appears to be increasing rapidly.[2]

Another concern is blood transfusion, should that be necessary. The blood supply (and needles and syringes) in developing countries may not be safe and there is the risk of improper cross-matching of blood as well as the possible transmission of hepatitis B and C, syphilis, and HIV. You can obtain information on transportation in the country you are visiting by contacting the Association for Safe International Road Travel (see chapter "Resources for the Traveling Medical Professional").

Modifying Your Risk

There are general measures you can adopt to modify and decrease your motor vehicle risk. Most involve just good common sense. Riding a motorcycle in the developing world is considered extreme risk. The motorcyclist may be experienced in the US, but road conditions are different in the developing world. In some countries, road etiquette is nothing less than bizarre. In one country, people run across the road in front of cars and motorcycles to test their "fate." It is a good sign or omen if you are not struck by the car (or motorcycle); it is likewise good for the driver. Accidents frequently occur from unanticipated (or unimaginable) events, like dogs, cows, goats or children on the roads. Often crops like coffee, corn or lentils are dried on the road making them a hazard. In one country in Asia, it is common for people to sleep on the roads at night since the surface is warm during the night in winter months and relatively clean. An unsuspecting driver in this country may find himself driving into a line of sleeping villagers. For these reasons, no matter how experienced, operating a motorcycle in the developing world should be discouraged.

The following are some helpful suggestions for road safety. (Adapted from Rose)[3]

1. Always wear a seat belt and use age appropriate child restraints. If the country you are traveling in may not have appro-priate restraints for children, consider taking them with you on your trip.
2. Consider hiring a qualified driver in an unfamiliar country. If he/she drives recklessly or too fast, do not be afraid to tell them to slow down. Consider an extra tip for a driver who is courteous and safe and let them know at the beginning that they will get something extra for being careful.
3. Rent a larger rather than smaller car. Size does count in an accident.
4. Know the road signs and local driving practices. Driving in foreign countries may be peculiar, (e.g. driver who honks his horn first has right-of-way) so stay alert and drive defensively.
5. Do not drive a motorcycle or moped, even if experienced. Traffic patterns that include cows, chickens, pigs and small children may not be part of your normal driving experience.
6. Avoid riding on overcrowded buses, trucks and trains. In South Asia, when the inside of buses and trains fill up, people stand on the outside rails of the vehicle and also sit on the roof. An overhanging tree branch or tunnel has been known to clear the roof of the bus or train.
7. Do not drive in rural areas at night except in an emergency and with an experienced driver and local resident. Accidents are more frequent at night as vision is limited.
8. Robbery is common in the developing world. If you are traveling by car, you are by definition "wealthy" and worthy to be robbed.

The best way to reduce risk of accidents, injury and infectious diseases overseas is not only to know the risks but to plan ahead and prepare well BEFORE travel. An emergency ceases to be an emergency if properly anticipated. Every traveler to underdeveloped countries should be familiar with the basics of at least these seven skills:
1. Know what water sources are safe and know how to disinfect water
2. Know how to eat to stay healthy

3. Know and follow basic immunization schedules
4. Know how to diagnose and treat travelers' diarrhea
5. Know the country-specific risk of malaria and know how to protect against, diagnose and treat malaria
6. Know how to protect yourself from blood-borne infectious diseases (HIV, hepatitis, etc.)
7. Know how to protect yourself from tuberculosis[4]

There are chapters in this book addressing all of the issues above. However, one or two require special mention. Many infectious diseases can be prevented altogether by proper attention to immunization schedules and self-protection techniques. Every year American travelers die from vaccine preventable illness. Some of this is from ignorance and some from poor advice and some from noncompliance. There is no excuse for not knowing and obtaining appropriate vaccinations. There are many immunizations available that should be considered routine prior to travel to the developing world. These include tetanus, diphtheria, measles, polio, hepatitis A and B, and influenza vaccine. Under special considerations travelers may also want to be vaccinated against yellow fever, typhoid, rabies, Japanese encephalitis and meningococcal disease depending on risk of travel and location [See chapter on "Immunizations" for further information]. Likewise, there are many serious infectious diseases that may be prevented by attention to protection from biting insects. These include malaria, dengue, yellow fever, hemorrhagic fevers, leishmaniasis, filariasis, and many others. Rabies can be prevented by staying away from all animal contact in endemic areas. Schistosomiasis can be prevented by not swimming in fresh water in endemic zones. Lastly, HIV infection is highly endemic in many regions. In some sub-Saharan countries, up to 20% (1 in 5) of men and women may be HIV infected and this may be an underestimate. Careful attention to universal precautions is essential to the individual health care worker and

a drug prophylaxis regimen should be carried in the emergency pack and considered in most cases involving exposure to blood or body fluids in highly endemic zones. (See chapter on "Post-Exposure HIV Prophylaxis"). These recommendations involve just good practical common sense and underscore the need for competent counsel and preparation ahead of time.

Travel Medicine and Information Resources

The specialty of travel medicine is growing and many major cities now have physicians specially trained to provide expert advice to the traveling public. Most of these physicians will belong to the American Society of Tropical Medicine and Hygiene and will have diplomas in Tropical Medicine and Travel Health or specialize in Infectious Diseases. The American Society of Tropical Medicine and Hygiene (ASTMH) web site publishes a list of recommended travel clinics around the world. These travel clinics provide up-to-date information on recommended vaccinations and travel related medical problems, if and when they should occur. The CDC in Atlanta also provides information including current malaria advisories, immunization schedules, disease risk and prevention, etc. In addition to these resources there are many other resources available to help the traveling public with information and services (see chapter "Resources for the Traveling Medical Professional").

Likewise, all medical team leaders and career medical missionaries on the field should be prepared to deal with the most common causes of morbidity and mortality should they occur—cardiovascular emergencies in those over 55 and traumatic emergencies in the younger travelers.

Travel Tips

(Adapted from Tsang Reginald)[5]

1. TRAVEL LIGHTLY: Remember that you are not traveling for people to see you. Take only what you need, and leave

your fancy clothing at home. A good judge of your load is if you can carry your luggage the distance of a football field and up three flights of stairs.

2. TRAVEL EXPECTANTLY: Every place you visit is a surprise package waiting to be opened. Untie the strings with an expectation of high adventure.

3. TRAVEL HOPEFULLY: "To travel hopefully," wrote Robert Lewis Stevenson, "is better than to arrive."

4. TRAVEL HUMBLY: Visit people and places with respect for their traditions and ways of life, as different as they may be from your own. You are a guest in their community.

5. TRAVEL COURTEOUSLY:
Consideration for your fellow travelers and for all you meet along the way will enhance your pleasure.

6. TRAVEL GRATEFULLY: Show appreciation for the many things done by others for your enjoyment and comfort.

7. TRAVEL WITH AN OPEN MIND: Leave all your prejudices at home.

8. TRAVEL FLEXIBLY: Have a flexible attitude especially when you experience unexpected delays or changes in your travel plans.

9. TRAVEL WITH CURIOSITY: It's not how far you go, but how deeply you go that mines the gold of the experience.

10. TRAVEL PATIENTLY: Take time to understand people in other countries especially when there are language barriers. Learn a few words, if only to say "hello" and "good-bye". Everyone will love it.

11. TRAVEL WITH THE SPIRIT OF A WORLD CITIZEN: You'll discover people are basically much the same the world over. Appoint yourself an Ambassador of Good Will wherever you go, after all, we are Ambassadors of Christ and come in the Spirit of Christ.

Classifying Your Physical Fitness

It is obligatory for every team member to realistically assess his or her skills and fitness level in comparison with the anticipated difficulty of the trip. One compromised team member can hinder the mission of the team and put other team members' safety in jeopardy. Since not all trips are equally difficult or dangerous, be realistic about your capabilities and the capabilities of your team members.

It is easy to classify participants into one of six groups:[6]

A. Demonstrated high performance individuals (world class athletes).

B. Healthy, vigorous individuals.

C. Healthy, but "deconditioned" individuals.

D. Those with health risk factors but no current evident disease (smoking, obesity, increased cholesterol, history of reactive airway disease).

E. Those with chronic illnesses who are well controlled (hypertension, diabetes, emphysema, coronary artery disease, etc.).

F. Poorly controlled chronic diseases.

Remember, the strength of your team is only as strong as the weakest member. Individuals can usually classify themselves according to this simple risk stratification. Careful consideration, soul searching and realistic appraisal of risk verses benefit should proceed before accepting "D" and "E" individuals onto a team where significant physical or psychosocial stress is anticipated. Except in very unusual circumstances, "F" category individuals are excluded from international travel.

Stratifying the Risk

Likewise, travel in the developing world can conveniently be categorized into four distinct risk levels—Low, Moderate, Substantial and High risk. Inquire ahead of time as to the level of risk your travel involves. Also realistically address your physical ability as stated above.

I – Low Risk

Travel to a western country or to a major city in the developing world with medical and social standards similar to western countries. No political or environmental uncertainties. Project requires only minimal exercise. Ground support team well established and experienced with previous teams.

II – Intermediate Risk

Travel to the developing world to cities with medical and social standards similar to western countries but with anticipated travel outside those cities. No political or environmental uncertainties. Project involves a moderate degree physical effort. Ground support team well established and experienced with previous teams.

III – Substantial Risk

(Any one applies.)

Travel to the developing world with few western amenities, poor social support and a marginal medical delivery system. Travel outside major cities. Political unrest sometimes present in country. Country at risk for environmental problems (earthquakes, hurricanes, tornadoes, floods, etc.) Infectious diseases may be a problem. Participation on team involves moderate psychosocial stress, physical fitness and physical effort. Ground support team new and/or inexperienced in handling teams.

IV – High Risk

(If any one of the following applies.)

Travel to the developing world with few western amenities, poor social support, and a poor medical delivery system. Anticipated travel to remote areas (All disaster response teams are in this category). Travel involves environmental extremes (altitude, cold exposure, high heat or humidity). Political unrest often present in country. Country at risk for environmental problems (earthquakes, hurricanes, tornadoes, floods, etc.) Infectious diseases are a problem. Participation on team involves significant psychosocial stress, physical fitness and physical effort. Ground support team new and/or inexperienced in handling teams.

The author's bias is that only low and intermediate risk travel be attempted by team members with chronic medical problems or risk factors—(e.g. "D" and "E" individuals as above—see chapter "Travelers With Chronic Medical Conditions") and team members new or inexperienced with work in the developing world. Likewise, when participation on a team involves substantial or high risk travel, this should be undertaken with a moderate to high degree of fitness (e.g. "A" and "B" individuals and in special circumstances, experienced "C" individuals) along with seasoned team leaders with special expertise, training and experience involving the conditions of travel.

Is God Calling You to This Ministry?

Finally, if you are considering traveling on a mission team, volunteering for an extended stay in the developing world or considering a career in missions, I suggest that you follow these four simple rules for determining whether or not this is something you should undertake.

1. Do you feel a personal sense of calling and is this calling strong enough to justify the degree of risk to your health and personal safety (and your family's health and safety)?

2. Is there corporate agreement with this calling (praying friends, elders, church leaders, sending organization, etc.)? Your "call" should always be validated by the Body of Christ.

3. Is there a scriptural imperative to undertake this mission? The Great Commission notwithstanding, not all mission endeavors may be scriptural. Unrepentant sin, unresolved conflict, family responsibilities and financial debt, an unprepared heart, or medical conditions that place you or your family or the team at increased risk may need to be resolved prior to undertaking a mission.

4. Is there an opportunity to participate that is in keeping with your call, your home life, your physical well-being, timing, your work, finances and personal responsibilities?

If God indeed does want you on the field, He will work it perfectly in His time and in His way. If any of the above answers is "no," then I suggest that you continue to pray and reevaluate your participation.

If all four of the answers are "yes", then embark on this great adventure knowing that what you are undertaking is a worthy endeavor and precious in the sight of God.

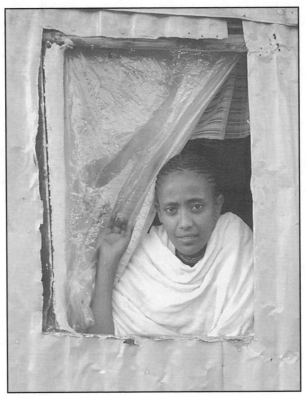

Ted Kuhn/
"The Risk of Travel"

References
1. Rose SR: *International Travel Health Guide*, 12th ed., Northamptom, MA, 2001, Travel Medicine, Inc., p 4.
2. Poudel-Tandukar K et al: Traffic Fatalities in Nepal, *JAMA*, 291(21):2542, 2004
3. Rose SR: *International Travel Health Guide*, 9th ed., Northamptom, MA, 1998, Travel Medicine, Inc., p 472.
4. Excerpted from lectures at the Wilderness Medicine Conference, Santa Fe, New Mexico, 2001.
5. Tsang Reginald in msips.org faq. #90, 2004.
6. Adapted from Wilderness Medicine Conference, Whistler, B.C, 2003 from workshop by Drs. Erb and Berghold, "Medical Suitability of Individuals for Wilderness Ventures: Ambition verses Ability."

4 Immunizations

Sharon C. Kuhn

Anyone planning international travel should contact their physician, travel clinic, or health department to determine the appropriate immunizations as soon as the itinerary is planned. Specific recommendations are based upon the geographic destination, length of stay, style of travel, purpose of trip, underlying health of traveler, and access to medical care during the trip. All travelers should seek appropriate counseling at least 4–6 weeks prior to departure and those planning prolonged stays or stays in rural areas may need to allow 2–6 months for immunizations if hepatitis B or Japanese encephalitis vaccines are needed. In case of emergent travel plans, it is possible to receive multiple vaccinations on the same day, injected at different sites, and provided the traveler is willing to tolerate possible side effects.[1]

Inactivated vaccines generally do not interfere with the immune response to other inactivated or live virus vaccines. An inactivated vaccine may be given either simultaneously or at any time before or after a different inactivated vaccine or a live virus vaccine.[1] Live virus vaccines, however, should be administered on the same day or at least 28 days apart in order to obtain the best immune response.[1] "Except for oral typhoid vaccine, it is unnecessary to restart an interrupted series of a vaccine or toxoid or add extra doses."[1]

Sources of Immunization Information

Comprehensive, up to date information on immunizations can be obtained from several sources including the Centers for Disease Control (CDC), the World Health Organization (WHO), the American Medical Association (AMA), and several private organizations (see "Resources" for this chapter).

The CDC publishes the annual guide, *Health Information for International Travel,* which provides a country-by-country listing of vaccination requirements. Travel immunization information can also be obtained from the CDC web site or by phone. WHO publishes the required and recommended immunizations for travelers each year in International Travel and Health which can be accessed through its web site. *Physicians' Guide to Travel Abroad* is available through the AMA. Private organizations that provide immunization information include International Association for Medical Assistance to Travelers (IAMAT), Travel Health Information Service, and Immunization Alert.

International Certificate of Vaccination

The World Health Organization is a voluntary association of member countries who agree to abide by mutually acceptable policies on immunizations for international travel and on quarantined diseases. Currently, the only vaccination regulated by the WHO is yellow fever which must be validated with an official stamp in the International Certificate of Vaccination (the yellow health card).[3] The card is provided to the traveler at the time of immunization at a government approved immunization site (usually a county health clinic or travel clinic). The yellow card has a separate page for documenting date, brand, and lot number of yellow fever vaccination. Space is also provided to document allergies, medical diagnosis, medications, blood type, eyeglass prescription, and records of non-regulated vaccines.[3] This is a very handy place for the traveler to keep an up to date listing of his immunizations.

Countries with specific requirements will have customs officials check the yellow card for verification of immunization. If the required vaccination against certain diseases cannot be validated, the traveler may be quarantined, denied entry, or required to be immunized on the spot[1] (often in less than optimal conditions).

Medical Waivers

Yellow fever is the only internationally required vaccine at this time. If someone who is allergic to the vaccine must travel to a country requiring it for entry, he must obtain a letter from his physician stating the reasons why the vaccine can not be given. The embassy or consulate of the country of destination should be provided with the physician's letter (written on letterhead stationary and bearing the official validation stamp used by the immunization center). The CDC recommends that travelers contact the embassy or consulate for specific advice about written waivers before departure.[1]

Routine Immunizations

The Advisory Committee on Immunization Practices (ACIP) of the CDC advises that all Americans should have up-to-date routine immunizations regardless of travel.[3] Routine immunizations are usually given in childhood with adult boosters given in adulthood or to immigrants and refugees upon entry into the United States. "Routine immunizations" for children in the United States include tetanus, diphtheria, acellular pertussis, measles, mumps, rubella, polio, hepatitis B, *Hemophilus influenza* type b, varicella, pneumococcal conjugate, and influenza and hepatitis A vaccines.[4] Varicella is given to adults who have not had chicken pox. Pneumococcal polysaccharide vaccine is routine for all those over the age of 65 and for younger adults with chronic pulmonary conditions, asplenia, or other immune compromise.

Diphtheria, Tetanus Toxoid and Acellular Pertussis vaccines (DTaP or DT) are given to children in a series of 3 doses 4–8 weeks apart usually beginning at 2 months of age. A fourth dose is given 6–12 months after the 3rd dose, and a booster at 4–6 years of age. For boosters in adolescents and adults one of the new Tdap vaccines (tetanus toxoid, diphtheria toxoid and acellular pertussis) are recommended. The FDA has approved Adacel® for persons age 11–64 years and Boostrix® for 10–18 year old children.

Inactivated Polio Vaccine (IPV) is now the recommended vaccine for use in childhood in the United States, and is given in a 3 dose series beginning at 2 months of age with dosing intervals of 4–8 weeks. A booster is given between 4–6 years of age. Previously, live attenuated oral polio vaccine (OPV) was utilized in the US and it is still in use in the developing world. OPV provides intestinal immunity for the individual and, because the immunized person sheds the vaccine virus in the stool for several weeks, "herd immunity" can occur.

There have been no cases of wild poliovirus infection in the Western Hemisphere since 1991 and the Western Hemisphere was declared polio free in 1994. In 2000 there was a small outbreak of vaccine-derived polio in Haiti and the Dominican Republic.[1] The only recent cases of polio in the US were in children who had received oral polio vaccine and had developed vaccine-related paralytic poliomyelitis (VAPP) infection, a very rare but troublesome complication of OPV. For this reason the Advisory Committee on Immunization Practices (ACIP) recommended the use of IPV exclusively for routine immunizations in children and in unimmunized adults. There have been no cases of VAPP in the US since 1999.[5] The schedule for unimmunized adults is 3 doses with the first two separated by a 4 week interval and the final dose 6–12 months later.

The global eradication of polio is now a priority of the international community and the incidence of the disease has dropped dramatically. As of 2001 there were only 10 countries in the world where polio was still endemic with most transmission occurring in the African countries of Nigeria and Niger, and in Afghanistan, Pakistan, and India.[1]

IPV boosters for adults who have received their primary series in childhood are recommended for travelers to those areas of the world where polio is still endemic. One booster dose of the vaccine in adulthood is sufficient.

Hepatitis B Vaccination has been routinely recommended for health care workers for many years and for children since 1991. The series includes 3 doses, with the second being given 1–2 months after the first, and the third at no less than 4 months after the first dose and at least 2 months after the second dose for best immunity. Infants should receive their third dose after 6 months of age. Seroconversion is greater than 95% after the third dose. Protection against hepatitis B persists despite loss of detectable antibody over time and neither retesting nor boosters are generally recommended except in health care workers. Protection probably persists at least 13 years.[6] Health care workers who are exposed to blood and body fluids and are at risk for needle sticks or injury from sharp instruments should have antibody titers checked following immunization and if the titer is negative, the 3 dose series should be repeated and titer rechecked after 1–2 months. If the HCW is still negative, he should be checked for HBsAg status. If this is also negative, the HCW will be considered susceptible to hepatitis B should he be exposed.[5]

Hepatitis B vaccine is recommended for travelers who will be visiting or living in countries where hepatitis B is endemic and this includes most of the developing world. Risk of exposure in these areas could occur through emergency medical or dental care or blood transfusion. Body piercing and acupuncture should be avoided.

Hepatitis B Post Exposure Prophylaxis. If a high risk blood or mucous membrane exposure should occur, cleanse the area and obtain identification, pertinent medical history and consent from the person who may be the source of infection and obtain blood for serologic testing for hepatitis B, C, and HIV. Hepatitis B immune globulin is administered to an unvaccinated individual with a high-risk exposure and vaccination initiated.[5]

Measles, Mumps and Rubella Vaccination (MMR) is routinely administered to those born after 1957 without prior evidence of vaccination after the age of 12 months. Before 1957, it is assumed that most individuals were exposed and developed immunity to the disease. In susceptible adults, at least one dose of the MMR should be given. If the individual is at high risk for measles exposure a second dose should be given at least 28 days after the first.[5]

MMR is a live attenuated vaccine. It is therefore contraindicated in pregnancy, but not in breast feeding. Severely immune-compromised individuals and those on high dose steroids (greater than 2mg/kg or more than 20 mg daily of prednisone) should not receive the MMR vaccine. Though the vaccine viruses for measles and mumps are grown on chick fibroblasts, the vaccine can be safely administered to individuals with egg allergy.[5]

Measles is endemic in developing countries and a leading cause of morbidity and mortality especially among malnourished children. All travelers to developing countries, especially health care workers should be fully immunized against measles.

Influenza Vaccine is routinely recommended for all travelers as well as the non-traveling public. While most influenza occurs during the winter months in the Northern Hemisphere, it is opposite in the Southern Hemisphere with influenza occurring May through August. Influenza occurs year round in the tropics. Vaccination is recommended not only to protect the traveler, but to avoid the spread of infection during air travel and for the safety of isolated indigenous populations.

Required Vaccinations

Yellow Fever Vaccine

The only required vaccination is yellow fever (YF) for those traveling to or from a YF endemic zone. The vaccine must be given at least 10 days before travel. The yellow fever areas are listed in the CDC Yellow Book[1] and are mainly the central regions of South America and Africa. YF is a very serious arbovirus infection with a mortality rate of 20–50%. It is spread by mosquito vectors. The yellow fever vaccine is a highly effective live attenuated and long lasting vaccine that produces a significant antibody response in 90–100% of recipients. Contact your local health department for the location of your nearest designated YF vaccination center. There you will receive the vaccine and the necessary International Certificate of Immunization ("yellow card") to carry with you as proof of vaccination. The yellow fever certificate of immunization is valid for 10 years at which time reimmunization is necessary for travelers to countries requiring this. However, immunity has been shown to last much longer, up to 30 years in the majority of recipients.[2]

The dose is 0.5 ml SC. Side effects are uncommon and usually limited to mild headache and myalgia. It is contraindicated in infants under 9 months of age (except during an epidemic when infants ≥6 months of age may be immunized). In the 1950s 13 of 15 cases of post vaccine associated encephalitis, which is now termed yellow fever vaccine associated neurotropic disease (YEL-AND) occurred in infants under 4 months of age. This necessitated the change in administration to only those infants over 9 months old except in epidemic situations. The risk of YEL-AND is approximately one in eight million. More recently, 13 cases (out of approximately one hundred million vaccine recipients) of another rare but serious vaccine-associated complication has occurred. It is known as yellow fever vaccine associated viscerotropic disease (YF-AVD). It is characterized by fever and multi-organ system failure. This adverse event occurred only in first time YF vaccine recipients and most often in those over 70 years old.[2] YF vaccine is contraindicated in those with anaphylactic egg allergy. Skin testing and desensitization are possible if the situation demands. Pregnancy and altered immune status are also contraindications since this is a live attenuated virus vaccine.

Meningococcal Vaccine

Meningococcal vaccine is required for travelers to Mecca, Saudi Arabia for the Hajj and is not required by any other country for entry. The vaccine must have been given not more than 3 years and not less than 10 days prior to arrival in Saudi Arabia.[7] It is recommended for travelers to sub-Saharan Africa (the meningitis belt), especially in the dry season of December to June and during outbreaks of meningitis caused by *Neisseria meningitidis*. This disease is transmitted from person to person via respiratory droplets or direct contact as through kissing or sharing a drinking glass. With modern care it has a mortality rate of approximately 10% and a 13% risk of serious sequelae.[1] The vaccines available in the United States are active against serogroups A, C, Y, and W-135 with serogroup A being the most common cause of epidemics out-

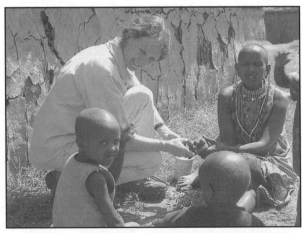

Ted Kuhn/
**"Dr. Sharon Kuhn,
Masai Village, Kenya"**

side the U.S. Serogroup B can also cause epidemics but there is no vaccine currently available for it.

Two quadravalent vaccines are available in the US. Menomune® is a polysaccharide vaccine which is given subcutaneously in a single dose of 0.5 ml to individuals 2 years of age and older. A booster is recommended at 3–5 years if exposure risk continues. Menactra® is a new conjugate vaccine which is approved for ages 11–55 and should soon receive approval for younger children and those over 55. It is given intramuscularly. It should have the advantages of preventing nasal carriage of the bacteria and providing long term immunity.

If a high likelihood of exposure has occurred, even the immunized individual should receive either ciprofloxin or rifampin to eliminate nasal carriage and further spread of the disease.[2] Side effects are mild, usually just redness at the injection site or low-grade fever in young children. The vaccine is not recommended in pregnancy unless in an epidemic situation;[2] however, no adverse effects were reported in pregnant women who received the vaccine during an epidemic in Brazil.

Recommended Vaccinations

Hepatitis A Vaccine
(Strongly recommended)

Hepatitis A virus occurs throughout the world. It is shed in the feces of infected persons and transmitted by the fecal-oral route through close personal contact (household or sexual), through contaminated food or water, and rarely through blood exposure. Symptomatic disease is more prevalent in adults. Though it is rarely a cause of death (0.3% overall, almost 2% in those over 50 years of age), morbidity can be significant.[5] Occurrence of symptomatic infections in all susceptible travelers is approximately 3 cases per 1000 travelers per month, but in adventure travelers in one study it was 20 per 1000 per month,[2] making it the most common vaccine preventable disease. Prior infection confers life long immunity.

In the US there are two inactivated vaccines available: Havrix® and Vaqta.® They are interchangeable and licensed for everyone not allergic to the vaccine itself or components of it and who is over 2 years of age. Immunity following one dose of vaccine is approximately 94–100% by 4 weeks following immunization. The second dose at 6–12 months is necessary for long-term protection.[1] Other than soreness at the injection site there are few side effects (occasional malaise or headache), and no severe adverse events have been attributed to this vaccine. Safety in pregnancy is unknown, but risk to the fetus is felt to be low. There is no need to check for vaccine response because conversion rates are so high. Vaccine immunity is thought to be long term and there are no recommendations at the present time for boosters beyond the original 2 dose series. This vaccine may be given concurrently with all live and inactivated vaccines commonly used in travelers.[1] It may be given simultaneously with Immune Globulin though this may slightly decrease the level of effectiveness of the first dose of vaccine, but full immunity will be achieved after the second dose. This vaccine will be recommended for most individuals going on short-term medical mission trips because of the considerable risk of acquiring the disease and the excellent efficacy and safety of the vaccine.

Havrix®
2–18 years (pediatric formulation)
720 EL.U.   0.5 ml IM   2 doses at 0 and 6–12 months

>18 years (Adult formulation)
1440 EL.U.   1.0 ml IM   2 doses at 0 and 6–12 months

Vaqta®
2–17 years (Pediatric formulation)

25 U   0.5 ml IM   2 doses at 0 and 6–18 months
>18 years (Adult formulation)
50 U   1.0 ml IM   2 doses at 0 and 6 months

Twinrix® (Combined Hepatitis A and B Vaccine) may be used in those over age 18. The dosage is hepatitis A dose 720EL. U/hepatitis B dose 20 micrograms per 1 mL.

3 doses are required for immunity given a 0, 1, and 6 months.[1]

Immune Globulin

Immune Globulin (IG) is a short-term alternative that provides passive protection against hepatitis A for children under 2 years of age or others in special circumstances. It can provide immediate protection that can last from 3–5 months depending on the dose given. IG is made from pooled human plasma, but there have been no reports of transmission of blood borne pathogens through the use of the IG produced in the US.[1] It is a pregnancy category C drug and use in lactation has not been studied for safety. If administered at the same time, IG may be given with all inactivated vaccines and with OPV and yellow fever vaccines. IG may be given 2 weeks following MMR. However, after IG is given, other live virus vaccinations must be postponed for several months because adequate immunity will not occur.[5]

Pre-exposure

0.2 ml/kg IM - 3 month's protection with an efficacy of approximately 90%

0.6 ml/kg IM - 5 month's protection with an efficacy of approximately 90%

Post-exposure

0.2ml/kg IM - 3 month's protection.

If given within 2 weeks of exposure, it has an efficacy of 85%

Typhoid Vaccine

Enteric or typhoid fever caused by *Salmonella typhi* or *paratyphi* can be a serious illness involving fever, abdominal, and systemic symptoms.

Untreated this disease carries a mortality rate of 10–30%. There is growing resistance to antibiotics used to treat typhoid. Currently the quinolones, chloramphenicol, or trimethoprim sulfamethoxazole are usually effective. If treated appropriately, mortality should drop below 1%.

Typhoid vaccines are recommended for travelers to developing countries, especially when they will be staying for longer periods in areas where contact with contaminated food and water is likely. No currently available typhoid vaccine is 100% effective; however, in view of the rising number of multi drug-resistant strains of *S. typhi*, any method of reducing the risk or severity of disease should be taken advantage of. Therefore, take the vaccine and use precautions in regard to food, water and sanitation.

There are two formulations of typhoid vaccine currently available in the United States: Ty21a oral vaccine manufactured by Vivotif Berna® and the Vi capsular polysaccharide vaccine (Typhim Vi® from Aventis)

1. The live attenuated Ty21a oral vaccine is administered as 1 enteric-coated capsule every other day for a total of 4 doses. It can be used in individuals 6 years of age and over. Capsules must be kept refrigerated. They must be taken on an empty stomach (1 hour before a meal) with a cool liquid. They may not be taken within 48 hours of a dose of antibiotic or other sulfonamide, mefloquine, or alcohol.[2] Typhoid vaccine may be given at the same time as other vaccines. The live vaccine should not be given to immune-compromised individuals or those infected with HIV or to pregnant ladies (there are no data on the use of this vaccine in pregnancy). The Ty21a vaccine causes very few side effects, indeed they were comparable to placebo. Currently it is recommended to repeat the full 4 capsule series every 5 years if exposure to typhoid continues.[1]

2. The new parenteral Vi capsular polysaccharide (ViCPS) vaccine appears to be just as effective with far fewer adverse reactions than the old whole cell inactivated vaccine. Only one IM dose of this vaccine is required to induce immunity and it can be given to children as young as 2 years. A booster should be given every 2 years if needed. The older inactivated parenteral whole cell vaccine, which was associated with a high frequency of local and systemic side effects is no longer used in the US. The parenteral (ViCPS) vaccine is probably safe to use in immune-compromised travelers and those who are HIV positive.[1] The only contraindication to the parenteral vac-

cine is a history of allergy to the vaccine itself or one of its components.

Oral Live-attenuated Ty21a Vaccine
age ≥6 years
1 capsule every other day for 4 doses
  Repeat 4 dose series every 5 years if needed.
Vi Capsular Polysaccharide Vaccine
age ≥2 years
0.5 ml IM   Boost every 2 years

Rabies Vaccines

Rabies is a fatal viral illness which can be acquired from the bite of an infected mammal (usually a dog, a bat, a cat or a raccoon in the US), or occasionally through an aerosol of the virus such as in a bat cave. The Indian subcontinent, Southeast Asia, and most of Africa are major foci of rabies today.

Rabies Pre-exposure Prophylaxis

In recent years safe and effective vaccines have become available for pre-exposure prophylaxis. Travelers and those planning long term residence in remote areas in high-risk countries should consider availing themselves of this vaccine, particularly considering that it may not be possible to obtain immediate access to post-exposure treatment of the quality available in the US. The rabies vaccines available in the US are safe and effective for children of any age and are recommended for children traveling to remote endemic areas or living in areas with a high incidence of rabies.[4]

Vaccines currently available in the US are Human Diploid Cell Vaccine (HDCV), Purified Chick Embryo Cell (PCEC) and Rabies Vaccine Adsorbed (RVA). All of these are inactivated or killed vaccines. Side effects are generally mild injection site soreness and/or malaise. Occasionally a delayed hypersensitivity reaction can occur after a booster. This is more common with HDCV.

HDCV, PCEC, and RVA are each given as a series of three doses of 1.0 ml each. They should be administered IM in the deltoid area on days 0, 7, and 21–28. Routine boosters for recipients of the tissue culture derived vaccines are recommended only for those at constant high risk of exposure. Antibody responses to these vaccines are nearly 100%.[2] However, if a vaccinated individual has a potential rabies exposure, two doses of vaccine must be administered three days apart beginning as soon as possible following the exposure to insure disease prevention. Rabies immune globulin is not given to previously immunized people.

Rabies Post-Exposure Prophylaxis

Perhaps the most critical means of preventing rabies in a bite wound is to first thoroughly cleanse the wound with copious amounts of soap and water and, after washing, to apply 0.1% benzalkonium chloride, 70% alcohol or 1% povidone iodine.

Human Rabies Immune Globulin (HRIG) at a dose of (20 IU/kg) is given as soon after exposure as possible on the day of exposure. If possible, the entire dose should be injected locally around the bite wound. If this is not possible, the remaining HRIG should be given IM at a site distant from the location where the rabies immunization will be given.[6] This binds the virus at the site of inoculation and keeps the virus from being absorbed into the nerve cells. Secondly, 1 ml of HDCV, PCEC, or RVA is administered IM on days 0, 3, 7, 14, 28 for a total of 5 doses.[1] Chloroquine and probably mefloquine taken for malaria prophylaxis may decrease the efficacy of rabies vaccine and these medications should be stopped if post exposure prophylaxis is necessary.

In some countries the only available rabies vaccine is the Semple vaccine. It is not advisable to vaccinate individuals with this animal nerve cell derived vaccine which is derived from rabies infected animal brain tissue. These vaccines are of questionable efficacy[6] and there is a possibility of post vaccination myeloencephalitis because of contaminating tissue residues. Evacuation of the individual for proper vaccination should be considered if safe, effective alternatives are not available.

In the developing world, if HRIG is unavailable and prophylaxis is considered imperative, **Equine Rabies Immune Globu-**

lin (ERIG) can be substituted for HRIG. This gives rabies protection essentially equal to the human immune-globulin but may cause serum sickness. The newer formulation of ERIG is much more highly purified than the older one and has a much lower incidence of serum sickness.[2]

If an individual has had the pre-exposure rabies immunization, then he will not need HRIG or ERIG. He will need 2 doses of vaccine, the first as soon as possible after the exposure, and the second 3 days later.

Cholera Vaccine

Vibrio cholera is a gram-negative bacillus that may produce severe, life-threatening, watery diarrhea. It is acquired through contaminated food or water (fecal-oral), hence, proper precautions will decrease the likelihood of disease substantially. The risk to most travelers of getting cholera is quite low. Morbidity and mortality from cholera are a result of dehydration from the diarrhea, and fluid replacement is the therapy of choice. The cholera vaccine previously used in the US has been discontinued. It had been only partially protective and only for a few months, and it had many side effects. WHO currently does not require cholera immunization, though some countries may require it during epidemics. Two new cholera vaccines which are more effective have become available in other countries. A killed whole cell oral vaccine, Dukoral® is available in Europe and Canada. It is given in a 2 dose series. A single dose, live attenuated oral vaccine (CVD-103 HgR) that is safe and very effective is also now available outside the US.[2]

If possible, give cholera and yellow fever immunizations at least 3 weeks apart. Otherwise give them on the same day and know that immunity may not be quite as high.[2]

Japanese Encephalitis Vaccine (JEV)

Japanese encephalitis (JE) virus is transmitted to man via the night-biting *Culex* mosquito. These mosquitoes breed heavily in rice paddies. Pigs are the predominant animal reservoirs though birds may also carry the virus. The disease is endemic in Asia (from India to Japan) including Southeast Asia, and Indonesia. Mortality rates range from 5–30% with young children being the most affected. For this reason several Asian countries include JE vaccine in their childhood immunization schedules. Basic mosquito precautions including use of a mosquito net, long sleeved shirts and long pants, and application of insect repellent are essential to preventing disease. JE vaccine is recommended for those who will be living in endemic areas and for travelers who will be staying 2–4 weeks or more in rural endemic areas, especially where rice paddies and pigs abound and when outdoor evening exposure is likely.[1]

The vaccine against Japanese encephalitis is a killed vaccine (formalin inactivated mouse brain) with an efficacy of nearly 100% after 3 doses and 91% after 2 doses.[8] Those who continue at risk for JE should receive a booster in about 3 years.[2] For persons over 3 years of age 1.0 ml of vaccine is given subcutaneously on days 0, 7, and 30. The dose for children ages 1–3 is 0.5 ml SC using the same schedule as for adults. These youngsters should be boosted at 2 years if needed.[1] Patients should be observed for 30 minutes after injection. The series should be completed no less than 10 days before departure because of the possibility of delayed hypersensitivity reactions.

Reactions may occur after any dose, but especially after the second dose. Persons who have a history of allergies, asthma, urticaria, or reactions to hymenoptera stings, may be at greater risk for an adverse reaction and may choose not to be vaccinated for JE.[1] Persons allergic to any vaccine component or who have had a reaction to a previous dose of the vaccine should not be vaccinated. Side effects include local swelling and tenderness, myalgias, malaise, etc. in one-fifth of patients to the very rare, but serious, acute encephalomyelitis or anaphylaxis in a very few individuals (1–2.3 per million vaccinees).[2] Urticaria and angioedema are also possible and may be treated with antihistamines, steroids, and/or epinephrine. A booster may be given in two to three years if exposure continues.[1]

Plague Vaccine/Treatment/Prophylaxis

The plague is caused by *Yersinia pestis*, a bacterium, which is transmitted via bites from infected fleas, direct contact with body fluids or aerosolized infectious material of an infected animal (usually a rodent), or from person to person through respiratory secretions. In general, travelers are at low risk of exposure to this disease.

The vaccine which was used previously is no longer commercially available in the US. Current guidelines recommend that travelers take preventive measures to avoid areas where plague has recently occurred, to avoid contact with sick or dead animals, and areas where there are rodent populations, and to overnight in clean accommodations. The use of permethrin treated clothing and DEET repellent for the skin to avoid insect bites is also wise.[1] If likely exposure can not be avoided, begin chemoprophylaxis with tetracycline 500mg four times a day, or doxycycline 100 mg twice a day during the time of exposure.

Children under age 8 may take Trimethoprim-sulfamethoxazole for prophylaxis. In case of an unexpected exposure, any of these three antibiotics can be taken for one week as post-exposure prophylaxis.[2]

Bacillus of Calmette Guerin (BCG) Vaccine

BCG is a live-attenuated vaccine that was created to protect against tuberculosis (TB). There are widely varying reports of its efficacy. It offers little protection against pulmonary tuberculosis, but a single dose may help prevent disseminated TB in children under one year of age. BCG is part of the routine childhood vaccination schedule in most countries where TB is highly endemic. In infants and children under age 5 who will be traveling or residing in highly endemic areas and who will likely be exposed to the local population, the vaccine may be considered.[4]

Since TB is spread by respiratory droplets, risk of acquiring the disease is highest when spending time in enclosed space with infected persons.

Unpasteurized dairy products are another potential source of infection. In the US BCG is rarely recommended for either children or adults. Those traveling to areas of high prevalence who will be working or living in close contact with the local population, such as health care workers or individuals working in the crowded conditions of refugee camps or slums should receive a PPD skin test to rule out infection prior to travel.[1] This test should be repeated after the traveler returns or yearly if potential exposure continues. If the PPD converts to positive, prophylactic medications may be recommended to prevent disease.

Tick-borne Encephalitis (TBE) Vaccine

TBE is a viral infection of the central nervous system that is transmitted through the bite of infected ticks and from drinking unpasteurized milk from infected cows or goats. The disease is found in forested areas of much of both eastern and western Europe and the former Soviet Union. There is no vaccine available in the US for this disease.

Currently there are 2 inactivated vaccines available in Europe: the Austrian-made FSME-IMMUN® vaccine which, in individualized cases, may also be obtained in Canada; and the Encepur® vaccine produced in Germany. Both vaccines have pediatric formulations for children ages 1–11[4] and the adult vaccine for persons age 12 and over.

The three dose schedule for children is given at 0, 1–3 months, and 9–12 months with a booster in 3 years. The adult dosing is similar at 0, 4–12 weeks and a booster at 9–12 months followed by boosters every 3–5 years. Immunity begins several weeks after the second dose. There have been allergic reactions to the vaccines and individuals should be observed for 30–60 minutes following immunization.[2]

Everyone hiking or camping in potentially tick infested areas should protect themselves from tick bites by dressing appropriately, using DEET containing insect repellent on their skin, and spraying clothes and boots with permethrin.

References

1. Centers for Disease Control and Prevention, Health Information for International Travel 2003–2004, US Department of Health and Human Services, Public Health Service, 2003.
2. Virk A, Jong E: Adult Immunizations, *Travel Medicine,* edited Keystone JS, Kozarsky PE, Freedman DO, Nothdurft HD, Connor BA, Philadelphia, PA 2004, Mosby, pp 87–122.
3. *Health Hints for the Tropics,* 12th ed., edited Wolfe MS, Northbrook, IL, 1998, published by the American Committee on Clinical Tropical Medicine and Travelers' Health of the American Society of Tropical Medicine and Hygiene, pp 8–21.
4. Makell SM, Pediatric Vaccinations, *Travel Medicine,* edited Keystone JS, Kozarsky PE, Freedman DO, Nothdurft HD, Connor BA, Philadelphia, PA 2004, Mosby, pp 123–130.
5. Atkinson W, Wolfe C, *Epidemiology and Prevention of Vaccine Preventable Disease,* 7th ed., Department of Health and Human Services, Centers for Disease Control and Prevention, 2002, Public Health Foundation.
6. Jong EC, Immunizations for Travelers, *The Travel and Tropical Medicine Manual,* 3rd ed., edited Jong EC, McMullen R, Philadelpia, PA, 2003, Saunders, pp 34–51.
7. Jong EC, McMullen R, Immunizations, *The Travel and Tropical Medicine Manual,* 2nd ed., edited Jong EC, McMullen R, Philadelphia, PA, 1995, WB Saunders Co. pp 28–49.
8. Halstead SB: Japanese Encephalitis, Lecture Handout from the Travel-Related Vaccine Preventable Diseases Course sponsored by the American Society of Tropical Medicine and Hygiene in November, 1999.

Resources

1. *Health Information for International Travel* by the CDC may be ordered from the Public Health Foundation at 1-877-252-1200 or online at http://bookstore.phf.org.
2. CDC web site for international travel is http://www.cdc.gov/travel/ or call the CDC automated travelers' hotline at (404) 332-4559.
3. WHO publishes the required and recommended immunizations for travelers each year in International Travel and Health. This information can be accessed through the WHO web site www.who.int/ith.[2]
4. *Physicians' Guide to Travel Abroad* is available through the AMA, 535 N. Dearborn Street, Chicago, IL 60610.
5. International Association for Medical Assistance to Travelers (IAMAT), 417 Center Street, Lewiston, NY 14092, telephone 716-754-4883;
6. Travel Health Information Service, 5827 W. Washington Blvd, Milwaukee, WI 53208.
7. Immunization Alert, PO Box 406, Stovis, CT 06268.

5 Getting There– The Stress of Travel

W. "Ted" Kuhn

Getting to the Airport
Aircraft Cabin Environment
Passenger Health

The decision to travel to a foreign country is the beginning of a complicated set of troublesome, stressors that we willingly inflict upon our minds and bodies. It is instructive to remember that the root of the word "travel" is "travail"—meaning to labor (literally the pain of childbirth). The stress of travel may begin as early as several days before departure during trip preparation.

There may be anxiety about the intended trip and last minute planning, causing sleep disturbances and the disruption of daily routines. Many times when the actual travel day arrives, the traveler is already fatigued, stressed and irritable.

Getting to the Airport

"Airport tumult" is the name given to the circumstances the traveler faces in just getting to the airport and settling on the plane.[1] Airports are often located in or near large busy cities. The traveler often finds himself or herself on congested unfamiliar roads with unanticipated delays. Sometimes getting to the airport means several hours of travel from home with concerns about getting lost, delays or car problems all of which cause anxiety. Since air travel is becoming more and more common, airports are often under construction resulting in ground transportation delays, parking problems and inaccurate signage and frequent delays secondary to increased airport security. Travel to and from an airport in a foreign country may be more troublesome since the traveler must rely on local transportation, may not speak the language and may not be familiar with the currency and local customs of tipping, etc. If you are running behind schedule, rushing to the airport creates time pressure. Once inside the airport, there are crowds, lines at ticket counters, security checks and concern about baggage. There may be long distances to the gates, with additional security checks. You may have heavy carry-on luggage and extra, unanticipated, charges for overweight baggage. Flight delays and cancellations cause stress when they involve missed connecting flights or missed meetings or plans to link-up with additional travelers at other destinations.

Aircraft Cabin Environment

Pressurization

Once inside the plane cabin, there are multiple physiologic stressors. The most noticeable is the change in barometric pressure.[1] Cabin pressures are adjusted to range between 5,000 to 8,000 feet above sea level once cruising altitude is attained. A normal healthy individual with a PAO_2 of 98 Torr at sea level would be expected to have a PAO_2 of 55–60 Torr at 8,000 feet. Most people tolerate this fall in PAO_2 without difficulty because of the favorable oxygen-hemoglobin disassociation curve.

However, problems occur in travelers with acute or chronic pulmonary disease, anemia, CV disease, seizure disorders or hemoglobinopathies. Anyone with a PAO_2 of less than 70 Torr at sea level, or who will have a calculated PAO_2 of less than 50 Torr in the air, will need supplemental oxygen in

31

order to maintain an acceptable O_2 saturation of no less than 85% at altitude. Oxygen ordered for a traveler by a physician must be provided by the airlines. However, most airlines require 48 hours advance notice and charge between $40–60 per flight segment. Oxygen used between flights on the ground is the responsibility of the passenger and can be arranged by local oxygen suppliers.

Barometric pressure changes can cause problems due to the expansion and contraction of gas. At 8,000 feet cabin altitude pressure, the volume of gas will be approximately 40% greater than at sea level. This expansion can cause a problem with trapped gas in various body cavities. A serious problem can occur in patients with a pneumothorax, pulmonary blebs or in post operative patients with trapped gas.

Less serious but disturbing problems can occur with trapped gas in the middle ear, sinuses or tooth. When the plane descends from 8,000 feet to sea level there will be a pressure gradient across the tympanic membrane which can be problematic particularly if there is congestion. Ascent of greater than 500 feet per minute or descent of greater than 300 feet per minute causes almost universal problems with pressure equilibrium in the ears, sinuses and air trapped in the cavities of teeth. The human ear is exquisitely sensitive to pressure changes and pain can be produced by as little as a change in cabin altitude of 250 ft. Problems with the ears and sinuses can be relieved with the use of vasoconstricting nasal sprays like Afrin® or Neosynephrine® or a sympathomimetic decongestant like pseudoephedrine if used 30 minutes before descent. Infants and children unaccustomed to clearing their ears can be heard crying in discomfort on almost all flights just before and during descent. Breast or bottle feeding small infants during descent can help alleviate the pressure gradient and thus relieve some of the painful ear symptoms.

Trapped bowel gas can expand causing bloating, abdominal cramping, belching and the embarrassing passage of flatus. Avoidance of carbonated beverages while traveling and the use of simethicone (Gas-X®) can help solve the problem of uncomfortable bowel gas.

Humidity

Low humidity during air travel may be another stressor. Air outside the cabin at an altitude of 30,000 feet typically has a temperature of -40°C and a relative humidity of less than 1%.[6]

The aircraft environmental packs that control airflow remove water to prevent contamination. Humidity on flights may be as low as 2% but usually not higher than 20% (below that which is normally accepted as comfort level). This will cause drying of mucous membranes which may be exacerbated by respiratory illness. The drying of the mouth, mucous membranes and eyes, as well as the sensation of thirst is due to drying of the pharyngeal membranes, not dehydration.

Fluid losses typically are no more than about 100 ml on long flights—not a major source of dehydration and can be easily replaced. One recent study demonstrated that fluid was in fact *retained*. The average surplus of fluid roughly corresponded to a 1 kg increase in body weight, which mainly accumulated in the lower extremities.[7]

Nevertheless on longer flights taking a moderate amount of fluids and avoiding the diuretic effects of alcohol and caffeine may be useful. Drinking large amounts of fluids during a flight for presumed dehydration only leads to longer lines at the lavatories and does little to alleviate the dryness experienced in the eyes and mucous membranes.

Travelers should consider using saline nasal spray for nasal congestion and dryness on long flights and ocular lubricants for dry, irritated eyes.

Noise Pollution

Noise can also cause stress in flight. Noise is capable of causing fatigue and both temporary and permanent changes in hearing particularly if there is an exposure above 85 decibels over time.[1] Most modern aircraft are well below this level with the exception of the turbo-prop aircraft used by some commuter airlines and helicopters.

Vibration

Vibration causes discomfort which is determined by the cycles per second and the G-level (gravitational forces). At low levels of vibration, any gravitation force above 1-G will cause discomfort. Vibration in helicopters is noteworthy as the vibration causes the maximum discomfort within the human body. Vibration, like noise, can cause fatigue; however, vibration can exacerbate the pain of chronic degenerative disease of the back, and has recently been implicated as the cause of leg edema. Recently, noise "canceling" headphones became commercially available. The effect these might have on flight fatigue is still unknown.

Turbulence

Turbulence can cause fatigue, motion sickness and injury. Turbulence is measured in G-forces. Moderate turbulence is 0.5 to 1.5 Gs and severe turbulence is greater than 1.5 Gs.[1] The turbulence in the rear of the aircraft may be up to 50% greater because of the rotational forces.

Turbulence occurs in poor weather conditions but clear air turbulence is not uncommon. Each year, the US reports both major and minor injuries in passengers caused by trauma from turbulence. This includes broken bones from loss of balance and falling or being struck by baggage and flying objects secondary to turbulence. Fracture of the spine—especially the C-spine—has been reported in heavy turbulence as well as death from trauma in heavy turbulence.

Airborne Disease & Air Exchange

There may be a temperature gradient in the cabin with cooler and warmer air settling out. With airflow of 10 feet per minute, air feels stagnant.[1] Above 60 feet per minute, there are uncomfortable drafts. There are usually between 16–33 air exchanges in the cabin per hour and about 50% of the air is recirculated. This is achieved by extracting air from the cabin (excluding kitchen and lavatory air) and mixing it with conditioned air from outside. This has the advantage of maintaining some of the humidity in the recirculated air and maintaining a high airflow in the cabin without cold drafts from cold outside air.

However, contaminants in some of the recirculated air may be retained. Recirculated air is filtered through a 0.3 micron HEPA filter. This removes the larger contaminants but may not filter all small bacteria and viruses. Thus, there is a small, but important, risk of acquiring bacterial and viral infections during air travel especially on long flights when mucous membranes are dry, thus encouraging penetration of the virus or bacteria into the oropharynx.

The traveler should consider influenza vaccine or antivirals like TamiFlu® in preparation for travel during influenza season (winter months in the northern hemisphere, all year round in the tropics and US summer months in the southern hemisphere).

Unfortunately, there has been documented transmission of tuberculosis and other droplet mediated illnesses on long flights in passengers sitting several rows in front and behind a traveler with active pulmonary disease. SARS has also been transmitted during flight, however, the exact mechanism for transmission (fecal-oral from contaminated lavatory or airborne) is still being debated.

Pesticides

The World Health Organization and the International Civil Aviation Organization recommend that the aircraft cabin be sprayed with pesticides when arriving in the US from countries endemic for diseases spread by arthropods and mosquitoes.[6] This has become controversial and is usually not done on American carriers but may be experienced when traveling on foreign airlines. However, residual pesticides (like permethrin) may have been applied when passengers are not on board.

Mosquitoes carrying not only West Nile virus, but malaria, yellow fever and dengue are easily transported into the US on overseas flights and the diseases can easily propagate in native mosquito populations near major US airports.

There are few health risks to passengers from such residual sprays (excepting allergy) and the potential ill effects of carrying diseased mosquitoes is obvious when studying the epidemiology of the spread of West Nile virus in the US in recent years.

Passenger Health

Deep Vein Thrombosis (DVT) and Pulmonary Embolism (PE)

Physical immobility during long flights is particularly troublesome when it leads to deep vein thrombosis and pulmonary embolus "the economy class syndrome."[1] A large number of cases of sudden death during flight or immediately after long flights have been determined to be due to pulmonary emboli. Pulmonary embolus is the second most common cause of death during flights, following the incidence of ischemic heart disease.[7]

Although healthy passengers seem to be at a very low risk, even during long flights, passengers with associated risk factors for thromboembolism seem to have considerable risk.[7] Most emboli occur during the first 24 hours after take-off, but emboli can also occur several days or weeks after travel. Pregnancy, obesity (more than 20% above recommended weight for age), a history of prior deep venous thrombosis (DVT) and vascular disease of the extremities are risk factors. Chronic heart disease, hormone therapy, malignancy, smoking and recent surgery may also place the traveler at increased risk.

It is suggested that travelers on long flights walk about the cabin at least once per hour and consider exercises while seated. A cramped position during flight with external compression of the popliteal veins is a risk factor for DVT. This can be partially relieved by wearing compression stockings. Compression stockings should be considered in all travelers with risk factors and in all passengers with a tendency for swelling of the lower extremities during travel.

Traveler's with one or more risk factors for pulmonary emboli or DVT should seek the advice of their physician before undertaking prolonged travel. The administration of a low molecular weight heparin (Lovenox® or other brand) every 12 hours may afford protection in the traveler with risk factors for DVT/PE and may be advisable. Although no study has been performed to date, many travel physicians advise taking one tablet of aspirin (325 mg) prophylactically every day for 3–5 days prior to travel for anticoagulation for the prevention of DVT for travel lasting longer than 5 hours.

Jet Lag

Circadian rhythms are adversely affected by flight, particularly when crossing multiple time zones. "Jet lag" is defined as "a combination of malaise, fatigue, derangement of sleep wake cycles, and poor performance which occurs when travelers cross several times zones rapidly and attempt to follow the time schedule of the new destination."

Sleep, mood, body hormones and body temperature are all affected. Resynchronization may take as long as 1 day per time zone. During this time the traveler experiences "circadian desynchrony." This is a significant consideration when traveling to and from Asia and Africa. It has obvious implications for vacationers as well as business travelers and athletes not to mention the health care professionals who must render a high level care in difficult circumstances once in the host country.

Conditions which contribute to or lessen "jet lag" are debated in the travel medicine community. However, it is generally accepted that interrupted sleep, excessive alcohol or caffeine and lack of exercise compounds the effects of "jet lag."

The role of diet in assisting the recovery of jet lag has been debated. To date there is no consensus among physicians as to whether special diets play any role in "resynchronization."

Bright light is known to help "reset" the internal clock in the new time zone and exposure to sunlight during the daytime at the new location is recommended.

Vigorous exercise is also known to help readapt to the new time zone and exercise after awakening in the morning at the new location can assist the jet lagged traveler.

Selective short "power naps" of less than 40–50 minutes may also assist in the adaptation process.[2,4] Longer naps may be counterproductive.

The role of medications in jet lag is more complicated. Melatonin is a chronobiotic that has received a considerable amount of attention in recent years as a potential treatment for circadian rhythm disorder.[2] Melatonin can indeed shift the body's sleep-wake cycle, but this depends on the time of administration. Because of the time sensitivity of the physiologic actions of melatonin, exogenous administration at incorrect times in the sleep-wake cycle may render the medication ineffective or, even worse, counterproductive. Melatonin used 1 hour before sleep at night in the new time zone combined with bright light exposure and exercise in the morning after arising may be the most beneficial. Dosages of 0.5 to 3 mg are usually sufficient to shift the body's sleep cycle.

The role of benzodiazepams (e.g., Ambien®) to augment sleep is also controversial. While benzodiazepams can induce sleep, they may also interfere with REM sleep and delta sleep so that the sleep that is induced may not be restorative. The traveler may awake after 8 hours in bed with a "hangover," irritability or difficulty concentrating.[3]

Radiation

Galactic radiation is usually not considered by most travelers and is of little consequence in altitudes below 25,000 feet because of the attenuating properties of the earth's atmosphere[7]. However, on long flights at a cruising altitude of 35,000 feet, radiation accumulation of several milli-REMS per flight is not uncommon.[1] Frequent travel over the course of a year may expose the traveler to the occupational exposure limit set by the government of 5 REMS per year.

This corresponds to between 100 hours of polar flight or 200 hours of trans-equatorial flight per year. This may be of concern especially for the pregnant traveler. The overall significance of this exposure is uncertain, notwithstanding, it is recommended that in pregnancy, exposure not exceed more than 50 milli-REMS per month (several moderate length flights).

In-flight Medical Emergencies

The incidence of true in-flight emergencies is quite low. These may range from minor inconveniences, such as headache, vasovagal syncope or earache on descent, to major life threatening emergencies like myocardial infarction, childbirth, pneumothorax and sudden death. One airline reported 3022 emergencies in 34 million passengers carried during 1 year.

Good Samaritans

Aircraft are subject to the laws of the State in which it is registered, although, when stationary, and not moving under its own power, as would be the case in an airport, it is subject to local law. Some countries require medical professionals to offer assistance during an emergency (e.g. France) whereas in other states or countries no such assistance is mandated (US and UK)[7]

Medical professionals offering assistance on board an aircraft when requested by cabin crew are referred to as "Good Samaritans." Many countries (US) have enacted "Good Samaritan" laws so that a medical professional offering assistance during an in-flight emergency can not be held liable for malpractice in case of an adverse outcome. Some airlines provide full indemnity for medical professionals assisting during in-flight emergencies.

To date, there is no case of a successful legal action against a medical professional providing emergency care during an in-flight emergency.[7]

At disembarkation, the patient is frequently transferred to a hospital at which point the care is no longer the responsibility of the "Good Samaritan."

Resuscitation Equipment

The FAA dictates a minimum standard of medical equipment to be carried onboard all US registered aircraft. In practice, many airlines carry more than the minimum standard, although there may be significant variation in foreign registered aircraft. The health care worker can not anticipate which emergency equipment may be available during an in-flight emergency and significant variation from airline to airline (and even within airlines depending upon route) does occur. Most airlines now carry AEDs (some with cardiac monitoring capabilities) and flight crew are trained in their use.

Oxygen

All commercial aircraft carry supplemental oxygen. The passenger supply is delivered through drop-down masks from chemical generators in case of cabin depressurization during an in-flight emergency. Flow rates of continuous oxygen at 4–8 liters per minute can be maintained for about 10 minutes to passengers throughout the cabin. Sufficient oxygen in "bottles" is carried in case of in-flight passenger emergency. Flow rates of 2–4 liters per minute can be maintained for a short time. Sufficient oxygen for an entire flight is not carried unless prear-ranged prior to take-off by the passenger of his/her physician.

Aircraft Diversion

Although at first consideration, it might seem prudent to divert an aircraft to a closer airport when presented with a sick or ill passenger, the reality is more complicated and the final responsibility for making the decision for diversion rests with the aircraft captain. Consideration must be given to time for descent from cruising altitude, jettison of fuel, landing weight, availability of appropriate medical facilities as well as the ability of the terminal to receive, repair and refuel the aircraft.[6]

Not all terminals can accommodate the number of passengers on board and crew duty time must be considered. Whether sufficient hotel accommodations are available for delayed passengers and onward flight connections are yet another consideration.

The cost to the airline of diversion can be substantial. If you are the "Good Samaritan" assisting in a life-threatening emergency in flight, communication with the airline medical advisor by radio or telephone may be prudent before recommending diversion. The captain will undoubtedly solicit advice from multiple resources before making a final decision.

References

1. Millett DP: Medical Aspects of Air Travel, *Audio-Digest—Family Medicine*, August 15, 1997.
2. Kuhn W, Wellman A: The Use of Melatonin as a Potential Treatment for Shift-Work Related Sleep Disorder, *Academic Emergency Medicine*, 5(8):842, 1998.
3. Kuhn W: Shift Work, Circadian Rhythm and Satisfaction: Surviving and Thriving in Emergency Medicine, *Emergency Medicine*, 29(3):80, 1997.
4. Jong EC, McMullen R: Disequilibrium: Jet Lag, Motion Sickness, and Heat Illness, *The Travel and Tropical Medicine Manual*, 3rd ed., edited EC Jong, R McMullen, Philadelphia, W B Saunders Co., 2003.
5. Ferrari E, et al: Travel as a Risk Factor for Venous Thromboembolic Disease: A Case Control Study, *Chest*, 115:440, 1999.
6. Bagshaw M; Aircraft Cabin Environment, *Travel Medicine*, edited JS Keystone, PE Kozarsky, DO Freedman, HD Nothdurft, BA Connor, Mosby 2004.
7. Arfvidsson B et al: Risk Factors for Venous Thromboembolism Following Prolonged Air Travel, *Hematology/Oncology Clinics of North America*, 14(2), 2000.
8. McLelland SLF: Jet Lag, *Travel Medicine*, edited JS Keystone, PE Kozarsky, DO Freedman, HD Nothdurft, BA Connor, Mosby, 2004.

6 Traveling with Children

Jim Carroll and Shirley Carroll

Medical Aspects
Accident Prevention
Long Distance Travel
Motion Sickness
Immunizations
Mosquito Protection
Malaria Prophylaxis
Malaria Treatment
Travelers' Diarrhea
Altitude Illness
Spiritual Aspects

Travel with children is quite rewarding, particularly in the context of missions. The keys to success have to do with adequate preparation from a medical, psychological and spiritual standpoint. Evaluation and planning in these areas for the trip should begin several months before departure. Depending on the length of the trip, short term or long term, and perhaps preparation for living in a new area and culture, thoughtful and elaborate arrangements may be necessary.

Medical Aspects

Planning should begin far enough in advance to achieve immunization appropriate for the trip. Contingency plans should be developed for any chronic illness the child may have, such as asthma, epilepsy or diabetes. Children may not adapt quickly to unfamiliar foods, so it is a good idea to bring items that the child will eat under any circumstances. Alternatively, foods from the host country can be prepared and offered to the child at home before departure. That way parents can anticipate which foods the child may consume on the trip, and which to avoid.

One should recognize that there is a close connection between the child's physical well being and the emotional aspects of the trip. Thus, it is wise to expend considerable efforts in making the child's experiences as pleasant and rewarding as possible.

Accident Prevention

Accidents are the most serious risk of travel, and safety-consciousness is lower in the developing world. If possible, try to obtain a vehicle with seat belts, and consider taking your own child's car seat. It is often best to have a local person as a driver. Don't hesitate to tell the driver to slow down. Make sure insurance policies cover care in the country and also pay for emergency evacuation.

Water safety is also a major consideration. Freshwater and saltwater each have their own risks. For freshwater swimming, be aware that schistosomiasis may be prevalent. For saltwater, the area may be inadequately guarded, and the tides may be unknown and risky.

Long Distance Travel

Like adults, children may suffer from alteration of sleep due to crossing time zones, but these travel-related sleep problems are usually less severe in children than in adults. Parents often ask about sedation for long travel times, but it is probably best to avoid this if possible. If sedation is desired, diphenhydramine (Benadryl®) 5 mg/kg daily divided into 4 doses may be used.

Infants can not clear pressure in their ears during aircraft descent. Breast or bottle feeding infants during descent will allow equalization of pressure in the middle ear.

For infants who are not yet toilet trained, diapers must be taken along. Disposable diapers, while convenient and lightweight are quite bulky and once used, must be carried until they can be disposed of. A clever trick which may extend the use of an individual diaper is to insert a women's panty liner into the diaper. Once soiled, the significantly smaller liner can be replaced and the diaper, if not significantly dirtied, can be reused.

Motion Sickness

Children under two years are rarely affected by motion sickness, and the peak susceptibility is between 4 and 10 years of age. Riding in the front of the vehicle, looking into the horizon may help. Small doses of dimenhydrinate (Dramamine®) 5 mg/kg daily divided into 4 doses may be administered. If vomiting is intractable, which is unusual, promethazine (Phenergan®) may be given, 0.25–0.5 mg/kg per dose, by mouth or intramuscularly.

Immunizations

Routine immunizations must be up to date. Yellow Fever Vaccine is required for endemic zones. The vaccine should not be given to those less than four months old. For those 4–9 months of age, one must assess the risk of exposure. The vaccine, which contains egg protein, may be given to all children older than nine months, unless there is a compromised immune system.

For influenza, consider the vaccine for children older than six months. For children <9 years old receiving vaccine for the first time, there should be two doses separated by one month.

Meningococcal vaccine may be given to children more than three months of age, particularly for travel in sub-Saharan Africa.

For Hepatitis A, consider the vaccine after two years of age, according to the area, with two doses. If less than two years of age or departing quickly, one should consider the need for immune globulin.

For typhoid, according to the area risk, use either oral Ty21a (six years or older), four doses every other day for four doses or intramuscular Vi CPS for those two years or older.

Rabies vaccine is recommended for those who intend to remain for prolonged periods in endemic areas. Use the human diploid cell vaccine with injections on day 0, 7, and 21–28. Pre-exposure immunization avoids the need for immune globulin, often difficult to obtain in developing countries, after a bite. Remember that post exposure immunization must be given after a potential rabies exposure.

Japanese Encephalitis Vaccine is recommended for prolonged stays in endemic areas of Asia. Since encephalomyelitis can occur as a complication of the vaccine, and safety data is not available for those less than one year of age, the need should be carefully evaluated. Doses are given on days 0, 7, and 30.

Mosquito Protection

Some of the diseases transmitted by mosquitoes include malaria, yellow fever, dengue fever, various types of encephalitis, and filariasis. Avoidance of mosquitoes is the most important factor. Wearing lightweight long-sleeved shirts and long pants, especially if they have been treated with permethrin, clearly helps to prevent mosquito bites. Staying inside a protected area at dawn and dusk, when mosquitoes are feeding, cuts down on bites as well. Nighttime permethrin-treated mosquito netting is often a necessity. Using insect repellent appropriately adds significant protection. DEET (10–30%) repellent is recommended for children[1, 2] and needs to be reapplied every 1–5 hours, depending on the concentration used. Be sure to follow the manufacturer's instructions on the label. DEET is not recommended in children under 2 months of age. Please see chapter on "Protection from Blood-Feeding Arthropods" for further details.

Malaria Prophylaxis

Because of the many medication risks and malaria complications in children, serious consideration should be given in taking a young child to areas where there is a high incidence of drug-resistant malaria. In areas where malaria is not chloroquine-resistant, chloroquine (Aralen®) should be used. The dose is 5 mg/kg base once per week up to the adult dose of 300 mg (the 500 mg tablet contains 300 mg base), with one dose taken per week one week prior to the trip, one dose each week during the trip, and for four weeks after the trip. For chloroquine-resistant falciparum malaria areas, the main choices are mefloquine (Lariam®) or doxycycline (doxycycline is not recommended for children less than eight years of age).

Mefloquine (Lariam®) 250 mg tablets

Child's weight	Dose	Dosing schedule
<15 kg	5 mg/kg	The dose is given once a week, beginning 1 week before the trip, weekly during the trip, and weekly for 4 weeks afterward.
15–19 kg	¼ tablet	
20–30 kg	½ tablet	
31–45 kg	¾ tablet	
>45 kg	1 tablet	

Another option for malaria prophylaxis may be atovaquone/proguanil (Malarone®). It is not recommended in infants.

Atovaquone/proguanil (Malarone®)

Pediatric tabs 62.5 mg/25 mg (respectively)
Adult tablets 250 mg/100 mg

Child's weight	Dose	Dosing schedule
<11 kg	Not recommended	
11–20 kg	1 ped tab	Daily beginning 1–2 days before the trip, daily during the trip, and daily for 7 days afterward
21–30 kg	2 ped tabs	
31–40 kg	3 ped tabs	
>40 kg	1 adult tab	

Consider administering primaquine terminal prophylaxis to prevent relapses of *Plasmodium vivax* and *Plasmodium ovale*

in children who are not G6PD-deficient and have had heavy exposure.

Malaria Treatment

For the treatment of malaria under field conditions in chloroquine-sensitive areas, chloroquine may be used, 10 mg/base/kg for the first dose, followed by 5 mg/kg at 6, 24, and 48 hours. Pyrimethamine-sulfadoxine (Fansidar®) may be used in chloroquine-resistant areas.

Malaria Treatment with Pyrimethamine-sulfadoxine (Fansidar®)

Child's weight	Dose	Dosing schedule
5–10 kg	½ tablet	Dose is given all at one time
11–20 kg	1 tablet	
21–30 kg	1½ tablets	
31–45 kg	2 tablets	
>45 kg	3 tablets	

Keep in mind that resistance to Fansidar® is widespread in parts of Southeast Asia, Africa and the Amazon basin. Mefloquine also may be given in resistant areas, 15–25 mg/kg as a single dose (Maximum dose in children is 1250 mg). Malarone® using the adult strength tablets is also recommended.

Malaria Treatment with Atovaquone/proguanil (Malarone®) Using Adult Tablets (250 mg/100 mg)

Child's weight	Daily Dose	Dosing schedule
<11 kg	Not recommended	
11–20 kg	1 tablet	Give daily for three consecutive days.
21–30 kg	2 tablets	
31–40 kg	3 tablets	

Finally, another alternative is quinine sulfate 30 mg/kg.day divided three times daily plus doxcycycline 2 mg/kg.day for 7 days.

Recommendations for malaria prophylaxis and treatment are frequently revised, so it is always wise to check the most up-to-date information before departure. (See references at end of chapter)

Travelers' Diarrhea

The management of travelers' diarrhea, as it applies to children, requires particular attention. Enterotoxigenic *E. coli*, *Campylobacter*, *Salmonella*, and *Shigella* are the main potential bacterial pathogens. Preventive medications are not recommended. The most important consideration is hydration. Regular drinks may suffice, but if there is dehydration, then fluid replacement should be accomplished. Alternatively, use prepared oral fluids such as Pedialyte,® Gatorade,® or home-made rehydration solution with eight teaspoons of sugar, one-half teaspoon of salt, and one-quarter teaspoon of baking soda (if available) in 1 liter of clean water. There are new WHO recommendations for composition of commercially produced oral rehydration solution, but these are generally too complex for home application.[3]

Generally, antimotility agents, such as loperamide, are not recommended for children. Systemic antibiotics are a reasonable choice, and perhaps the best choice is azithromycin, 10 mg/kg once and 5–10 mg/kg on the following one or two days. While in the past there were concerns about joint cartilage toxicity, ciprofloxacin, 10 mg/kg twice daily for one to three days, also is safe in children. Diarrhea that persists should be investigated for other organisms including *Giardia*.

Altitude Illness

Altitude sickness may occur at altitudes as low as 7,000 feet, but more commonly at altitudes above 9,000 feet. The best prevention is slow ascent. A history of asthma is not a contraindication to high altitude travel. Symptoms include headache, nausea, or shortness of breath. Remember that the signs and symptoms of altitude illness are even less clear-cut in children than in adults. High altitude pulmonary edema is more common in children. Small dosages of acetazolamide (Diamox®), 62.5 mg twice a day may help, but the drug is not clearly indicated in children. If altitude sickness is suspected, then the child should be taken to a lower altitude.

Spiritual Aspects
Preparation

Several months before beginning a mission trip with children you should start to talk about and plan the trip. Of course, the plans must be age appropriate. Infants and very young children will need the necessary equipment and items for their entertainment. As the children grow older, you can learn about the country together. A map of where you will be going as well as the customs of the people would be included in your study. A discussion of the climate and living conditions of the places where you will be staying is necessary. The appropriate type of clothes to wear on a mission trip may need some thought and discussion particularly among teenagers. Perhaps some attention could be given to the language of the country. An attempt to learn a few basic phrases might be most beneficial.

Perhaps the most important part of the preparation is the praying about the trip. Pray for right attitudes, especially when we are tired and hungry. Remember that only the Lord can give us his "Fruit of the Spirit" under perhaps uncomfortable conditions, and that we must trust in Him to supply us with His Spirit. Apart from the physical needs of good health during the trip and a willingness to accept conditions which might at least stretch us, we can begin to pray for the people we meet.

Pray for receptive hearts, and that we will be filled with words and actions that are meaningful to the people we meet and a glory to Christ.

Pray for a real vision of our purpose in going: that all people may come to know the love of Christ and know Him as their personal Lord and Savior. The chief aim of man, as stated in the Westminster Catechism, is to glorify God and enjoy Him forever. Our primary concern is to lift the name of Jesus among others and among ourselves. Participate in the privilege God gives us to enjoy Him and to tell others about him. The privilege of going on a mission trip is God's plan and blessing to us.

For our family we also pray that each member of the family will have something to do. Since we may not know what we will be doing, we ask that we will each have a specific assignment, which we will be able to fill.

We also remember past mission trips. We think and talk about the times when the Lord has been there for us even when circumstances were difficult. We thank Him for His promises and His care over us. We remember personal Bible verses and Scripture that the Lord has given us. It has been good to refresh our memories about the poverty we have seen and will see again, and remind ourselves that God's care and love is for everyone, even those who live in very poor conditions

The Actual Trip

It is good to talk about what has happened to each person during the day. Again, poverty might be discussed and Scripture which the Lord may have given in a particular situation. Specific prayers are offered for the needs for each day. There are needs to pray about...fatigue, jet lag, loss of sleep, change in schedules, and just being hungry or sick. A time needs to be put aside for private devotions for older children. If the family can be a part of the prayer time with the rest of the team, this is beneficial. As much time spent with the rest of the team as possible will certainly add to the experience. Each child needs his own devotional book.

When a set time is arranged for prayer for the whole group, it is important to be punc-

tual, even when this time might be 5:00 a.m. and you didn't get to bed until midnight.

A spirit of thankfulness should continually be remembered. Be thankful that God cares about the people everywhere just as much as He cares about us. The Lord is most concerned about the spiritual growth of and His relationship with His people. Be thankful that God has a perfect plan and purpose and nothing happens by accident, especially our being on the trip. By God's grace, each person must decide not to complain. We can rest in the fact that God does it all, and the trip and His purpose are not carried out just because of our preparation or activity.

After the Trip

There must be time to talk and express "why's" and "doubts." It also helps to remember that salvation is in the Lord's hands. This is a time, too, that we can rejoice together over what we have seen God do and His grace to us. Many times on a mission trip our children have led someone in the sinner's prayer or made salvation more clear to someone. It takes continual effort to persist in quiet time and build our relationship with the Lord. Be sure that the Lord will use every experience in our relationship with Him and in that of our children.

Finally, it is fun to get the pictures developed relive the experience, share memories, and to look forward to the next mission trip.

References
1. Fischer PR, Pediatric, Neonatal and Adolescent Travelers, *Travel Medicine*, edited Keystone JS, et al., Philadelphia, 2004, Mosby, pp 217–227.
2. Stauffer WM, et al., Traveling with Infants and Children, Part 4: Insect Avoidance and Malaria Prevention, *Journal of Travel Medicine*, 2003: Vol. 10, pp 225–240.
3. www.cdc.gov/travel/travel.html
4. *2003 Red Book, Report of the Committee on Infectious Diseases*, American Academy of Pediatrics.

Resources
1. http://aapnews.aappublications.org/cgi/content/full/e200399
2. http://www.aap.org/advocacy/releases/summertips.htm
3. http://rehydrate.org/ors/who-unicef-statement.html

7 Travelers with Chronic Medical Conditions

Sharon C. Kuhn

Asthma
Sleep Apnea
Hypertension
Gastrointestinal Disorders
Severe Allergies
Deep Vein Thrombosis
Cardiovascular Disease
Diabetes

Traveling as part of a medical mission team will involve more strenuous activity and more challenging environmental conditions than are experienced in normal tourist travel. Those individuals who desire to participate should be in good general health and have fair to excellent cardiovascular fitness. There are several chronic stable medical problems that will not significantly interfere with an individual's ability to enjoy and contribute to the success of such a team. However, any condition must be stable and well-controlled. It must not interfere with fairly vigorous physical activity or require an inflexible schedule.

When considering an overseas medical assignment, whether short or long term, the individual with a chronic medical condition should first consult with the team leader concerning the details of the mission and how these might impact his health. He should also consult with his personal physician. Together, they can determine if there is a likely increase in risk relative to the other travelers and whether or not the level of risk is low enough to allow confident participation by the individual. If further consultation is needed, the team leader or participant should contact the medical director of the sending agency.

All travelers should compile a brief health history to be carried on the trip . It should be carried in an easily accessible location such as with the passport. This will be helpful to health care providers in the event of an emergency. Include an up-to-date immunization record and a list of current medications including the generic name, the dosage and frequency of administration. Also have a list of all ongoing medical problems such as hypertension, asthma, and diabetes; include any pertinent medical history such as appendectomy, myocardial infarction (bring a copy of a recent EKG), spontaneous pneumothorax, deep vein thrombosis, etc. Be sure to include any known drug or insect allergies and their manifestations and severity, and blood type. The traveler should write down the name, telephone, and fax numbers of his personal physician and of a close relative or friend in the United States who could help in an emergency. The team leader should receive a copy of this document from all team members, not only those with chronic conditions, well ahead of departure. (See chapters on "The Medical Team Leader", and "The Risk of Travel" and the "Health Questionnaire" in the appendix.)

As a general rule, persons using prescription drugs should carry all that they will need for the trip in their carry-on luggage. In addition, they should pack an equal amount in their checked luggage, just in case. Persons who take medications infrequently, such as for mild asthma, motion sickness, or migraine, should take their medicines along since the stress of travel and unexpected conditions may necessitate the use of these medications. Persons with surgically implanted metal devices (e.g. artificial hip replacement) should carry a letter from their physician stating this fact and this note should be carried with the passport to avoid delays at airport security checks.[1]

Asthma

Travelers with mild to moderate asthma that is well-controlled will be able to participate on most medical teams. Asthma does not put one at greater risk when working at altitude,[2] but there are other issues of concern for asthmatics. Air pollution in some large cities can be quite severe. Allergens such as dust mites, mold, cigarette smoke and diesel fumes may cause unexpected trouble, and there is the increased risk of contracting an upper respiratory infection, especially on long airplane flights. These factors need to be evaluated in light of the traveler's asthma status.

Before travel the individual should acquire and learn how to use a peak flow meter. This will help gauge any subtle aggravations of his asthma while traveling and will allow for timely adjustment of medication. Extra medication should be packed in case of an exacerbation. If necessary, plans can be changed to serve on a medical team in a more asthma-friendly location.

Sleep Apnea

Individuals with sleep apnea are more likely to have problems at altitude[2] and such trips are not recommended. If an electronic device (e.g. C-PAP machine) is used at night, one must be sure that there will be stable electricity and that proper transformers or plug adaptors are available.

Hypertension

Stable well-controlled hypertension is not a problem for most travel. Travel to higher altitudes may, however, cause an increase in blood pressure, and beta blocking medications may not be as effective in controlling blood pressure as at home.[2] When traveling to altitude the hypertensive individual should monitor his blood pressure regularly and increase his dose of medication

as needed. This eventuality should be discussed with his personal physician before travel and with the medical team leader. Resting and reducing salt intake for the first few days at altitude may be helpful.[2]

Gastrointestinal Disorders

Individuals who are taking H2 blockers or proton pump inhibitors are at increased risk for travelers' diarrhea due to the inactivation of the stomach acid's protective effect against pathogens. Food and drink safety precautions should be carefully followed and medications for prompt treatment be available.

Severe Allergies

Travelers who have experienced a severe allergic reaction to medications, insect stings, foods, or anything else should discuss the risk of travel with their physician and the medical team leader. This is critical because in many areas where medical teams minister, access to emergency medical care is difficult and will depend on what the team can provide themselves. The team leader should be fully informed of the exact nature of the allergic reaction and the nature of prior episodes.

If travel is decided upon, the individual must carry with him at all times several EpiPens® or an Anakit® so that sufficient doses of epinephrine will be available should an emergency arise. Antihistamines and a short course of prednisone should probably also be packed in an accessible location.[3] In addition to the team leader, other teammates need to know where the EpiPens® are and how to use them. While traveling, special attention must be paid to avoiding exposure to the allergic trigger.

Deep Vein Thrombosis (DVT)

Travelers with a history of thromboembolic disease are in the high risk category for recurrence during long air flights,[3] or prolonged travel by other means. Prevention strategies for those not on anticoagulation therapy include wearing graduated compression stockings on the plane, taking aspirin, getting up and walking around and doing leg exercises intermittently during the flight and remaining well-hydrated. Using low molecular weight heparin during travel is also an option. If the individual has a history of frequent recurrences of DVT, many medical team destinations would be too risky. If the history of DVT is remote and there are no other complicating factors, participation on a team, preferably in this hemisphere would be possible.

Cardiovascular Disease

Symptomatic, even mildly symptomatic, cardiovascular disease is probably too great a risk for most medical teams, primarily because of the lack of accessible, western standard of care hospital facilities in many developing countries. Asymptomatic individuals should receive careful counseling concerning the nature and demands of the trip and should review their current cardiovascular status with their cardiologist before making the decision to participate on a medical team.

Diabetes

Diabetics may experience a number of disruptions during travel which will require a change in their medication dose or frequency. Unfamiliar foods, irregular schedules, varying amounts of exercise, and travelers' diarrhea can all wreak havoc with glycemic control. These factors are most significant to the insulin dependent traveler.

The diabetic who is controlled on oral medication will not need to make major adjustments in his medication. He should begin taking his medicine on the daily time schedule in the country of destination on arrival.

Both type II diabetics and insulin dependent diabetics need to monitor blood glucose more frequently than at home (every 6 hours if daily routine is disrupted). This will allow timely adjustment of insulin doses or snacks. In addition to packing sufficient insulin, diabetics need to take adequate quantities of needles, alcohol wipes, and syringes for the trip. Take supplies for testing blood glucose including a blood glucose monitor, extra batteries, lancets, etc. (Check with the airlines to obtain information on bringing necessary syringes or monitoring equipment through airport security in your carry-on luggage.) Be sure to include glucagon, and verify that the medical team leader will be carrying antibiotics, antidiarrheal medication and antiemetics.

Alert the team leader if any symptoms of illness occur as soon as they start. Bring a supply of snack foods such as crackers, cheese, peanut butter, something sugary (glucose tablet or candy), juice boxes, etc. Keep some of these with you at all times to prevent or treat low blood sugar in case of travel delays.[2]

Travel across more than 5 time zones will also necessitate changes in insulin requirements. There are several ways of making these adjustments. One fairly easy method suggests that travelers flying west (making a longer day) increase their daily insulin dose by 2–4% per hour of time shift or, if traveling eastward (making a shorter day), reduce their daily insulin dose by the same percentage.[3] On a long westward flight this would be accomplished by one or two extra doses of short-acting insulin during the flight. On the eastward journey an extra dose of short acting insulin would be given to cover the late evening meal with a subsequent reduction in the breakfast dose of intermediate acting insulin.[2]

A Note of Caution Is in Order

Blood glucose monitors perform differently, tending to underestimate blood glucose, at altitudes above 6800 feet.[2] Diabetics should test their glucose standards and correct their blood values accordingly.

The American Diabetes Association (ADA) has several helpful resources for the diabetic traveler which can be accessed from their web site. Another valuable resource is a booklet prepared by the International Association for Medical Assistance to Travelers which lists clinics and English-speaking doctors in many countries. (See "Resources" at the end of this chapter.)

References

1. Sullivan MC, Jong EC, Travel with Chronic Medical Conditions, *The Travel and Tropical Medicine Manual*, 3rd ed., edited Jong EC, McMullen R, Philadelphia, 2003, Saunders, pp 234–245.
2. Bezruchka SA, Altitude Illness, *The Travel and Tropical Medicine Manual*, 3rd ed., edited Jong EC, McMullen R, Philadelphia, 2003, Saunders, pp 129–141.
3. McCarthy AE, Travelers with Pre-existing Disease, *Travel Medicine*, edited Keystone JS, Kozarsky PE, Freedman DO, Nothdurft HD, Connor BA, Philadelphia, 2004, Mosby, pp 241–247.

Resources

1. The American Diabetes Association (ADA): web site: www.diabetes.org Diabetes Day by Day series #3, *Guide to Eating Out*, #13 *All about Insulin* and #29, *On the Go.* The ADA also publishes a "Buyer's Guide to Diabetes Supplies" which addresses types of insulin and supplies available abroad as well as in the US.
2. International Association for Medical Assistance to Travelers (IAMAT) has a booklet which lists clinics and English-speaking doctors in many countries. Website: www.iamat.org

8 Cultural Sensitivity and Cross-Cultural Communication

Susan Benesh

Picture, if you will, the eager missionary stepping off a plane in India. He, anxious to establish a good relationship, wants to greet his new friends. Being from Texas, he waves vigorously to his in-country hosts, "HOWDY!" he says. Greeted with stares of confusion he waves again, "HOWDY!" A few chuckles erupt from the locals and a local interpreter finally tells him that in their language "howdi" is the local word for prostitute. Luckily, this is a good natured group and the whole episode breaks the ice with a hearty laugh enjoyed by all.

This illustrates the first lesson of cross cultural sensitivity and communication. One must understand that the most important thing to bring on a trip is an accommodating nature, a good sense of humor and the realization that, "we aren't in Kansas anymore."

We are "on-duty" for God at all times, but our behavior is particularly conspicuous when we are traveling abroad. Many people will be watching us and judging our words and actions. How we present ourselves will reflect not only on ourselves, our team, our hosts and our home county, but also on our Lord.

In order to be a positive ambassador for Christ, we must first seek to understand the foreign culture, and then to create a caring relationship with its people based on mutual respect, concern and trust. Only then can we begin to share the Word effectively.

It is impossible to cover every aspect of international travel in this manual, but there are a few main points which will help in every part of the world.

A Good First Impression

Research shows that in every culture, people make a generally positive or negative impression within the first minute of interaction. This impression is formed by an analysis of facial expression, body language, attire and accessories. We do not want the way we are dressed or the way we behave to be offensive to the people we seek to serve. Inappropriate clothing or unintentional impoliteness may block or severely delay our ability to build positive relationships in a new culture/community.

Attire and Accessories

Think hard before packing and do some research on both the weather and the culture at your destination. You will want to be comfortable, but also well in keeping with the local customs, and you will want to travel light. Ask your national contact for specific advice on the most appropriate clothing for the different activities that you will be involved in. Consider the reason for your trip and the people with whom you are likely to be interacting. Will you be hiking through the jungle and working in remote villages or will you be lecturing at a prestigious medical school?

Once on a trip to Africa a young woman, despite clear direction from her team leader, brought only pants and shirts to wear. The day after arrival in the village where the team would be working, the local pastor presented her with a long skirt which he had paid for from his own meager funds and instructed her to please wear it. Her careless disregard for local custom was an embarrassment to the local church, and finally to her.

Attire Tips

1. *Loud colors tend to be quite conspicuous* (as well as attract mosquitoes in some countries!). Remember that dignity is always an asset. Loud golf or polo type shirts for men, easily accepted in the US may be ridiculed in a foreign country. Neutral tones of browns, blues, greens and black are generally preferable. Pastels in soft hues are typically considered correct for women in all countries. However, there are some definite "no-no's" for women. All white outfits should generally be avoided in many Far East and Asian countries, since this is a sign of mourning. Bright red is a bridal color in some Middle Eastern countries.

2. *Extreme styles should be avoided.* For men who may be lecturing, preaching or meeting high level officials, a dark suit with matching jacket and pants, white shirt, conservative tie and black shoes and socks is considered acceptable in every part of the world. A long skirt and conservative blouse is appropriate in most places for women. Pants for women may or may not be acceptable. Loose pants with long tunic are a recognized outfit in many Muslim countries and in India. In some locations a scarf or head cover is needed. Modesty is the rule. Clothing that is too tight fitting and bare shoulders are offensive and convey the wrong message in conservative cultures. Shorts for men and women should be reserved for the resort, not for working.

3. *Pretentious jewelry is a bad idea!* A simple wedding band, conservative watch, and small earrings (if any) are quite adequate for most occasions. Loud or excessive jewelry marks you as a target for thieves in many areas and can be seen as an indication of sexual promiscuity in some parts of the world. However, in other countries, multiple bangle bracelets are worn by women as a symbol of marriage.

4. *Accessories.* Keep briefcases, luggage and purses modest and unassuming. Expensive accessories may make you a target for kidnapping, thieves and pickpockets. Travel light. If you don't absolutely need it, leave it at home.

5. *Hair styles.* Men and women should be neat and well-groomed at all times. Women with long hair should keep it in a scarf or bun. Watch what the other women are wearing in a hair style and behave accordingly. In some countries, women's hair takes on a sexual significance. In others, only young, unmarried women wear their hair loose. The ubiquitous American baseball cap should be left at home unless you are a young boy or working in the sun.

Language

Americans in general are louder than almost all other human beings in the world. Further, it is a well recognized fact that when we are attempting to communicate with someone who speaks another language, we get even louder as though shouting will somehow make us more easily understood. We also have the unfortunate reputation of being impatient and insistent on having things our way.

Please recognize that a low, pleasant voice is more suitable when communicating. Calm, polite, respectful speech and behavior are powerful tools in building relationships, especially in times of stress.

Make every attempt to understand at least a few words in your host language. A sincere attempt, no matter how clumsy, to understand and communicate in the other person's language is appreciated by a foreign host. It is a humble sign that you are there to learn as well as to teach. Learn the most common phrases in the new language. (See the web site at the resource free online translator at the end of this chapter.)

1. Hello.
2. Good-bye.
3. Please.
4. Thank you.
5. Thank you very much.
6. No, thank you.
7. I am pleased to meet you.
8. I hope you are well (healthy).
9. That is very impressive, that is wonderful. (Do not praise personal possessions excessively, in some countries the host may feel compelled to give it to you.)
10. Where is the...? (the American Embassy, airport, hotel, for example).
11. I am sorry.
12. Please forgive me.
13. You have a beautiful country.
14. I am having a wonderful time.

Never use profane language, never use slang, colloquialisms or idiomatic terms ("howdy"), and always speak slowly and clearly.

Relating to and Working with an Interpreter

If you are quite unfamiliar with the language you will need an interpreter who is trustworthy and reliable. The national contact for the medical team will be arranging for the best interpreters that he can find. In some countries, fluent translators are available, but often some team members will be working with translators who will struggle, especially with medical vocabulary. Patience and a good sense of humor will usually lead to a good working relationship. Do make sure your interpreter has breaks for rest, food, water and personal needs. Your interpreter should always be treated courteously and with respect. Invite him/her to join you

at lunch. Learn more about the country and culture from him. You will find getting to know this invaluable team member very rewarding.

When using an interpreter, always look at the person to whom you want the message given, not the interpreter. Often, facial expression can convey a sense of your message. Similarly, look at the person who is doing the talking, even when their remarks are being translated. Do not assume the interpreter knows what you are saying at all times. Even the best interpreter has language difficulties, especially when you are using technical jargon such as is used in medicine and health care. Ask the interpreter frequently and without impatience if he understands what you are saying. If the conversation is delicate, explain the situation to the interpreter and ask them what the best way to phrase something might be.

Dining in a Foreign Country

Safety of food is well covered in other places in this text. Dining is another matter entirely and the "breaking of bread together" is of extreme importance in almost every culture. Dining rituals in most countries involve a slower, more deliberate pace. Eating together is generally more leisurely and business is typically never discussed when eating. You will see many customs and foods that we may consider awkward, odd or even distasteful. It is up to your judgment in those situations to respond most appropriately and graciously. Sometimes the food offered to you in one meal will be more than your hosts have had all week. You may be presented delicacies that the host would never buy for his own family.

In the sincere and deeply ingrained tradition of hospitality your in-country hosts will honor you with the best they have to offer. Let them know how much you appreciate their welcoming you and honoring you in this way.

There may be times when you and your team will be served with food which you deem risky from a health perspective. If there is no polite way to avoid eating it, a few individuals may be chosen (select these individuals ahead of time if possible) to sample the risky food, rather that risk the entire team. This is clearly a delicate issue and great care should be taken to avoid offending one's host.

Gift Giving

The exchanging of gifts is an integral part of the cross-cultural dialogue. It is important to have small, easy to carry tokens of esteem, honor and thanks. Gifts should never be too costly or they may be considered bribes. Presentation is quite important. A small, well wrapped gift shows that you have thought about the person in advance.

When meeting someone of high rank, try to do as much research about that person as possible to understand what might be of significance to them. Do not give a gift at the first meeting, or at the beginning of a meeting if this is to be the only time you meet a person of rank, it seems overly anxious. Confer with your national host about the appropriate use of gift giving when meeting with officials.

Most teams like to thank the pastors and their wives who have hosted them as well as their translators and others who have helped make the mission a success. Small gifts, especially those with a personal touch, are very welcome. One may ask in advance of the trip if the host has any special request for something available in the US but not in his home country.

Requests may range from theological books to peanut butter to specialty chocolates.

Gift Ideas

1. The "latest" small gadget such as a business card flashlight or pen.
2. A small book of an appropriate topic.
3. A small box of stationery.
4. Appropriate tapes of music.
5. Gifts of local interest or hobbies, such as golf balls.
6. Gifts that are useful such as shoes, small articles of clothing, or hats.

Region-specific Gift Giving

Arabic Countries

Appropriate:	Inappropriate:
Books	Liquor
Stationery	Blue or white
Gifts for children	(religious and
often elaborate	mourning significance)
	Gifts for the office
	Gifts for a spouse
	Food or any gift at the first meeting
	Gift given with the left hand

Latin America

Appropriate:	Inappropriate:
Gifts for a family	Knives
Gifts for children	Black/purple
Logo gifts	(death and
Perfume	mourning)
Chocolate	NO-gift
	Excessive gifts

India and Hindu Areas

Appropriate:	Inappropriate:
Flowers	Leather or cowhide
Chocolate or	Liquor
cookies in a tin	Pigskin items
Small logo pens	Lavish gifts
& calculators	Gifts to members
Perfume	of the opposite
Photo frames	gender

Japan and South Korea

Appropriate:	Inappropriate:
Let host initiate	Gifts of flowers with
gift giving	yellow or white
US brand names	(death)
Company products	Numbers 4, 6 or 9
Hand made gifts	Things made in
Books	Japan
	Ribbons, bows. Use only paper to wrap.
	Humorous gifts or surprise gifts

ALWAYS present gift to only one or two people in a group. Present business cards with both hands almost everywhere in Asia.

China and Hong Kong

Appropriate:	Inappropriate:
Company or logo product	Clocks (strong assn. with death)
Regional US gifts	Money
Books	Lavish gifts
Sets of items in even #s only	Food, tips
	White flowers

NOTE: Tipping in Hong Kong is acceptable in most places. Tipping in China was formerly TABOO, however, tipping is now catching on quite quickly. When in doubt, ask hotel staff, host, etc.

Singapore, Taiwan, Philippines

Appropriate:	Inappropriate:
Quality pens and pencils	Clocks
Paper products or books	Appointment books
Food	Anything made in Asia

Social Customs

Protocol comes from two Greek words, "protos" meaning "the first" and "kolla" meaning "glue." Countries have unique social customs which are either conspicuous by their absence or presence. For example, the hand gesture we use in the US to indicate OK, by making a circle with our thumb and forefinger, with the remaining three fingers outstretched literally looks like the letters OK in our alphabet. But in other cultures it has a sexual and even offensive meaning. In general, avoid using hand signs including the automatic reflex "thumbs up." When beckoning someone to come to or to follow you, most countries use a hand motion with the palm down as one flexes the fingers rather than the American way with palm facing up (which they consider quite rude). Pointing with the finger can also be frowned upon.

When in doubt about any custom, ask your host and watch what the nationals do. Being aware of these gestures and customs will give you a bit more confidence and polish in a foreign country, at least it will help avoid an embarrassing moment.

In some places shoes are removed prior to entering the home or place of worship. Do not neglect to comply with this.

Africa

Africa is a complicated continent. South Africa tends to be British and Dutch in its customs and not too different from the US. However, the northern nationals tend to be more Arab and Islamic, abstaining from alcohol and having a very conservative attitude toward women and the mixing of the genders. French speaking countries tend to be more formal and may kiss a friend on both cheeks when greeting. In all parts of the continent, expect to shake hands constantly, this is an important part of their culture. They also tend to hold the handshake a bit longer than in the US. Meetings may need to be confirmed many times as plans tend to be fluid with some cultures.

The Middle East

Again, be prepared to wait on meetings as this culture tends to be polychronic. What we think of as late, may be totally acceptable in some cultures. Do not use your finger to point at or beckon people in this part of the world as this is a gesture used to call dogs. The left hand is considered unclean and should never be used in public. Also considered offensive is the showing of the bottom of the shoes or feet. Be cautious not to cross your legs and show the bottom of the feet. When individuals of the same gender meet their good friends, they will kiss on both cheeks, and men who are friends often walk holding hands. It is considered quite rude to ask questions about spouses or the children of an acquaintance unless you know them quite well.

Women in this part of the world are typically covered completely when in public. Women do not shake hands with men, and women do not generally maintain eye contact with men. As a foreign visiting woman, one may be more included in the company of the men and certain rules may be bent. Still a woman should be accompanied by a suitable male escort in public, and even as a foreigner, she should comply as much as possible with local dress and behavior codes. Only women can meet with other women in this kind of culture.

It is a unique opportunity for the foreign lady to go back to the kitchen to speak with the women of the house, to thank them for their hospitality, and to begin to form relationships. When women are together with women, the rules are more relaxed and discussion of children and home are welcome.

Be careful how you treat your Bible. In the Muslim world the Koran is never laid on the floor. That would be disrespectful. As Christians we should be at least as careful with the Word of God.

India

The traditional social greeting is called the *namaste* and is made by putting the fingertips of your hands together in an almost prayerful gesture and bowing slightly. The handshake may only be used in a business setting. If someone does not extend their hand, look for the *namaste* greeting.

Many items of clothing are loose and light colored because of the heat. Even business men may forego a jacket and tie in very hot climates. The *bhindi* or small red dot on a woman's forehead indicates that she is married.

In India and Bangladesh, the right hand is used for giving people things both formally and informally. The left hand is considered unclean.

Japan

A greeting will almost always consist of a standing, formal bow, bent at about a 30 degree angle. Hands are lowered, palms down at your side, pause, then lift your head. If you are a guest in someone's home, be prepared to remove your shoes, and you may or may not be given slippers to wear.

The low dining table is traditional and you will be asked to kneel on a *tatami* mat. Do not sit cross legged. You may sit with your knees bent and your lower legs angled away from you. Keep your hands clasped on your lap or at the edge of the table.   Hot moist towels are almost always offered. These are for your hands, not your face or neck unless

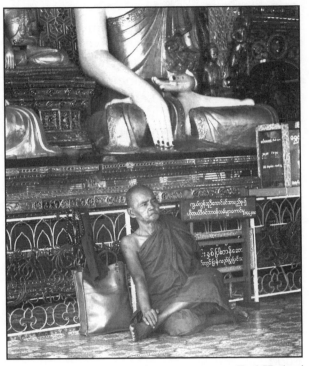

Ted Kuhn/
"Yangon Monk"

the weather is quite hot and you are grubby from outdoor activities.

Unless you have been invited to a formal dinner, stay no longer than 60 to 90 minutes. They may try to urge you to stay longer, this is customary, but they probably are just saying this to be polite. Leave, after making arrangements for another visit either to your home or a restaurant. It is impolite to eat on the street. Never leave chopsticks in a bowl (signifies ill will toward the host or someone at the table). There is a whole body of etiquette regarding Japanese dining customs. It is quite ceremonious and interesting. The wise traveler will acquaint themselves with these customs which are too elaborate to detail in this chapter.

Alcohol consumption tends to be excessive and the local liquors are quite strong. Watch out!

Always remember that there is great respect for the elderly in Asian countries. Always defer to an elder.

White is the color of mourning and yellow signifies death. Mums also signify mourning and death. Flashy or loud colors are also no-no's on all except the very young.

Tipping in most Asian countries has been somewhat frowned upon, but this practice is becoming more commonplace. When in doubt, ask your host.

China

Noisy, conspicuous behavior is frowned upon. The Chinese tend to dress in subdued tones. Again, white is the color of mourning.

Punctuality is quite important and even the slightest bit of lateness is considered quite rude. Even the smallest decisions may require many meetings and much discussion. Relationships take time to develop.

Political discussions are considered rude. Tipping is largely prohibited if known, but subtly and privately, the practice is catching on and almost always appreciated. Letters of praise are considered the height of good taste.

You will likely be served tea at almost every meeting. It is important to smile at everyone. Occasionally, the more rural people clap at people they meet as a sign of greeting or welcome, clap back.

If you are the guest of honor, you must begin to eat first and you must leave first. Watch for cues on this. Occasionally, someone may take something off of their plate and place it on your plate, this is a sign of respect. They think you are more worthy of this than they are.

Alcohol, Tobacco and Card Games

Societies vary widely in their attitudes toward alcohol. Some prohibit it, while in others social drinking to excess is common. Organizations typically discourage their personnel to partake of alcohol while working abroad. It is rare that one will offend by politely refusing to drink if the host understands that it is for personal religious, or health reasons. Within the Christian communities of many countries the use of alcohol and tobacco and sometimes playing cards are all negatively associated with life in secular society. Many people give these habits up when they become believers. It would be offensive for one who comes to help in these communities to display these behaviors which their hosts feel are dangerous or wrong.

Other Tips When Traveling in a Foreign Country

1. Know the holidays.
2. Know the top political parties and figures.
3. Know the top local stories and news items of the day. If sports are important, know the sport and the top teams.
4. Be humble about what we have in the US, do not make comparisons between their country and the US in a disparaging manner.
5. Many things may be different in the host country from what you are accustomed. Do not make jokes or "humorous" remarks about these differences that might be negatively perceived by persons overhearing you (e.g. driving on the "wrong" side of the road).
6. Be interested in the culture, history and stories about your host country. Listen attentively to your hosts.
7. Acknowledge everyone in a greeting and with a handshake when appropriate.
8. Be aware that eye-contact, especially prolonged OR between men and women may be unacceptable.
9. Display a patient attitude.
10. Never sit before your host sits in any country UNLESS they indicate that you should sit first. Sit only on the edge of a chair and then slide back to "settle in" only after the host does so.
11. Always be aware of the people around you and observe their behaviors. Especially watch who defers to whom, this can be an indication of rank and authority which you will want to honor.

Women Traveling Abroad

The status of women in many foreign countries is not the same as for American or "western" countries. Even in many Latin American countries, women can be more at-risk when traveling alone. Even more restrictive, women may be totally unable to travel alone in countries such as Saudi Arabia and other strict Islamic countries. In all cases, women should adhere to local customs when traveling abroad.

Resources
1. MTW trip information packets.
2. Country specific travel books.
3. Department of Commerce (DOC) www.doc.gov
4. International Trade Administration (ITA) www.ita.doc.gov
5. The US based Embassy of country to which you will be traveling. An internet search will yield this information.
6. http://ets.freetranslation.com/

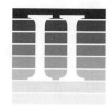

Section II:
Team Preparation for International Travel

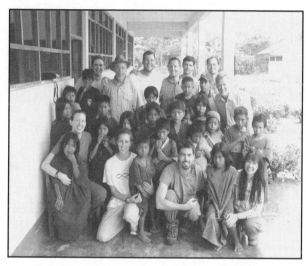

Ted Kuhn/
"Amazon Team"

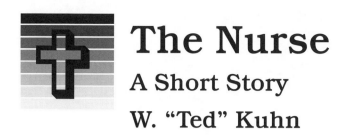

The Nurse

A Short Story

W. "Ted" Kuhn

Her light, sandy-brown hair fell easily over her right shoulder as she knelt on the concrete in front of the old man. Her gloved hand, wet with sweat, was extended toward his black callused foot. He leaned heavily on an ancient stick he used as a cane. His white hair tussled, his face deeply lined from the years. The wound on his foot, covered with flies, was a deep red-purple with a yellow coating reminiscent of melted cheese. Her delicate fingers brushed aside the flies as she painstakingly and gently cleaned the wound. The aroma of her love filled the little clinic-the sweet fragrance of the knowledge Christ. Several generations apart and from two vastly different worlds, sharing the same healing moment. Both consumed for the time in their own private thoughts, unaware of the more than 200 Haitian onlookers who watched silently in astonishment.

I have watched those hands care for other wounds on other feet at other times and in other places. First as a student, then as a nurse. There had been the infected shotgun wound on the foot of a pastor in a remote area of the Amazon. And a tattered cast on a broken ankle high in the Andes. There had been imbedded thorns and open sores on the feet of children and flies that were brushed away from a foot that had been wrapped in a dirty cloth. The same light-brown hair, the same simple smile, the same tender touch. A bright-faced girl kneeling on concrete and mud at the feet of others. God's hands reaching down through her hands. A letter written by the Spirit of

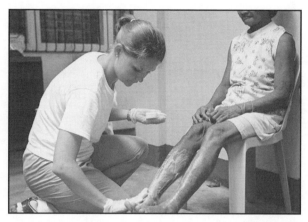

Ted Kuhn/
"Nurse Washing Feet."

God on a human heart. Grace, mercy and healing dispensed with a smile, with sweat drenched gloves and a bent knee. A gentle touch, a simple gesture -a girl, somehow now a woman. Love kneeling on concrete in a hot steamy jungle.

Thousands of years ago, another woman knelt to clean a man's feet. She washed them with her tears and dried them with her hair. She anointed them with a costly ointment, and the fragrance filled the room. A simple act indelibly burned into the collective consciousness of mankind for over two millennia. He, like the old Haitian man of today and the hundreds who watched, had been stunned by her offering. Love, kneeling down and not counting the cost. A declaration mightier than the edicts of governments. A force sufficiently strong to alter the course of history. A gift more precious than gold and healing lasting for eternity.

Reference

1. Kuhn, W., *My Eyes, His Heart*, Winepress, 2002.

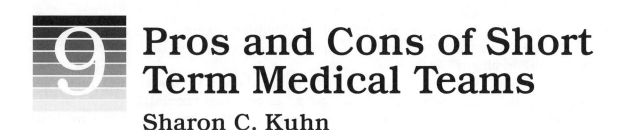

Pros and Cons of Short Term Medical Teams

Sharon C. Kuhn

Negative Arguments
Supporting Arguments and
    Accomplishments
Lasting Public Health Interventions
Medical Teams Can Open Doors
Can the Positive Turn Negative?

There are overwhelming, ongoing, unmet medical, emotional, and spiritual needs in many areas of the world today. The HIV/AIDS epidemic, natural disasters, famine and political strife compound the burden of illness and despair. Help is needed. Currently large numbers of faith-based and humanitarian teams are being sent out to destinations around the world. Is their contribution effective? Are such teams worth the investment of time and money required?

Negative Arguments

1. *Medical needs are too vast.*
   In the face of such incredible need in both curative and public health arenas, the care provided for a few hundred individuals by a 1–2 week medical team seems like trying to put a band-aid on a gaping wound. Such a team cannot make a dent in the acute health problems, let alone chronic disease. Because of poor public health measures, many will just get sick again. So, what is the use?
2. *Financial investments are great.*
   Short term teams require a large investment of money for airline tickets, room and board and transportation in the field. Could that money not be used more effectively by sending it directly to the field without the team?

3. *Time investments are significant for many individuals.*
   The missionary or national pastor hosting the team must take time to arrange the logistics for the team. This may involve travel to the remote villages where the team will practice medicine or hours spent in offices obtaining medical licenses and permission to work in the country. Other work will also be interrupted for 1–2 weeks while the team is in country. The team leaders and the team members likewise spend time preparing and must take off from their work or school to participate on the team.
4. *Cultural and language barriers decrease effectiveness.*
   Most short termers do not know the language or the culture at the destination. This may make medical care more difficult. Can the Gospel be shared effectively?

Supporting Arguments and Accomplishments

Curative medicine for the masses is admittedly not possible on a short term mission. Not everyone will be helped, but some will be helped.
Examples from the author's experiences:
- On nearly every team a life is saved, either a child with pneumonia, a lady with cholera, etc.
- Many acute illnesses are relieved.
- Chronic pain sufferers are given at least temporary relief.
- Sometimes a remarkable intervention is facilitated: a referral of a blind man for a successful corneal transplant.

- The provision of reading glasses for pastors and elders and those whose livelihoods depend on clear near vision.

In addition to physical relief, emotional and spiritual support is given in patient encounters, especially when the patients are put in contact with the local church and community sponsors who will continue to visit and encourage them when the expatriate team has gone. Providing hope and the knowledge that one is not alone in facing these burdens of suffering is a powerful healing tool.

Lasting Public Health Interventions

In even one intense clinic day, public health problems can often be identified for the village and attempts to help them find solutions can be initiated.

Actual examples of public health interventions by short term teams:

During a village clinic a large number of patients were diagnosed with bloody diarrhea from *E. histolytica*. Villagers showed the team the hurricane damaged water system and stated that they were now using the river as their source of drinking water. Local officials with the help of a subsequent international team made the necessary repairs.

A localized cholera outbreak was contained by recommending a change in the location of the latrine relative to the water source.

A discussion with village leaders concerning the malnutrition and high incidence of TB identified during a 2 day clinic in a remote area ultimately led to government health officials traveling to the village to verify the problems and then to intervene.

Villages in a mountainous area of Southeast Asia where malaria was found to be very severe were assisted by providing and teaching how to use permethrin treated bed nets.

Health teaching can be done in the context of short term teams. This can be general or targeted to specific community needs.

Local health workers as well as the general population can benefit from this.

Medical mission teams are not just going as medical teams!!!!

Jesus was the first short term medical missionary and we look to his example:

"Then Jesus went about all the cities and villages, teaching in their synagogues, preaching the gospel of the kingdom, and healing every sickness and every disease among the people." (Matthew 9:35)

Many people came to Jesus. Some came because they wanted to hear him preach with authority, but many came to be healed. Yet, while they were with him, they heard the good news and many were saved. This is the key to medical missions. The teams are not there just to provide medical care. They are there to meet people's needs, medical, spiritual, and emotional, and to build up the church. Jesus had compassion on the crowds and he met their physical need for healing, but he also met their more vital need for a Savior.

How can short term teams follow the example of Jesus and provide tangible help to the national pastors and missionaries? How can teams reach the people with the Good News of Jesus and help the church to grow when they lack language skills and cultural finesse?

Teams only go at the request of a pastor or missionary who believes that a medical team would help his church planting effort by demonstrating the love of Jesus for the people. The medical team is a part of the overall outreach of the church not an independent entity with its own agenda.

Medical Teams Can Open Doors

People who wouldn't ordinarily enter a church, who never thought of going to a Bible study, who were afraid that Protestants were a cult, will come to the church building for a clinic. They will experience compassionate medical care and concern for them as individuals, whatever their faith or lack thereof. Often the fear or hesitation disappears, and some will return for worship and study.

Act as a "wedge": An unreached community may be willing to host a Christian medical team because they desire the medical care. The team can build a bridge into the community as relationships are begun through the giving of health care that can be continued by the missionary or church planters.

Academic teams: Through lecturing and teaching, academic teams can also begin relationships and establish the credibility of national believers.

Encourage the local church: Believers in remote areas or in countries where they are a small minority are encouraged to know that they are not alone. It is a comfort to know that the Body of Christ in another part of the world knows about you and is praying for you.

Can the Positive Turn Negative?

Whether or not a team has a positive impact for the ministry of those they go to help will depend to a large extent on their attitude, behavior and relationships among themselves and with their national colleagues. A careless comment could damage a relationship that the missionary has been working on for years. A loving act may bring someone into the Body of Christ. Team members must remember that they are ambassadors of Christ. They should be respectful of customs, always speak courteously and positively about the culture and country in which they are a guest. They should treat every one they meet honorably, and maintain a patient, humble, servant's attitude in all situations.

Summary of the positive effects of short term missions on the church:

1. New believers are born into the family of faith, the church grows and its witness in the community is enhanced.
2. The church is encouraged and strengthened by its relationship to the Body of Christ in other parts of the world.
3. People experience physical healing and the compassionate touch of Christ through his church.
4. Team members' faith grows, lives are challenged by the work and by the faith of the national believers.
5. Prayers increase for the field as the team members and churches at home are now aware and praying.
6. There is increased awareness, prayer and giving by the churches at home for the work of the Lord around the world.
7. Through these experiences God will call some individuals to long term or further short term international ministry.

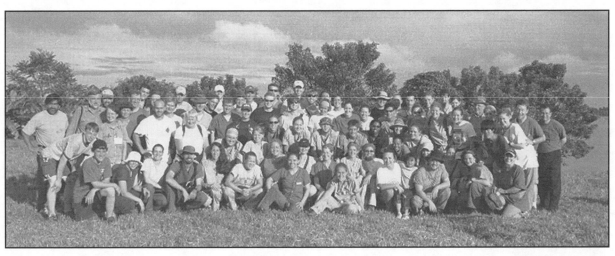

Clark Newton/
"Medical College Team in Amazon"

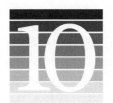

Medical Team Leader Responsibility

Sharon C. Kuhn and W. "Ted" Kuhn

Medical Team Leader Responsibilities
Pre-Travel Communications
Guidelines for Medical Evacuation
Special Situations on the Field
On the Field

To be the leader of a medical team is at once an honor and a great responsibility. Before accepting that responsibility, prayerfully consider the substantial amount of time that will be involved in coordinating with the field, in preparing team members and in organizing supplies before the trip in addition to the time to be spent on the field. The team leader will be responsible for the physical, emotional and spiritual health of the team while on the trip, and he or she will be responsible to see that the ministry is carried out in a way that honors Christ and encourages the church.

Consider these questions: Are you able to commit to pray for each team member? To spend time communicating with each one? Will you be able to work with the national church partner or missionary in the place you will be ministering and are you willing to submit to his direction? Are you able to humbly assume the role of servant leader? Are you able to make unpopular decisions for the good of the team? Are you willing to take sufficient time with the Lord for your own spiritual growth and preparation?

"If we undertake work for God and get out of touch with Him, the sense of responsibility will be overwhelmingly crushing; but if we roll back on God that which he has put on us, He takes away the responsibility by bringing in the realization of Himself."[1]

No one of us is perfectly equipped to bear this responsibility. Even though we train and prepare as well as we can, we can not imagine every situation which will arise. We will have to depend upon the Lord, whose work this is, to direct us through his word, his Holy Spirit and the wise counsel of Christian brothers and sisters. Remember that "we have this treasure in earthen vessels to show that the all-surpassing power is from God and not from us." (II Corinthians 4:7)

Medical Team Leader Responsibilities

Pre-departure

The national or missionary team in the field that has invited the medical team will be in charge of the in-country logistics of the trip. Day to day decisions about where the team will go, where they will stay and sleep and eat and the budget for the trip are usually made by this leadership team in consultation with the leadership in the United States (team leader and medical department staff). The designated medical team leader will be responsible for the overall health of the team and assist the national leaders with the medical outreach in the field.

The team leader is responsible for being sure that each team member has completed his application forms and submitted his deposit and ultimately the cost of the trip within the established time frame. *"A commitment to thorough preparation is absolutely necessary. This commitment will be tested by [the team leader] meeting a series of [established] deadlines.... Failure to meet these deadlines is usually a true indication that the leader is not taking his task seriously. Failure to adequately prepare one's group could result in forfeiting the group's participation."* [2]

Overseeing Team Health and Safety

1. The medical team leader should be aware of medical risks involved with travel in the destination country and plan ahead for possible emergencies. For example, will there be travel at high altitude or excessive heat or humidity or rigorous exercise involved in the mission? What are the risks of individual infectious diseases? Will there be clean water and food available for the team and if not, how can these be safely provided? If the team leader is traveling to a country where he/she has not worked before, information can be gathered from the sending organization's medical director, the CDC, World Health Organization (WHO), the US embassy and other resources listed in the "Resources for the Traveling Medical Professional" chapter. People living in the country and recent visitors may also be a source of information.

2. The medical team leader needs to learn about the general health and fitness and any medical problems of team members before arrival on the field. Certain health issues may be of greater concern in certain parts of the world and these should be evaluated in advance. The medical team leader should also be certain that each team member has received his or her recommended immunizations by their private physician and that each team member carries individual supplies of prescription medications that may be needed on the field, including malaria prophylaxis.

3. The medical team leader will be responsible for carrying and maintaining an emergency medical bag equipped to provide medical support for ill or injured team members as appropriate to the country and risk involved. What is included will vary from one team leader to another and from one country to another. For example, travel to and from locations that are low or interme-

diate risk (see chapter on the "Risk of Travel") may need few additional medical supplies. Since by definition these countries or areas have the availability of western style medical facilities, it is reasonable to use local in-country resources if an emergency arises. Travel to locations classified as "substantial" or "high risk" will involve extended preparation and supplies to assure the safety of the team. A list of supplies that the authors carry for "substantial" and "high risk" travel is included in the chapter on "The Emergency Medical Kit."

4. The medical team leader will be responsible, in consultation with other team leaders and the sending organization, for decisions regarding hospitalization of team members and evacuation from the field if the need arises. (See "Guidelines for Medical Evacuation" later in this chapter.)

Preparation for the Medical Outreach

1. The medical team leader will be responsible for making sure that there are sufficient and appropriate medicines and supplies for the trip to assure success in the medical outreach. The medical team leader will be ultimately responsible for the quality of care provided by the team.

2. The medical team leader will be responsible for all aspects of the medical outreach of the team including set up of the clinic and logistics of patient care: triage, patient numbers and flow, decisions on hospitalizing patients, etc. These logistics are worked out in cooperation with the national pastor or missionary at whose invitation the team has come. (Details on clinical logistics can be found in the "Logistics of Outpatient Medicine in the Developing World" chapter.)

Composition of the Team

Though a medical team may come from only one church, this is the exception rather than the rule. Most teams are made up of individuals from different churches in different towns and include a variety of health professionals, students, pastors and other non-medical folk. Each team is unique with individuals possessing gifts and skills especially suited for the ministry the team will undertake. It will be the job of the team leader to encourage the unity and building of positive relationships within the team. If feasible, have as many team members as possible meet together for pre-field training and orientation. If this can not be achieved, then time should be taken early in the trip to help the group get to know each other.

To help assure team unity and good will, it is a good idea to have each team member agree to work together under the principles outlined in the Team Covenant (See Appendix). Discuss the content with each would-be team member and be sure that they agree to live and work by these biblical principles of behavior while serving on the team. Many potential interpersonal conflicts can be avoided or dealt with easily if this Covenant is used.

Recruiting for a team may be done by the team leader and/or the sending agency.

Medical teams can be composed of all types of medical, dental, and allied health professionals, students, and nonmedical individuals. Each team member must have a role in order to feel that they are contributing to the ministry. It is a good idea to discuss different possible roles with nonmedical people before the trip so that they can prepare for them. (See chapter on "The Role of Nonmedical Individuals")

Share Leadership Responsibilities

Team leadership is a great responsibility covering multiple areas. It is almost too large a job for one person. Ask for help. Share the responsibility. Delegate to those who are willing and able to help. Begin to involve others early in the planning stages.

Helpful suggestions include:
1. Request a co-team leader.
2. Request that a mature team member of the opposite sex assist you in the care of team members of that sex. For example, young women may feel uncomfortable discussing certain health concerns with a male team leader.
3. If the team leader of a medical team is not a physician, he should appoint a medical director for the team. This individual will be responsible for making final medical decisions including those concerning team members.
4. Designate a reliable, organized team member to be your financial assistant on the trip. This person can be in charge of the team finances, gathering the receipts and compiling the accounting sheet at the end of the trip. This is especially helpful on large teams.
5. Encourage different team members to sign up before the trip to be responsible for giving a devotion or sharing their testimony with the team or to help to plan the worship music. Depending on the request of the national church, have 1–2 team members be prepared to give a short message/sermon for the local church. The team should prepare a couple of worship hymns or songs that they can sing together for the church.
6. Request a volunteer to make the daily work assignments for the team. This volunteer can solicit job preferences from team members and may plan to rotate some of the more stressful (triage) or less glamorous (water purifying) jobs.

Pre-Travel Communications

Logistics

Good communications between the team leader, the sending agency's home office, and the field are critical for a successful mission. All teams go at the invitation of a field and at a time that is either requested by or suitable to the field. The size of the team may have to be limited in certain areas due to available accommodations and transportation.

Medical teams should not go out with their own agenda. The on-site team has invited the team to help with specific outreaches that will enhance the ministry of the gospel in that area. The field (missionaries and/or national pastors) will set the schedule with input from the team leader. The team leader needs to gain a clear understanding of the vision for the work and for what is expected from his team. For example, if the expectation of the field is that the team would see

500 patients per day for 10 days in a row, it will be the job of the team leader to honestly communicate the actual capabilities of his team and the need for quality, compassionate care. With good, open discussion, most of these differences in expectations can be easily resolved.

Depending on the size and composition of the medical team, several different medical outreaches are possible. Large village clinics can be done if the team is well-staffed. Smaller clinics by appointment only work for smaller teams. Health screening for children or adults work well when doctors are few but there are sufficient ancillary providers. Home visits are another option, as are teams that do community health teaching. Specialized teams for physical therapy, academics and disasters may be requested and these are covered elsewhere in this book.

The team leader must work with the field in planning the daily and weekly schedule both before and upon arrival. Clinic hours and travel time must be decided upon.

The team will probably need a half or whole day off after 3–4 days of work. Travel, work in the heat, jet lag, the emotional stress of poverty and disease all accumulate. Team members need a break to rest and reflect so that they can then continue to work with renewed strength and enthusiasm. Avoid skipping meals. If your team is able to eat well (at least regularly) and sleep well, they will be able to handle the rigors of the trip.

On two week teams, it is wise to plan a recreational activity on the weekend. The team will also want to participate in the worship of the local congregation. Provide the best tentative schedule that you can for your team before leaving, but remind them that they will need to be flexible because the schedule will most likely change.

Pre-travel Communication with the Team: Preparation and Education

A team meeting is the easiest way to build team unity and to be able to share vital information easily and efficiently with the team. If, however, members live far from one another communication will be primarily by E-mail and telephone prior to the trip. Several weeks before the anticipated travel, the medical team leader should contact every team member.

This is a time to answer questions and handle concerns. Clarify any items of concern from the team member's health form and find out if the team member will be carrying prescription medications. Be sure that travel immunizations are being received and that malaria prophylaxis, if needed, is obtained. Verify that the individual has essential paper work (medical license, passport and visa) and the packing list for proper gear and equipment. (See "Health Questionnaire" and suggested "Packing List" in the Appendix).

The team leader needs to share the vision with his team for the work they will be participating in. The team needs to understand how their contribution will fit in to the overall mission of the church in that area. Once in the field, encourage team members to take the opportunity to hearten the missionaries and pastors and church members at their destination by getting to know them, by listening to their stories, their testimonies, and their hopes for the church. Building relationships with brothers and sisters in Christ and with patients and others will strengthen not only the team's faith, but also the church.

Prepare your team for the challenges they may face physically, emotionally and spiritually. Review the basics of food and drink safety and protection from insects. Let team members know ahead of time if they need to get "in shape," if they need to be prepared for outdoor latrines, or more seriously, for grinding poverty and disease. The fewer the surprises, the better. Strongly encourage each team member to enlist the support of at least five committed intercessors who will pray daily before, during and after the trip for the individual, the team, the national believers and the outreach.

Guidelines for Medical Evacuation

There are guidelines to aid in the decision-making process if the question of evacuation of an ill or injured team member arises. The medical team leader must not only consider the health and welfare of the ill or injured team member, but also the impact the evacuation may have on other team members left behind and on potential incoming rescuers. Everyone's safety is a concern.

Teams going into very remote areas should be prepared to accomplish self-rescue should the need arise, since assistance from the outside may be difficult to obtain or be delayed if available at all. Once a decision has been made to evacuate a team member, usually the evacuation should take place immediately without waiting for further deterioration of the patient or deterioration in weather or climatic conditions. Most often this will involve ground evacuation and not air evacuation. It is wise to remember that evacuation by litter or stretcher is agonizingly slow. It will require a minimum of 6 team members to carry a litter over smooth trails and up to 8 over rough terrain. It is physically demanding to carry a litter for more than 15 to 20 minutes and additional team members will be needed if progress is to continue without significant breaks. Aeromedical evacuation has its own problems and limitations. Take off and landing may be hazardous and attention must be paid to the effects of in-flight conditions, including comfort, cold and the effects of the reduced atmospheric pressure in flight on both the patient's condition and medical devices. Also, access to the patient may be limited during flight making procedures or life saving medical interventions difficult or impossible. In general, aeromedical evacuation should only be undertaken by medical personnel familiar with the unique problems that flight involves.

The Wilderness Medical Society has provided a list of conditions requiring emergency evacuation from a remote location.[3] This list is taken directly from their text.

1. Sustained or progressive physiologic deterioration, manifested by orthostatic dizziness, syncope, tachycardia, bradycardia, dyspnea, altered mental status, progressive weakness, or intractable vomiting and/or diarrhea, inability to tolerate oral fluids, or the return of loss of consciousness following head injury. In other words, if patients are not improving, they must get out!
2. Debilitating pain.
3. Inability to sustain travel at a reasonable pace due to a medical problem.
4. Passage of blood by mouth or per rectum, if not from an obviously minor source.
5. Signs and symptoms of serious high altitude illness.
6. Infections that progress despite the administration of appropriate treatment.
7. Chest pain that is not clearly musculoskeletal in origin.
8. The development of a dysfunctional psychological status that impairs the safety of the person or the group.

Travel may continue if it is towards definitive care in the case of points 3, 4, and 8 or when descending in the case of point 5 above.[1]

Special Situations on the Field

Occasionally, teams from different locations or countries will come together for a special project such as a disaster response. Each team may have their own team leader. If at all possible, the leader who will have the ultimate decision making responsibility should be identified before the teams are deployed. Certainly, as in every situation, the servant leader must seek the wisdom of those around him, all should pray, and if possible, a consensus should be reached.

The persons in authority over the teams should also be clearly designated before deployment and contact information obtained. For example, the leader for the career team in a country might be contacted by a short-term team leader, or a regional director might be the next line of authority over a disaster relief team, or the question may need to be referred to someone in the sending agency's main office.

In some cases the team leader is not the most "senior" medical person on the trip. Should a medical emergency arise, the team leader would be expected to consult with the senior medical person.

In many cases the team leader will be a very capable woman. Even though she will make all the team decisions, in certain societies, she will need to designate a mature male team member to be her spokesman when meeting with community leaders.

On the Field

Soon after arrival the team leader should give the missionary/pastor an opportunity to speak to the group to orient the team to the culture and to cast the vision for the work. Encourage him to share what God is doing, future plans, how the short-term team fits in, etc. Be sure to introduce other nationals and missionaries who will be helping with the team: church members, elders, translators, cooks, and drivers. Let them share a bit about themselves, their testimony and their work to the whole group. Invite the missionaries and nationals to join in your team worship and devotions and debriefing. They are a vital part to your team.

As team leader, make a conscious effort to build a relationship of respect and trust between yourself and your host missionary or pastor. Pray for unity in the Holy Spirit. Schedule regular times to meet daily for "business", i.e. to review or revise the schedule, how the clinic is going, etc. Also make time for personal, informal chats. Keep each other informed. The better you understand each other, the current situation and its implications, the smoother and more effective the ministry will be.

While on the field the team leader's responsibility for the team's physical, emotional and spiritual well-being continues. The daily devotions and prayer time will help the team maintain their focus on the purpose of the trip. In the evening a time of debriefing should be held. Logistical issues and frustrations can be addressed by the team, but more importantly individuals need time to share the joy, the challenge and the pain of the day's ministry.

The team leader and his co-leader or helpers need to be sensitive to cues from team members concerning perhaps unspoken physical or emotional needs so that they can be addressed quickly. "Checking in" with each team member every day or two will help the leader support and encourage his team so that each one has the best experience possible.

A week or two after the team returns home, the team leader should once again contact each member and debrief concerning any physical complaints, any troubling thoughts and any praiseworthy events. The team leader should leave the door open for the individual to get back in touch with him. The team leader should also send a note or E-mail of thanks to those who hosted the team. Ask them for follow-up on patients and the mission as a whole. Ask them to offer suggestions for improving or expanding the ministry of future teams. Be sure to thank the individuals and organizations who helped the team with supplies, prayer and preparation. Continue to pray for the team and those you have worked among.

References
1. Chambers O., *My Utmost for His Highest*, © 1935 by Dodd Mead & Co., renewed © 1963 by the Oswald Chambers Publications Assn, Discovery House Publishers, Grand Rapids, MI.
2. *Leader's Manual for One to Two Week Projects*, Missions to the World (MTW) / IMPACT staff, 1999.
3. Forgey WW: *Wilderness Medical Society Practice Guidelines for Wilderness Emergency Care*, Old Saybrook, Connecticut, 1995, Globe Pequot Press, p 70.

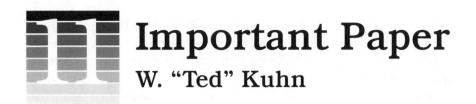

11 Important Paper

W. "Ted" Kuhn

While no one really enjoys a paper shuffle, whether or not you have the correct form or paper resources can mean the difference of practicing or not practicing medicine in a host country or the difference between a large customs/importation fine and receiving your supplies on time, duty-free. On a recent trip to a country in Southeast Asia, I was detained at the airport by customs officials. While I had a general list of which medicines the team was carrying, they wanted every pill in every container counted. It took all day to comply. They confiscated (held in customs) a significant portion of the teams medicine. I spent (read "wasted") 1 day to "find" the appropriate office (visiting many other "customs" offices in different parts of the city on the way) to formally "declare" the medicines. It took another day to fill out forms and actually locate the officials in their office at the appropriate time and another 8 months of leg work to get the medicines "released" at which time most of the medicines had been damaged by water (in the secure customs storage) or were expired. Unfortunately this story is not unique. Everyone working in a developing country has had a similar experience (if not many such experiences). If I had carried the correct piece of paper on the day I entered the airport, all of this time, energy and frustration (and waste of good medical supplies) could have been avoided.

The suggestions below have been developed from more than 30 years of experience in traveling to and from developing countries and practicing medicine. While it is unlikely that you will need all of this documentation on any one trip, you will need some of it on every trip. Of course, the problem is, you never know ahead of time which piece of paper will prove to be the critical link! Fortunately, paper is both light and cheap.

Gathering Your Team

You will need to encourage your team members to complete their organizational applications. These are typically due 3 months before the target departure date. This is critical for several reasons. Not everyone who wants to be on the team, is appropriate for membership on the team. There may be valid health concerns, psychosocial problems or theological issues which would make participation by an individual inappropriate. You can not screen out these individuals until you know that a problem exists. The time to deal with issues is ahead of time, not in a remote field setting. Frequently medical licenses must be procured or permission to travel to a remote location in the host country must be obtained. This may take months in the host country. These can not be accomplished until you know exactly who is on your team.

Before You Go
1. Each team member will need to copy his/her passport and visa form. These should be kept separate from the original should the original be lost. It is easiest

to obtain another passport if you have a copy of the old one—most embassies will issue another in 1–2 days. However, it may take a week or longer to obtain a new passport if you do not have a copy of the old one and passports DO get lost.

2. You will need to distribute copies of all emergency contact numbers to every team member in case the team becomes separated. This includes emergency numbers in the US as well as hotel and contact information on the field. During a recent team to Central Asia, bad weather caused the delay of several flights out of the US The result was that there were team members stuck in 3 different American airports, one European airport and 1 Asian airport and no one knew where the others were.

3. Copy your credit cards so that if they are lost or stolen, you can report them immediately before charges are accrued. The simplest way to do this is to place them all together, face down on a copy machine and make 1 copy of them all. Turn them over and copy the other side. The reverse side usually includes the emergency contact number in case of lost or stolen credit cards.

4. Do the same as in 3 for all traveler's checks, medical licenses, driver's license and photo ID.

5. Team leaders will need to carry a copy of each team member's health forms. This allows you to remember who is taking which medicine for which disease, and also allows emergency medical treatment should a team member become incapacitated.

6. Carry "clean" money. Many times banks and exchange counters in developing countries will not exchange U.S. bills that have been torn or have pen marks or look old. Ask your local bank before you go for clean, fresh bills.

7. Copy your airline ticket and carry it separate from the original. If you have paper tickets, you will need to unstaple them and make a copy of each segment of your journey. This is NOT the same as the itinerary and does not include the

"front" of the ticket—but the actual part that is exchanged for the boarding pass. Airlines will issue a new ticket without charge if you have a copy and lose your original. If you don't have a copy of the original ticket, at best you will be charged a heavy fine; at worst, you will have to buy a new ticket for the remainder of the trip at whatever charge the airline decides to impose (often many thousands of dollars on the day of travel). If you are traveling with "e-tickets" lost tickets are not a problem. You will need a copy of your itinerary in case the computers are "down" in the airport (often the case in developing countries).

While Traveling

1. People love business cards, especially in Asia. Carry a sufficient number to hand out—but only to those people who you might want to have contact you in the future. Remember not to hand out "mission" related cards in "sensitive" countries.

2. Carry your travel insurance card and a copy of the policy brochure if you have one. This gives the emergency telephone number should the need arise and will explain your coverage and the limits of your policy. In an emergency, you don't want to have to "wonder" if you are covered!

3. Keep a copy of your expense receipt book handy in your carry-on so that you can track all your own and your team expenses. If a receipt is not available, have a team member sign a receipt from your expense book.

4. You need your vaccination record to clear immigration in some countries. If they want to give you a vaccination in a developing country, unless you are absolutely sure the vaccine is safe and they are using sterile technique and clean needles, "just say no"!

5. If you are carrying medicines and supplies into a country, you will need documentation that you are in compliance with the laws of the country. This may

mean that you need to be licensed to practice medicine in that country, or that you have a letter of invitation from the Ministry of Health or a letter from an organization under whose umbrella you will be practicing. Without such documentation, you may not be allowed to enter with your supplies, or your will be forbidden to continue your work. Non-compliance may have an impact on future teams and work in this particular country. You will also need a copy of your US medical license (State license) and carrying a notarized copy of your medical school (or nursing school) diploma can sometimes be helpful.

6. Your sponsoring organization will prepare an official letter for your team stating that you are organizationally working under them. This is what we call our "get out of jail free" letter—the name taken from the game Monopoly® since this letter is helpful in many situations. The letter will carry a stamp and yellow seal—very impressive—and the signature of one of the agency's senior staff. See a copy of this letter in the appendix Organizational Letter.

7. To get your medicines and supplies safely through customs, you will frequently need a listing of everything you are carrying. You also need this list when returning to the US. If you have gotten medicines from King Pharmaceuticals, they will send you a letter stating that all medicines have been donated and are not for sale. They also send you a copy of the list of all medicines they have provided. International Aid and MAP will do the same if requested.

8. If you are carrying the "emergency bag," you may need a copy of your DEA license since there are controlled substances in the emergency bag. US Customs officials have been asked if there is a problem with licensed physicians carrying a small amount of controlled substances for team use. There is no problem with this from the US customs perspective as long as the quantity is small and clearly for non-commercial use.

9. If given a "hassle" about your medicine, supplies or equipment, or if customs wants to charge you a large sum of money (or bribe) to bring supplies into a country, just "bond" the items in question at the airport. Every international airport has a "bonding" warehouse where travelers can leave items and pick them up on the way out of the country. Thus the items never officially enter the country and are not liable to tax or duty. Sometimes the threat of "bonding" will result in the "official" releasing your property as it becomes apparent to them that you know what are doing and their bluff won't work.

While in Country

1. Copies (minimum of 5) of a list of all team members with passport information—needed for security checks and for checking into hotels. Likewise you should carry copies of team members emergency contact information, should sickness or injury occur on the field.

2. Extra passport photos for lost passports, licenses etc. Photos should be "face-on" like a passport photo and measure 2×2 inches—the size of passport photos.

Returning to the US

1. If you are carrying expensive equipment or supplies (laboratory equipment, microscope, laptop computer, LCD projector, camera, ultrasound machine, I-STAT's etc) out of the US, you will undoubtedly be returning with them on your return home. US Customs requires that you register all equipment BEFORE leaving the US on Form 4455. You can take this form, with a list of serial numbers, to the customs office at the airport (or any US customs office) when you leave and have the forms stamped by the US customs officials. Although this only takes a few minutes, be sure to allow sufficient time before your departure to accomplish this. Equipment, once registered, can be carried in and out of

the US indefinitely, as long as you have your form 4455.

2. Since it is our practice to return all unused medicines back to the US for reuse in another country, you will undoubtedly be carrying medicines back into the US with you. US customs requires a listing of all medicines you are returning with. This should be the responsibility of the person in the pharmacy the last day of clinic. It will be the list of what you carried out of the US, minus what you used.

Summary

The difference between having the required paper and not having the required paper is the difference between having a delightful travel experience and having a very, very bad day in a strange city in a far-away country. A few minutes of time before travel and gathering a few pieces of paper can mean all the difference.

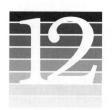

Medical Malpractice in the Developing World

W. "Ted" Kuhn

The threat of malpractice litigation is a major concern for almost all practicing American physicians. Nearly everyone in the US health care system has been adversely impacted by the current litigation crisis. There seems to be little hope of a solution in the near future. It is increasingly uncommon to find physicians and nurses who have not been sued at least once and multiple suits are unfortunately becoming common. Some specialties are affected more than others—but everyone is impacted. What is the current risk of practicing medicine in the developing world? What is the liability to the health care worker who volunteers for service on a medical mission team for either short term or long term service assuming that his/her US based malpractice insurance is not valid outside the US, which is almost always the case?

The author's own experience in cross-cultural medical ministry dates to the early 1970s, before malpractice became such a major concern. An apparent trend began to emerge in the mid to late 1990s, when nongovernmental organizations (NGOs), medical schools and missionary organizations began deploying an increasing number of medical professionals overseas to assist in volunteer medical ministry in "Word and Deed" ministry. Volunteer American medical teams have been and continue to be deployed to the Caribbean, Central America, South America, Asia, South Asia, SE Asia, Central Asia, former Soviet Union, Africa and the Middle East and many organizations have long term health care workers ministering in many of these same places. In other words, American physicians and

nurses, and allied health professionals can be found in every corner of the world.

This virtual army of American medical professionals has used their medical skills to provide compassionate care, to advance church planting, and assist missionaries and national church planters in their individual areas of service. This work involves the entire spectrum of health care professionals participating in both short and long term capacities in clinics and hospitals, in community development projects and public health programs. Many are involved in disaster relief, specialized surgical teams and academic teaching in medical schools. Many thousands of patients have been cared for, hundreds to thousands of hours of teaching has been provided and millions of pounds of medicine and supplies have been distributed.

At the same time, American physicians have staffed various hospitals and clinics involving "for profit" ventures with American or other entrepreneurs. This is distinctively different from medical volunteerism in developing countries and needs be considered separately for malpractice purposes.

During these same years the world has become a less friendly place for volunteers and missionaries. The risks involved in present day travel are more pronounced secondary to war in the Middle East and the ever present concern about the possibility of terrorist attacks and hostage taking both at home and abroad. During this same time, the litigation crisis in the United States heightened and awards appear to have no limit. Since the increased risk of travel coincides with the increase in malpractice litigation and liability in the United States, it is no wonder that health care workers are concerned about malpractice liability while traveling.

Before 2002, malpractice coverage for volunteer health care workers providing free care to indigenous populations in the developing world was available as a "rider" onto general liability packages. This was available through several insurance carriers and was considered inexpensive and was comparable to coverage most physicians carry in the US (1 million/3 million occurrence with "tail" coverage).

In 1999, the author conducted a survey of the risk of malpractice by contacting over 20 international agencies involved in health care in the developing world.[1] No agency that year (1999) responded with knowledge of any suits brought against them or their providers and none could recall a lawsuit ever brought against an American health care worker providing free humanitarian services in the developing world. That corresponded with the author's experience dating back to the 1970s. No malpractice suit had ever been filed according to the author's knowledge and none had ever been filed against any medical professional in the history of missionary work around the world.

The availability of inexpensive malpractice coverage rapidly changed after September 11, 2001, and few insurance carriers were interested in malpractice coverage for volunteer health care workers and those willing to provide coverage began "drying up" by January of 2002.

In February 2002, a repeat survey was conducted, with a larger sampling than that of the previous survey.[2] Over 50 medical schools in the US that had international medical involvement were surveyed by the author. There was not one verified report of a malpractice suit against an American health care worker providing free humanitarian services in the developing world.

Nevertheless, there have been reports of civil suits involving damage and/or injury, though none involving medical malpractice in volunteer or "not-for-profit" organizations. The author also found that by the spring of 2002, no one carried commercial malpractice insurance and no one knew of an insurance carrier that would provide coverage at any cost. Several medical universities did comment that they "self-insure." The author also spoke with several missionary organizations that conduct medical missions and several NGOs. None of these agencies carried malpractice insurance by the spring of 2002. Likewise, none had any knowledge of malpractice lawsuits, and no one knew of any insurance carrier that would provide malpractice coverage.

It is important to recognize the wording of the above paragraph. *"No malpractice claim has ever been filed against any American health care worker providing humanitarian services without charge in the developing world."* The operative words are "*malpractice*", "*humanitarian services*", "*without charge*" and "*developing world*". There have been claims against physicians providing care for American travelers overseas and claims in the developed world or "Western countries" almost all of which are against American doctors providing care for "western" travelers outside the United States and charging for those services. There have also been civil suits against American health care workers involved in road traffic accidents, accidental deaths or injury or similar disturbances—but these are not "malpractice" suits.

To summarize, Americans travel and carry their malpractice mentality with them, even though malpractice is not an issue in the country where they are traveling. The malpractice liability is in providing care for Americans traveling or living overseas, and charging for those services. There appears to be minimal to no risk in providing free medical care to the indigenous population in poor countries while doing "voluntary" or "humanitarian" service.

We can draw several conclusions:
1. Medical malpractice is a Western phenomenon and virtually unknown in the developing world. The risk for a medical malpractice suit against an American health care provider in the developing

world is exceedingly small to nonexistent if the practice of medicine is limited to the indigenous population and that care is provided free or at minimal charge.

2. There is a small but existent malpractice liability risk involving the care of American or "western" patients in "for profit" health care facilities overseas when billing or charging for services. (Most American "for profit" clinics and hospitals maintain and insure their health care workers through their existing malpractice policies in the US).

3. There is a small but extant civil liability risk apart from the malpractice risk. This appears to involve mostly traffic accidents and accidental injury and death when American health care workers are involved in an incident as an individual in a non-medical capacity.

4. No one is alone in their concern about liability or lack of coverage. The author could not find even one volunteer or missionary agency that will be providing malpractice insurance for their health care professionals from a commercial source after 2003.

5. NGOs and missionary organizations cannot provide malpractice coverage for their medical professionals since coverage is simply not available at any cost. For now, we are all in the uncomfortable position of practicing without malpractice coverage. Nevertheless, we can be comforted by knowing that we are all together and are in the best of company.

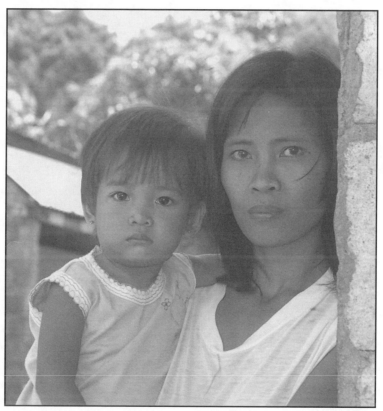

Ted Kuhn/
"Waiting for Medical Care"

References

1. Kuhn, WK: Unpublished data from 1999 survey.
2. Kuhn, WK: Unpublished data from 2002 survey.

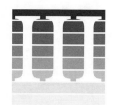

Section III:
Safety and Well-Being in the Field

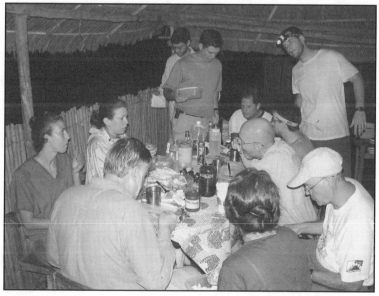

Hartmut Gross/
"Eating Well in the Jungle"

13 Food and Drink Safety

Hartmut Gross

When travelers return home and tell stories of their encounters, it seems common to hear about the gastrointestinal illness they suffered. In fact, it is accepted by many, that when traveling, they will contract some type of illness with vomiting and/or diarrhea as symptoms; indeed their medication supply includes enough medication to ease the symptoms for the duration of the trip. The reality, however, is that these illnesses are almost completely avoidable with a little preparation and care in what one chooses to eat and drink. With only a few supplies to carry along to decontaminate water and knowing which foods prepared properly are perfectly edible, you need not worry how far it is to the nearest pit latrine. Meals may still be very diverse and you may even gain weight during your healthy stay.

There are a few things which one must always assume in the developing world:
- Tap water is always contaminated. Don't drink it. Don't brush your teeth with it.
- Bottled water may be contaminated.
- Ice cubes are contaminated, no matter how many times the waiter says they are made from bottled water.
- Stream water, no matter how clean it looks, is always contaminated. Consider it contaminated everywhere in the US as well.
- No! Taking antibiotics (e.g. ciprofloxacin) does NOT protect you from all the organisms that cause gastrointestinal disease. You CANNOT eat and drink indiscriminately just because you are taking antibiotics.

A less harsh way of viewing these concepts is to look at the water (or food) you are about to consume and ask yourself, "Is it worth with the risk? To me? To my team if I should become sick and need care? To jeopardize the purpose of my traveling here?"

Water Safety

Waterborne illnesses are caused by a variety of organisms, including:
- Protozoa—*Giardia lamblia, Entamoeba histolytica, Cryptosporidium.*
- Bacteria—*Escherichia coli, Shigella, Campylobacter, Vibrio cholera, Salmonella.*
- Viruses—*Hepatitis A* and *E, Polio*, enteric viruses including *rotavirus.*
- Parasites—*Ascaris, Taenia, Fasciola, Dracunculus.*

While some of these illnesses require ingestion of a large number of the organisms, others require taking in only one or two infectious particles to cause illness! Consequently, these common illnesses in the developing world cause some 1 billion cases of diarrhea annually, and account for 10–25 million deaths each year.

Several methods for treating water are available, each with advantages and limitations. These include boiling, sedimentation/flocculation, prefiltration, filtration, chemical treatment, and adsorption. After describing each one below, some simple successful combinations will be recommended for field use.

Boiling

Boiling is considered by most as the "gold standard" for water treatment. Heat will kill all organisms, and most by the time 60°C is reached.

Old recommendations of boiling water for 5–10 minutes were made to destroy *Clostridium* species; however, these are not typically waterborne. Therefore, bringing water to a boil, and conservatively, boiling it for 1 minute is sufficient. Water may also be covered to prolong the exposure of any organisms to high temperature after the heat source is removed.

Questions about the lower boiling point of water at high altitude and the effectiveness of killing are often asked. As noted, since pathogen death generally occurs well before reaching 100°C, it is not a problem. The principle drawback to boiling is providing the large amounts of necessary fuel, which must be purchased or packed in. If electricity is known to be available, an electric immersion heater, set to the correct voltage, may be an option for small quantities of water.

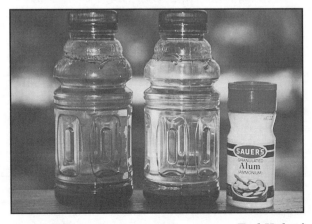

Ted Kuhn/
Figure 1. Alum

Sedimentation Using Alum

Sedimentation/flocculation is a water pretreatment. Water with considerable amounts of suspended sediment will quickly clog water filters. Removing this debris ahead of time will greatly lengthen the usefulness of ceramic and paper filtering devices. Sedimentation is nothing more than allowing turbid water to stand for about an hour to let larger particles settle by gravity. Obviously, the longer the water stands, the more debris will settle. If the water is already quite clear, there is no need for this step. The process can be accelerated and finer particles removed by addition of a flocculating or coagulating agent. Aluminum potassium sulfate (alum) is available in the grocery store and when stirred into cloudy water, will clump together the fine particles and some organisms and settle out over a few hours. (Figure 1.) The recommendation is a "pinch" of alum per gallon. The exact amount is not important as it is not toxic and excess will settle out as well. The clear water above the sediment is then poured off for further treatment. This process does not kill any organisms, nor precipitate out enough organisms to make the water safe to drink; additional purification of the water is necessary.

Prefiltration is another form of water pretreatment. It is a quicker method than sedimentation or flocculation and consists of nothing more than pouring the water through filter paper (e.g. coffee filter paper). A kitchen sieve holds the filter paper well and is easy to transport. This system will not remove any fine particles but will prevent any subsequent filter from clogging as quickly. Again, this process does nothing to kill any organisms and additional treatment of the water is required.

Filtration

Filtration devices are little more than fine mechanical barriers or traps to strain out small particles, including larger organisms. Personal units are about 3 inches in diameter and about 8–12 inches long. Larger units can be purchased for large groups. When selecting a water filter, a few points should be considered. The first is the pore size. Many filters will filter only to 1–3 microns; this will easily filter out parasite eggs, *Giardia, E. histolytica,* and *Cryptosporidium;* however, bacteria and viruses will easily pass through. Other filters will drop down to pore sizes of 0.2–0.4 microns and filter out bacteria too, but still let viruses pass. Filters may be paper or ceramic; ceramic filters are more expensive, but will last much longer provided some type of prefiltration is used. Be cautious when you read on the package that a filter removes 99.9% of bacteria. (If a million bacteria are present, removing 99.9% still leaves 1000 organisms to cause illness, and some illnesses only require consuming 10–20 organisms to cause disease.)

Keep in mind also that fine filters will clog sooner than coarse filters. Filter life expectancy is generally reported on the box in number of gallons the filter will treat before recommended replacement. Regardless of the filter you purchase, additional water treatment will be required to kill viruses and bacteria, depending on the filter size. Some filters have addressed this additional required step by including an iodine resin into the filter. Water comes in brief contact with the iodine resin to kill the residual bacteria and viruses (see below about chemical treatment). Some filters also include a unit with activated charcoal to help eliminate bad taste from the water (see adsorption discussion below). There are many different filters available on the market. These authors have personal good experience with Guardian,® Pur,® and Katadyn® units; however, no endorsement is intended towards these over other available filters. Filters may be found at larger sporting goods and wilderness outfitting stores. Tables comparing various filter brands and models may be found in several of the references at the end of this chapter.[1,3]

Chemical Treatment

Chemical treatment is a method of disinfecting the water with any of a variety of chemicals. The chlorine in your home tap water is an example. Similarly, chemicals may be taken along to treat water in the field. The effectiveness of each chemical is dependent upon temperature, concentration of the chemical, and duration of exposure to the organism. Additionally, sensitivity by the organism to the chemical also plays a major role. While bacteria are typically destroyed in minutes, viruses and some cysts require longer contact times and higher concentrations. *Cryptosporidium* cysts require 15 hours of contact time with halogens to be killed. Parasitic eggs are resistant! Cold temperature requires increased contact time, as does a large amount of debris in the water. These chemicals often have a somewhat unpleasant taste in high concentrations. Lower concentrations may be used but will require longer contact time for equal disinfection. The resistance by larger organisms to chemical treatment makes it clear why this method should be used in conjunction with some type of filter.

Chlorine

Halogenation is inexpensive and the most commonly used method for chemical treatment of water. Chlorine and iodine tablets or crystals are easily transported, but are susceptible to heat, air, moisture, and light. The chemicals may stain materials with which they come in contact. Filters with built in halogen resin release little of the free chemical into the water, but have been known to fail near the end of the filter's life expectancy. Halogens' unpleasant taste may be counteracted by running the treated water through activated charcoal (see adsorption below) or by binding the residual halogen with sodium thiosulfate or ascorbic acid (sold in separate small vials but also contained in powdered drinks such as Kool-Aid®). These neutralizing substances should be used only after sufficient time has elapsed to kill the contaminating organisms, as they render the halogen inert as soon as they are added. This order is critical to performing the chemical treatment correctly.

Chlorine is effective, but somewhat less reliable than iodine. A variety of chlorine supplements are manufactured. A household bleach solution may be used, but it is heavy and bulky to transport. Vials of tablets are available, but more difficult to find in stores; the Internet is a good source for these. Some find chlorine's taste more palatable than other chemicals; however, for effective concentrations, the taste and smell should be that of a strongly chlorinated swimming pool. For individuals not able to use or tolerate iodine, chlorine is a good alternative.

Iodine

Iodine is more stabile and more effective than chlorine. Many will argue that it tastes better at disinfecting doses than chlorine. Available tablets (EDWGT®—emergency drinking water germicidal tablet, Potable Aqua,® Tetraglycine,® Globaline®) typically are dosed at 1 to 2 tablets per liter of clear water. The dose for 2% tincture of iodine solution is 0.2 mL or 5 drops per liter while 10% povidone iodine solution requires 0.35 mL or 8 drops. Another option is 13 mL of iodine crystals in a saturated water solution (Polar Pure®) per liter or 0.1 mL of crystals saturated in alcohol. (Figure 2.) Twenty to thirty minutes of contact time is generally recommended provided the water is clear and not cold, otherwise the contact time should be doubled. If longer contact times are allowed, e.g. overnight, then lower concentrations may be used.

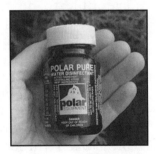

Figure 2.
Polar Pure

CAUTION: Use of iodine is contraindicated in anyone with any type of thyroid disease (even if under control with medication), pregnancy, or known allergy to iodine. Prolonged use of iodine is discouraged; however, if low doses are used, especially use of iodine resins, and the residual iodine is bound with activated charcoal or ascorbic acid, prolonged use may be possible. This is deliberately vague as individual tolerances vary widely, and no one knows the precise answer.

Chlorine Dioxide

A relatively new product for individual or group water disinfection is chlorine dioxide. Pristine® is a product which generates the chemical by mixing two solutions in the water. It has no taste or color, has no side effects and appears to be effective in killing everything except helminth eggs. Although not widely available yet, it may be purchased via the Internet at www.pristine.ca. Chlorine dioxide and other oxidants may also be generated via electrolysis with a small battery powered Miox® water purifier.

Charcoal

Adsorption is one more highly effective method of water purification; but, it does not destroy any organisms. Instead it removes odors, tastes, coloration, many toxins, and even nuclear waste from the water. Granular activated charcoal (GAC) is an inexpensive material which binds these impurities to itself and is generally one of the terminal processes in the water purification processes. It is built into, or attached, to a number of commercial water filters.

Miscellaneous

Other products are available but still with limitations of size or amount of water that can be disinfected quickly. Some new products include reverse osmosis filters, use of ozone, or use of ultraviolet light to treat water. A sports water bottle with a central filtering core and iodine resin and a drinking straw on top is available. While it advertised as ready to fill from any water source and immediately begin drinking, this conservative author is not yet convinced that there is sufficient contact time and cannot recommend it.

In summary, a combination of methods is necessary. Heat will kill organisms but leaves impurities and unpleasant color and residues behind. Filtration only works down to a limited particle size and permits viruses and bacteria (with coarser filters) to pass through. A number of important organisms are resistant to chemicals, both halogens or chlorine dioxide. Prefiltration, flocculation, and sedimentation do not remove organisms, but they do remove larger particles and prevent fine filters from clogging as quickly.

Recommendation for Water Treatment

No doubt, having read all these descriptions, the reader is now wondering what works and what they should do. The following is a general description of a water preparation process which has proven to work well for these authors.

1. Allow sedimentation and consider flocculation if water is very turbid.
2. Prefilter source water with coffee filter paper.
3. Filter water with a commercial water filter with a pore size of 1–2 microns to remove *Cryptosporidium* and helminth eggs. Smaller pore sized filters at the 0.2 micron level may be used and will remove most bacteria, but will still leave viruses in the water.
4. Treat with halogen (iodine or chlorine) or chlorine dioxide for 30 minutes to eliminate residual bacteria and viruses.
5. (Optional) Granular activated charcoal may be used before or after halogenation. If used before, it obviously will not be able to remove the halogen. If used after, it should not be used until after the water has had sufficient contact time with the halogen.
6. (Optional) Any residual unpalatable iodine may be inactivated with ascorbic acid, again after the water has had enough contact with the halogen. *Important*—this is always the last step, if used at all.

If a 0.2 micron commercial filter with an iodine resin is used, be aware that the contact time with the resin is very brief. If the water is very cold or the water is heavily contaminated, this may not be sufficient and additional halogen may need to be added to the water.

Food Safety

The number of foods and varieties of preparation you may encounter are as limitless as the human imagination. While many foods may look like something you are very familiar with and reflexly trust as safe, nothing may be farther from the truth. It is impossible to list every available dish and rank its safety. But it is possible to list some safe foods and guidelines by which to judge the risk of others.

Safe Foods and Drinks

- Drinks made with boiling water, including piping hot coffee (even with a small amount of potentially contaminated milk added if allowed to sit for 1–2 minutes).
- Bottled carbonated beverages (opened in front of you). Drinking surface should be considered contaminated and cleaned or drink from the bottle with a straw. No ice!
- Canned or other pasteurized milk. Do not accept an open glass of milk.
- Beer and wine.
- Meat and fish which have been completely cooked and are served piping hot.
- Hot, cooked vegetables, rice, potatoes, etc.
- Jams and jellies.
- Ketchup and mustard.
- Fresh bread which has not been left out in the open for flies to rest on.
- Hardboiled eggs in the shell.
- Fruit peeled by the traveler. Bananas are ideal when served unpeeled. Depending on the fruit, consider soaking in iodine solution before cutting (e.g. watermelon). A two knife technique is also recommended; one knife is used for the peel, the other to cut the fruit.
- Dried goods such as sugar, powdered creamer, salt, pepper, etc.

Foods to Avoid

- Ice
- Any food allowed to sit out and become infested with parasites or larvae.
- All food left uncovered or out in the sun.
- Leftover food unless it has been refrigerated in the interim. Remember, even if recooked, toxins may not be broken down. Avoid repeatedly handled and rewarmed foods.
- Anything which has come in contact with contaminated water.
- Locally bottled water or tap water. If treated with halogen for 30 minutes, it should be acceptable.
- Salad/lettuce.
- Uncooked vegetables.
- Unpasteurized milk and milk products including cheese. Check the label. If pasteurized, it should be safe.
- Raw meat or fish, including sushi.
- Aquatic plants in the orient as they have parasitic cysts (e.g. watercress or water chestnuts).
- Shellfish from polluted water.
- Any fruit whose surface can not be readily disinfected, e.g. strawberries and pineapple.
- Raw or undercooked eggs.
- Airline food not meeting the above requirements as well as ice cubes when returning from the developing world. Food served is prepared in the country from which the plane departs.
- Street vendor food is tricky. It should generally be considered contaminated. However, if it is prepared in front of you and thoroughly cooked, it may be consumed safely, no matter how bizarre it may be. Remember that cooking kills germs.
- Eating utensils should be considered contaminated. Many places will boil the silverware and present it at the table still in the hot water. Be careful not to burn yourself. Alternatively, you may use your bottle of gelled alcohol hand sanitizer to clean your silverware.

When dining in a restaurant, remember that the food you consume is as safe as the weakest link (Figure 3). Ask to take a look

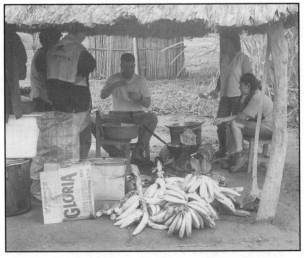

Hartmut Gross/
Figure 3. This is a safe kitchen.

at the kitchen. Is it clean? Where does the cook wash his/her hands? Does the food preparation meet your safety standards?

In the field, you must eat your food from a clean surface with some kind of utensil. A simple solution is a Tupperware® container with a tight lid and eating utensils which fit inside (Figure 4). After eating from the bowl

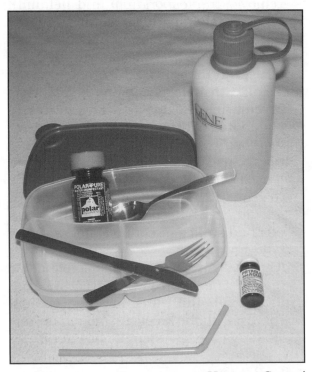

Hartmut Gross/
Figure 4. Water tight container and iodine.

or off of the lid, rinse the dish and silverware with the most clean water available. Then add a little water and iodine; then seal and shake the container. By the time of the next meal, the container and utensils will be disinfected and safe for use again.

Another method for cleaning dishes is a system of three large washing bowls with progressively decreasing concentrations of chlorine or bleach (Figure 5). Dishes are washed starting in the strongest bleach bowl and finally rinsed in the most dilute solution. This method also allows for safe cleaning and disinfecting of utensils.

The safety tips boil down to a simple saying, "Peel it, boil it, cook it, or forget it." While there is a good chance that food is actually safe to eat, each bite carries a risk, however small. You must ask yourself, "Do I feel lucky?" and "Is it worth the risk?"

Having said that, there come times when one must compromise to keep from offending your hosts, who may have gone well out of their way and even beyond their means to prepare a veritable feast, which you deem unsafe. Saying "No" is not an option. This may be the time to pick out a variety of items which are safer than others. Occasionally, some designated "volunteers" in the group may be asked to step forward to sample as little as possible of the high risk foods. That way only a few team members may become ill.

After utilizing all the suggestions and advice given in this chapter, when it is time to sit down and enjoy safe food and drink, it is imperative not to become one's own weakest link. Be sure you have washed or cleaned your hands. While tap water is considered contaminated, as is the bar of soap on the sink edge, they may nonetheless be used to wash off dirt and sweat. However, don't use the towel beside the sink to dry your hands; it is likely the most contaminated object you will encounter on your entire journey. Instead, finish cleaning your hands with gelled alcohol. It is recommended that you keep a small container in your pocket at all times to increase the chance that you will use it regularly. You can refill it from a larger bottle you keep with your other packed supplies.

Finally, it is time to eat. We toast to safe food and drink. Bon appétit!

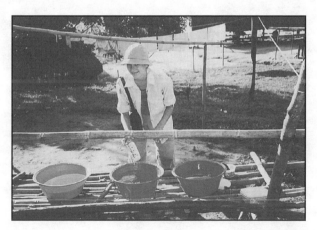

Ted Kuhn/
Figure 5. Washing dishes.

References

1. Backer HD: Field Water Disinfection, *Wilderness Medicine*, 4th ed., edited Auerbach PS, St. Louis, 2001, Mosby, pp 1186–1236.
2. Backer, HD: Water Disinfection, *The Travel and Tropical Medicine Manual*, 3rd ed., edited EC Jong, R McMullen, Philadelphia, 2003, WB Saunders Co., pp 87–111.
3. Backer HD: Water Disinfection for International Travelers, *Travel Medicine*, ed. Kestone JS, et al, Edinbaugh, Mosby, 2004, pp 49–59.
4. Ericsson CD, Mattila L, Prevention of Travelers' Diarrhea: Risk Avoidance and Chemoprophylaxis, *Textbook of Travel Medicine and Health*, 2nd ed., edited Dupont HL, Steffen R, Hamilton, BC Decker, Inc, 2001, pp 159–176.
5. Foodborne and Waterborne Health Risks, *International and Travel Health 2004*, World Health Organization, 2003. Also available online at http://www.who.int/ith/chapter03_02.html#4
6. http://www2.mf.uni-lj.si/~mil/praz2/praz2-e.htm
7. Risks for Food and Drink, *Health Information for International Travel 2003-2004*, Centers for Disease Control and Prevention, 2003, US. Department of Health and Human Services. Also available online at http://www.cdc.gov/travel/food-drink-risks.htm
8. Rose SR: Food and Drink Safety, *International Travel Health Guide*, 12th ed., Northampton, MA, 2001, Travel Medicine, Inc., pp 67–76.
9. www.pristine.ca
10. www.miox.com

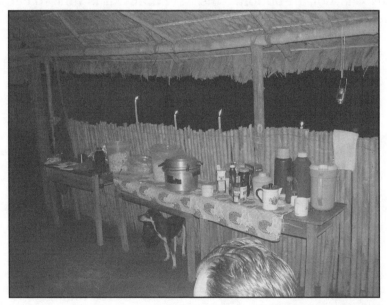

Hartmut Gross/
A safe meal by candlelight.

Protection from Arthropod-borne (Insects & Other "Bugs") Diseases

Hartmut Gross

There are many beautiful and interesting creatures to find and admire around the world if you take the time to notice. The fear most people have of insects and their kin is rooted only in their ignorance of them. Most of these creatures have no interest in humans and will in fact try to avoid contact. A small percentage of animals, unfortunately, may find you desirable for other reasons. These insects will actively seek out humans (and other animals) as food and/or hosts to raise their young. In this process, some insects become vectors for disease transmission. An awareness of these creatures and knowledge of a few simple measures of self-protection may make the difference between a miserable trip with illness, and a rewarding experience making you want to return again and again. In becoming more aware of the insects, you may start noticing more of them around you and actually enjoy their presence.

Why Protect Yourself?

Problems you want to protect yourself from can be grouped into a few simple categories.

Diseases including malaria, yellow fever, dengue fever, multiple kinds of encephalitis, trypanosomiasis, Chagas' disease, filariasis, onchocerciasis, leishmaniasis, various kinds of 'fever,' typhus, plague, and ehrlichiosis, are just a few you'd like to avoid. While there is not room to discuss each of these illnesses, it is good to review which illnesses are prevalent in the region to which you are planning to travel. It is also wise to see if there are any special vaccinations required for travel in that region. Awareness of the endemic illnesses will help you recognize, diagnose and avoid them.

Allergic reactions may be mild and localized such as the itching and redness of a mosquito bite, or severe, like the anaphylaxis individuals risk in their own backyard from a bee sting.

Host situations may arise when an insect, such as a fly, lays eggs in an open wound. The eggs hatch and the larvae grow in the wound and may be felt and seen wriggling under the skin. Botflies, scabies, and jiggers are examples.

Secondary infection of a wound may occur with any break in the skin, including minor bites and sting sites. Sanitation will generally not be what you are used to at home. Good wound care is essential to help avoid this complication; avoiding being bitten or stung is better.

Nuisance discomfort may be immediate and/or delayed. It is not fun when you spend much of your time swatting and waving away insects for fear of getting bitten, stung, or contracting some illness you can't pronounce. The initial assault may be painful, and later the wound may itch miserably for days.

Where and When to Protect Yourself

Distribution of illnesses around the world will give you a good clue about the presence of their vectors. This information can be found in travel guides, as well as in travel health information available from your local health department. The most authoritative and always up-to-date source is available free on the Internet from the CDC web site at www.cdc.gov. Additionally, some of the references at the end of this section contain several tables with this information. (Also see "Resources for the Traveling Medical Professional" chapter.) Travel agents are usually not well informed about health issues and it is unrealistic to assume that your local primary care physician is an expert on tropical diseases in every country. Fearing declining tourism, foreign embassies are sometimes less than honest about health risks in their country.

Timing and location of activities is an easily overlooked precaution. Dawn, dusk, and early evening are prime feeding times for many animals. It is wise to remove one's self from the smorgasbord during these hours. But other insects feed during the remaining times as well, so one should never go without some form of protection. Dark, damp locations and swampy or stagnant water areas tend to harbor large numbers of hungry insects. Look around your lodging and sleep area for insect droppings and empty molt shells; these may give you warning of what is crawling and flying around.

What to Protect Yourself From

There are a variety of biting and stinging arthropods:

Mosquitoes are by far the number 1 problem no matter where you go. They live every where except South Pole. Mosquitoes carry malaria which is responsible for the illness of 700,000,000 people annually and results in the death of 1 of every 17 people![2] They have only one pair of wings and are flies. It is true that only the female takes a blood meal; males only eat flower nectar. There are many different species of mosquitoes and various ones transmit different illnesses. Fortunately, the protective measures described later are effective against all mosquitoes.

Other flies (horseflies, deerflies, blackflies, midges, etc.) may carry onchocerciasis and the sandfly carries leishmaniasis. African sleeping sickness (African trypanosomiasis) is carried by the tsetse fly. Some bites, while not infectious, are simply very painful.

Fleas, lice, and ticks carry typhus, other rickettsial diseases, or bubonic plague. Some bites hurt, others itch. Infestations are very uncomfortable.

Chiggers and mites (e.g. scabies) are extremely irritating and itch like little else you've previously encountered.

True bugs (bedbugs, kissing bugs) bite and are vectors for disease; e.g. the cone-nosed kissing bug (Triatoma) transmits Chagas' disease (South American trypanosomiasis). Bedbugs simply sneak out of bedding at night and take a blood meal, leaving an itchy wound that may become infected.

Beetles (blister beetles) may squirt a caustic chemical in self-defense.

Wasps, bees, ants, and scorpions simply envenomate as they sting, usually by injecting venom, although some will spray noxious chemicals onto the wound they create by biting. These are all self defense mechanisms as humans are not on their menu. However, severe allergic reactions do occur and may be deadly.

Spiders tend to instill fear in more people than any other arthropod. The reality is that humans provoke spider bites, however innocently. These bites are all defensive; humans are not bitten for food. Fortunately, most spiders do not have mouthparts strong enough to break human skin.

While this is not intended as an entomology course, the more one understands the organisms, the less intimidating they become. For those readers curious to learn more about these interesting creatures, there are fascinating references listed at the end of the section.

Now What?

Now that I have your attention because you don't want to contract these illnesses, you surely want to know how to protect yourself. There are 2 options:

1. Don't go. Obviously, this is a ridiculous suggestion because you'd miss out on the greatest experience of a lifetime and you wouldn't be reading this.
2. Follow the easy prevention suggestions below to ensure you will be able to concentrate on things other than worrying about "bugs."

How to Prevent Getting Bitten or Stung

There are several methods to achieve prevention and no one method should be used alone. As you will see, each process continues where the previous one leaves off, so there is a full circle of defense around the clock.

Chemical Repellents

DEET repellent is clearly the first line of defense. DEET (N, N-diethyl-3-methylbenzamide, formerly N, N-diethyl-m-toluamide) is an effective insect repellent and works by forming a vapor barrier over the skin. This vapor cloud, for unclear reasons, seems to deter the mosquito from landing and feeding. Concentration of the DEET vapor, completeness of skin coverage, and pressure by mosquitoes to feed (e.g. huge numbers and voracious hunger) will determine if there is breakdown in the line of defense. There are many, many preparations available; so which one should you buy? Here are some guidelines to help with your choice. For adults, concentrations of 15–90% should be used. (Figure 1.) The higher the concentration, the less often you have to reapply it. The 30% preparation generally lasts 4–6 hours and is the recommended concentration for adults. The higher concentrations generally do not protect better, only longer. Although they exist, you generally don't need higher than 50% strength, just remember to reapply the 30% solution. The very high concentrations are often very irritating to skin, hence they are discouraged. DEET comes as a spray, lotion, towelettes, ankle bands, etc. A noteworthy product is a 29.5% long acting lotion (e.g. Sawyers,® Ultrathon®). This preparation may last 18 to 24 hours.

Slow release DEET employs molecular technology to slowly release DEET over time. Apply DEET lightly everywhere you have exposed skin or may temporarily have exposure (e.g. going to the bathroom). If you miss even one square inch, the surrounding application will not protect you. Avoid areas immediately around the eyes and mouth. Since you might lick your fingers, wash your hands afterward. Application several times 10 minutes apart increases the duration and DEET concentration for high-risk situations. For children > 2 months old, no more than 10–30% DEET is recommended[11,12] because of an extremely remote, although never proven, possibility of poisoning. However, a 10% solution of DEET needs to be reapplied every 1–2 hours! Skintastic® has 10% DEET and Skedaddle® has 15% DEET. DEET is safe in pregnant and nursing women.

CAUTION: DEET may damage plastics if it comes in contact with them. Many plastics and DEET do not mix!

Another chemical sometimes added to DEET is MGK-264 (N-octyl bicycloheptene dicarboximide). It works synergistically and potentiates the effectiveness of DEET. It is a larger molecule than DEET and is poorly

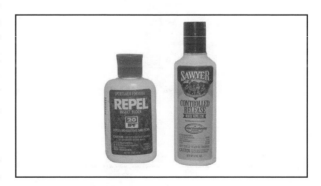

Figure 1.
Example of DEET Product.

absorbed through the skin. DEET does not protect against other flies. The best repellent for flies, gnats and no-see-ums is Di-n-propyl Isocinchomeronate (R-326). If flies and gnats are a concern, pick a repellent with several names on the label including DEET and one or two long names you can't pronounce.

Composite formulations are available containing all three chemicals (DEET, MGK-264, and R-326) (Figure 2). When the combination is also a slow release preparation, it would seem difficult to go wrong. Remember, ALWAYS READ THE LABEL! It was pointed out that DEET works by forming a vapor cloud directly over the skin. This is important in understanding why sun block must be applied before DEET is applied. Usually waiting 30–60 minutes after applying sun block allows the lotion to be absorbed into the skin sufficiently. The DEET is then applied on top so it can vaporize. Combined formulations of DEET with sun block exist and are effective.

It is noteworthy that in the US, DEET is considered the "gold standard" in safety and efficacy and until recently was the only repellent recommended by the Centers for Disease Control (CDC). The rest of the world does not embrace DEET as eagerly; concerned about the handful of reported adverse reactions, despite the fact that it used literately billions of times each year. The World Health Organization (WHO) recommends two other products as equally

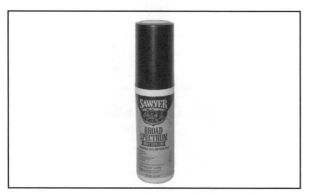

Figure 2.
DEET, MGK-264, and
R-326 composite formulations.

effective. The first is IR3535® (3-[N-acetyl-N-butyl]-aminopropionic acid ethyl ester), produced by Merck,® and was approved for use in the US in 1999. It is sold under a somewhat familiar name: Skin-So-Soft Bug Guard Plus IR 3535® (Figure 3) (not to be confused with plain Skin-So-Soft®). It is available in 10–30% strengths and with or without sun block. It is approved for use in children over 6 months of age. It is recommended to be applied every 4–8 hours. The other product endorsed by the WHO, and now also the CDC, has recently become available for purchase in the US. This product is Bayrepel® (1-piperidinecarboxylic acid, 2-(2-hydroxyethyl), 1-methylpropylester), also named icaridin or picaridin. Produced

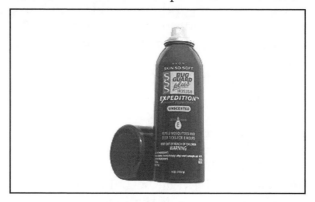

Figure 3.
IR 3535

by Bayer,® it is sold under the brand name Autan® (the older formulation with the same name used to contain DEET). Autan® (Figure 4) appears to have an excellent safety profile. Neither IR3535 nor icaridin exists as a long acting formula and therefore must be reapplied frequently.

Many other repellents such as Skin-So-Soft,® citronella, "natural" products, electronic devices are available. As great as they sound and as much as they are advertised, they are poor alternatives. Skin-So- Soft® works for about 40 minutes before reapplication is necessary; it is 10 times less effective than 12% DEET. Citronella oil is good for about 2 hours. The candles decrease the numbers of mosquitoes in the area, depending on the wind, but otherwise don't protect. Bite Blocker® (soybean, geranium, and coconut oils) seems to be effective for

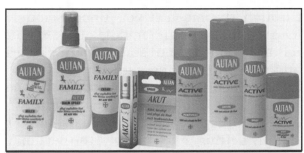

**Figure 4.
Icaridin (Bayrepel®)
Now available in US.**

is mixed with water (13.3% solution diluted 1 part to 26 parts water), and clothes are soaked to become impregnated. Clothes are then allowed to dry. This type of application may protect for months. On clothes, it is possible that permethrin may not work fast enough to keep mosquitoes from biting; you may need other protection on your skin (DEET or thicker clothing). Spray it on walls in closed off quarters (inside house, latrines, etc.) and the mosquito count will go down. Spray permethrin on mosquito

about 2–3 hours and is comparable to 6% DEET. These are mentioned mainly in case someone has an allergy to DEET. Finally, electronic gizmos don't work, period.[2]

CO$_2$ generating traps, with and without pheromones, are presently flooding the market. Scientific studies are limited, but the devices do show some promise. Presently, they require electricity or propane to drive them. They are quite large and bulky. These features make them less than desirable for fieldwork and not worth further discussion at this time.

Insecticides

Permethrin insecticide is the second line of defense. It kills insects within a few minutes of contact, even insects landing on a sprayed surface 2 weeks later! It can be applied to clothing, other fabrics, and to mosquito netting and bonds to the fibers. Permethrin is non-toxic to skin; but your skin harmlessly converts permethrin to an amino acid within 15 minutes of application. Thus it has no real use on skin. It is odorless and non-staining. It can be applied by spray or soaking clothing. At the concentration level of 0.5%, an application lasts about 14 days of exposure to light or up to five normal washings. If you store the clothes in a black plastic bag, you can extend the time of effectiveness. Spray clothes thoroughly for 30–45 seconds on each side and let dry for 2–4 hours before wearing. A typical can will treat two long sleeved shirts and two pairs of long trousers. Permethrin solution

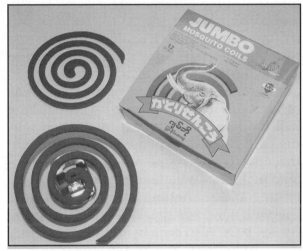

**Figure 5.
Mosquito coil.**

nets and mosquitoes die when they rest on the net. You can spray treat your mattress with 0.5% permethrin when you first arrive; allow drying and cover the mattress with a clean sheet to kill bedbugs. It is best to treat clothing and nets with permethrin before traveling. Aerosol cans might be confiscated in airports and liquids often spill or leak. Fabrics must be allowed to dry, as the chemical is quite pungent until dry. Remember, ALWAYS READ THE LABEL!

Another permethrin containing product is the mosquito coil. (Figure 5) It burns slowly and vaporizes the permethrin into the surroundings. Useless outdoors, it is effective in decreasing the insect count indoors. Electric versions exist too, but are useless if there is no electricity or the voltage is incorrect. Several similar products have been developed such as deltamethrin, tetramethrin, and cypermethrin. Some are already available as outdoor yard sprays. Some of these newer chemicals appear to be longer acting and may eventually replace the current shelf products. Keep an eye open for these changes.

Physical Barriers

Proper clothing cannot be stressed enough. The more you are covered, the less of you there is to get stung or bitten. Good shoes, long pants tucked into boots or tied off around the ankles, long sleeved shirts, and a bandana clearly cover you well. But this must be balanced against the heat and humidity, and the risks of being bitten, and how often you want, or will remember, to apply repellent. Keep in mind that areas of the body usually covered with clothing will have to briefly be exposed when taking care of bodily functions, i.e. bathroom. Insects will eagerly seize upon the vulnerable moment and at a minimum, leave you itching and scratching later on. Anticipate this with a little extra DEET before exposing these areas. Also keep in mind that brightly colored clothes and perfume tend to attract insects.

Mosquito netting is another critical tool in preventing bites and stings. (Figure 6.) You will no doubt work hard during the day and will not want to stay up at night swatting insects. The answer is netting. Nets are made with a standard weave as well as finer meshes called "sandfly nets." The finer the mesh, the smaller the insects kept out, but the trade off is less air movement. Finer nets are useful in zones with endemic sandfly or flea transmitted diseases (leishmaniasis, kala azar, bartonellosis, sandfly fever, plague, and murine typhus, etc.). A standard weave impregnated with permethrin effectively becomes the equivalent of a sandfly net and will keep out most everything of concern including sandflies. There are many shapes and sizes. It is important to set up the net properly, making sure no insects have been trapped inside and there are no openings left for insects to enter. It should be sprayed with permethrin; otherwise mosquitoes may bite you through the mesh if you unconsciously lean against it in the middle of the night. It is a good idea to put some of your clothes and shoes inside the net with you, so no creatures can climb into them during the night. Several foldable one man and two man tents are available with mosquito or sandfly netting. Alternatively, the nets may be purchased without a tent. Cost is quite low for the degree of protection afforded. See references and any camping equipment store.

Dangerous Areas

Try to stay away from any place where there are likely to be large numbers of biting insects. Swampy areas will have particularly large numbers of mosquitoes. Thatch roofs may hide kissing bugs in endemic areas of Chagas' disease. Open markets with pots and jugs may unwittingly harbor excellent mosquito breeding grounds. Don't go out during insects' prime hunting hours: dawn, dusk, and early evening. Be vigilant during the remaining times, when other insects feed. If you do go out in those times and areas, be sure to be maximally protected with repellents, insecticides, and clothing.

Medications

Medication is helpful and important because no matter how hard you try, some insects are bound to get through. Oral diphenhydramine (Benadryl®) and some type of topical anti-itching preparation (diphenhydramine, calamine lotion, hydrocortisone cream) may help sooth the irritation once you are bitten or stung. Antimalarials are discussed in the malaria chapter. Remember to take them and take them correctly!

So, without reading the whole chapter again, what should you buy before you go? Here is a simplified shopping list. Specific brand names are avoided because of local availability. This will discourage the urge to look all over for one specific product when there are ample excellent products on the shelf, if you know what to look for.

Shopping List

1. DEET 15–50% spray or lotion. Best is a long acting lotion 30% or higher. Look for a long acting composite with 3 drugs you can't pronounce. Remember to reapply as directed. DEET is safe in pregnancy and nursing mothers. Use 10% for children. It will melt many kinds of plastic. Apply sunscreen before DEET.
   a. IR3535. Contained in Skin-So-Soft Bug Guard Plus IR 3535.® Recommended by WHO as effective alternative to DEET.
   b. Bayrepel.® Contained in Autan® and Cutter Advanced®. Recommended by WHO and CDC as an effective alternative to DEET.
2. Permethrin. Spray or concentrate. Apply to clothes and nets before you leave. Consider taking a spray for closed off rooms you might be in.
3. Mosquito netting. One-man or two-man net. Mesh only supported by rods or hung by string. Also available as tents.
4. Clothing. Clothes to cover yourself as much as possible. Don't forget a hat, socks, and sturdy shoes. Treat all clothing (including socks and shoes) with permethrin. Avoid flowery, brightly colored clothes.
5. Anti-itch meds. Take diphenhydramine and any topical lotion of choice.
6. Anti-malarial. You'll need a prescription for this prophylaxis. Find out about resistance patterns to malaria to make sure you are taking the right medication.
7. Vaccinations. No matter how good your technique, the reality is that insects may manage to get through. Prevention of the disease is far easier than treating after it has been contracted. Get all recommended vaccinations well before you leave.

Any questions? Catch any interesting insects and need help with identification? Snap a photo or catch the critter and feel free to call Hartmut Gross at 706-721-4412 or send an E-mail to hgross@mail.mcg.edu. Happy travels and wishes for few bites and stings on your mission.

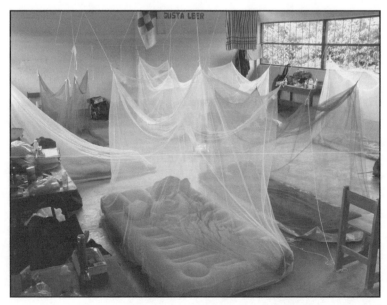

Hartmut Gross/
Figure 6. Mosquito net set up.

References

1. Bayrepel information is available at the Bayer website www.bayrepel.com

2. Fradin MS: *Mosquitoes and Mosquito Repellents: A Clinician's Guide,* Annals of Internal Medicine, 128(11):931, 1998. This article is also available at no cost online at www.acponline.org. Type "fradin" into the search box and you'll see the citation. More than most of you ever wanted to know about how to protect yourself from mosquitoes. A benchmark paper that team leaders should keep.

3. Fradin MS: *Protection from Blood-Feeding Arthropods, Wilderness Medicine,* 4th ed., edited PS Auerbach, St. Louis, Missouri, 2001, Mosby-Year Book, Inc., pp 754–768. Reviews of types of insect problems and how to treat each one. Tables of DEET and permethrin preparations and examples of netting. Excellent reference.

4. IR 3535 information is available at the Merck website http://pb.merck.de/servlet/PB/menu/1093160/index.html.

5. Peters W: *A Colour Atlas of Arthropods in Clinical Medicine,* London, 1992, Wolfe Publishing Ltd. An excellent reference if you love insects and want to learn more.

6. Peters W and Pasvol G: *Tropical Medicine and Parasitology,* 5th ed., London, 2002, Mosby. A pictorial text in full color. Easy to follow, concise review of tropical diseases, parasites, and their vectors.

7. CDC via Internet at www.cdc.gov. Check here for immunization requirements, endemic diseases, outbreak alerts, and precautions to take.

8. Rose SR: *International Travel Health Guide,* 9th ed., Northampton, MA, 1998, Travel Medicine, Inc., pp 95–124. Concise with examples of repellents and nets and their manufacturers.

9. WHO via Internet at http://www.who.int/ith/chapter03_05.html Current recommendations for protection from bites and stings, including alternatives to DEET.

10. WHO via Internet at http://www.who.int/ctd/whopes/ WHOPES (World Health Organization Pesticide Evaluation Scheme) and evidence behind the current WHO recommendations for protection against insects.

11. http://aapnews.aappublications.org/cgi/content/full/e200399.

12. http://www.aap.org/advocacy/releases/summertips.htm.

15 Dressing for the Job

W. "Ted" Kuhn

Sensitivity to Local Customs
Footwear
Dressing for Heat or Humidity
Dressing for the Cold

Many of the people who travel into the "hinterlands" and wilderness areas have a naiveté about the risks and proper preparation. Teams venture into the jungles of the Amazon basin, into the deserts of Central Africa and into the altitude of the African plains and Andes, into freezing temperatures and thin air. Appropriate dress and preparation may make the difference between effectively accomplishing the mission on returning having had a poor experience, or in the worse case scenario, needing evacuation or rescue.

Sensitivity to Local Customs

In many locations, dress will be dictated by local customs and team members will need to dress in locally purchased garments. Notwithstanding, Hudson Taylor[1] in China, who dressed according to the local fashion, was more the exception than the rule! In the vast majority of situations, clothing and supplies will be purchased in the US before travel. It is good to remember that if the local population is accustomed to a particular type of clothing or fabric, it is usually efficient for the local climatic conditions.

In many cultures, what you wear (or don't wear) says a lot about who you are. For example, in South Asia the dress standards for both men and women are very particular. Hair worn "loose" and unbraided by a woman implies a "loose" woman, not the impression we would want to make, but an easily made honest mistake. In some Middle Eastern countries, not wearing a hair covering by a woman is punishable by a jail sentence. Men in South Asia, who wear the "lungi", a wrap around skirt, make fun of men who wear "half-pants" or shorts. In other cultures the wearing of shorts is acceptable. Many countries require you to remove your shoes (sandals) upon entering a home or building—not an efficient environment for lace-up boots. It is best not to have a strike against you before you begin.

Footwear

Your feet will absorb more punishment than any other part of your body. Footwear may be the most important item of gear. There should be no compromise in the selection of appropriate footwear. Where the feet will not go, the body will not follow! A good rule of thumb is to never rely on footwear in the field that you have not traveled at least 100 miles in prior to leaving for the field. This assures proper fit and avoids the unpleasant surprise of friction blisters from swelling of your feet on long hikes.

Shoes should obviously be chosen according to the terrain. If muddy trails, ice, snow, or crossing streams will cause the feet to get wet, blisters will form within an hour of walking, halting all forward progress.[1] If the terrain is rough and necessitates travel over uneven ground or climbing on sharp stones or rocks, soft-soled shoes will cause foot pain and bruising of the bottom of the foot. If at all possible, it is recommended that a second pair of socks and a spare pair of shoes be carried if necessity may dictate changing shoes or socks. Socks made of Cool Max® are particularly useful because they dry quickly, will not chafe or cause blisters and can be washed out at night, dry and ready for use in the morning. Stores carrying running supplies carry a variety of Cool Max® socks (Road Runner Sports and others). A single layer rather than a double layer sock is recommended as the double layer sock may bunch-up in the shoe and cause a "hot spot" on the foot. Cotton and wool socks when wet will stay wet losing insulation and comfort. Wool socks are warmer in cold weather than Cool Max® socks and are preferable if you are sure that your sock will not become wet—but a wet wool sock will not insulate and is difficult to dry in field conditions. Socks made of Polar fleece® are now available

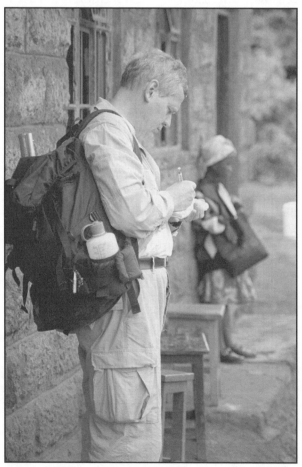

Ted Kuhn/
"Dr. Hartmut Gross in Appropriate Field Dress for East Africa"

and will insulate as well as wool, maintain insulating capacity when wet and can be easily dried in field conditions—something to consider! Prior to travel to the field, you can soak your socks in a 0.5–1% solution of permethrin and spray the same on your boots or shoes which will keep chiggers and ants from crawling up your sock and biting you on the ankle (or making their home in your crotch!).

Trail shoes that are just above the level of the ankle will provide some stability for the ankle in rough terrain. They also may provide some protection from snake bites and insect bites and a little higher protection for water, if water proofing is desirable. Shoes should be purchased slightly large to accommodate for swelling of the feet after long walks or hikes. When purchasing a trail shoe or boot, make sure your toes do not touch the front when standing on an incline. This causes painful bruising of the toes when descending a steep trail. Protective rubber toe caps help keep the big toes from being battered or bruised. Deep tread outsoles provide traction in muddy terrain but running shoes with high impact soles become slippery on logs and river rocks. Shoes constructed of nylon or Cordura® with split leather are resistant to abrasion and may be somewhat breathable and dry faster when wet compared to full leather shoes. Shoes or boots with "quick-lace" steel hooks can snag on vines or weeds causing the traveler to fall or stumble.

The following are some helpful suggestions for dealing with boot problems in the field[2]:

1. Bypassing some of the lacing rings on your boot will allow you to reduce pressure over sore spots while maintaining comfort in other nonsensitive areas. If you boot has "locking hooks" at the bend in the ankle, this allows different tensions above and below the hooks. Learn to use them.

2. "Boot "tongues" may migrate to one side or the other. Train them to lie correctly from the first time you put on your boots. Do this by taking special care to make the first folds in the tongue gussets in

the correct position. If the tongue still "wanders," stitch a button on the center of the tongue to block its wandering."[2]

3. The rubber strip around the sides of the boot is to protect your toes from injury and keep water out of the leak–prone junction of the boot upper and sole. This may peel back with time, rendering the boot no longer water resistant. Not overheating the boot, and not drying them quickly and not applying leather treatments along the edges which weakens glue over time will prolong the life and comfort of the boot.

4. Apply enough even tension to the laces to produce a good snug fit prior to beginning your day's journey.

5. Avoid putting on your boots with cold toes or wet socks. If your feet are wet from perspiration prior to putting on your boots, your socks will become damp and may stay damp all day permitting painful blistering. Carrying an extra pair of dry socks can be a real advantage if your socks become wet from water or perspiration. A breathable dressing like Tegederm® can be applied over "hot spot" areas to prevent blistering and for comfort.

Open toed sandals may be appropriate for walking around towns in the tropics but are usually not appropriate in jungle regions. Many worms penetrate the open skin of the foot in damp, moist soil including hookworm and strongyloides. Schistosomiasis can be contracted if walking through streams and water in endemic areas. Toes can be bruised or battered on uneven ground. Biting insects gain access to the foot and the jigger flea (Tungiasis) can jump onto exposed skin and burrow into the foot.

Dressing for Heat or Humidity

Dressing for the desert and jungle is somewhat less complicated than dressing for cold. In countries where there is a military dictatorship or in remote border regions, military type clothing or camouflage-style clothing should be discouraged as it may imply that you are a guerilla or foreign infiltrator or represent a foreign government. A hat should be carried to protect from the sun (and rain). Sunglasses, with shatter proof lenses offer eye protection and sun protection in both the tropics and at altitude and from snow glare. If sun protection is a high priority, for example at altitude or in areas near the equator, or on open water or in snow, polarized lenses can significantly reduce glare, although more expensive. A pullover may be helpful if a drenching rain is anticipated. A polyester fleece pullover will offer protection from the rain (although it eventually will get wet), can be wrung out, and yet will still offer thermal protection (L.L. Bean, REI, Patagonia, and others).

There are several new high-tech fabrics that have revolutionized travel in hot humid conditions (L.L. Bean, REI). I prefer a long sleeve shirt and long pants even in the most demanding hot environments. There are new tropical weight shirts and pants that offer protection from the sun, are lightweight (but expensive) and dry almost instantly. These offer protection from biting insects and can be impregnated with permethrin for extra protection. Garments can be soaked in a 0.5–1% solution of permethrin which will maintain some protection from biting insects for up to 20 washing and will not damage fabrics or cause an odor. Light colored clothing absorbs less heat and attracts insects less than dark colored clothing. They can also be washed and will dry in less than 1 hour and actually don't look too bad after washing in the sink or stream. Long sleeves can be rolled up in the day and rolled down at night for mosquito protection. Some pants can unzip to make shorts and several offer mesh linings obviating the need for underwear, making hygiene in the tropics less complicated.

Dressing for the Cold

While dressing for the tropics and warm climates usually focuses on comfort, dressing for cold not only focuses on comfort but also on the prevention of major life threatening problems including hypothermia and frostbite. In the cold, protection from both wind and water play vital roles. Your body heat warms the air inside your clothes and this in turn warms a thin layer of air just outside your clothes; this keeps your body warm. When the wind blows, it quickly dissipates this warm air and results in rapid chilling. For example, at 20 degrees F with a 20 mph wind, our body perceives the temperature as –9 degrees F; this is wind chill. Water can also be extremely dangerous. Water can come from outside sources, like rain or snow, or from inside sources, such as sweat and perspiration, causing the thermal protection of fabrics to fail. Moreover, fabrics like cotton and wool lose most of their thermal protective capacity when they get wet. To deal effectively with wetness, you must keep both your insulation and yourself dry. Outside water proof layers can keep you dry from the outside. Inside moisture can be reduced by venting, reducing the rate of physical activity, using a vapor barrier and reducing insulation layers.[3] Protection from cold is really the story of appropriate layering and this is a principle you must master to protect both yourself and your team.

The three clothing systems for cold exposure are the breathable system (good), the waterproof-breathable system (better) and the vapor barrier system (best).[4] The breathable system consists of an underwear layer, a middle insulating layer and an outer shell fabric. A waterproof-breathable system consists of the same layers but the outer shell is made of a waterproof fabric such as Gore-tex® (Thin-tech,® Helley-tech,® Ultrex,® etc). The vapor barrier system is a four-layer system and places a vapor barrier between the underwear layer and the insulation layer. The vapor barrier is made of polyethylene or a coated nylon to be waterproof and vapor proof. This reduces heat loss by reducing evaporating water from the skin. It also protects against sweat from damaging the thermal protection of the outer two layers.

Many materials are available for the underwear layer. Polyester (Thermax® by Dupont or Capilene® by Patagonia), polypropylene (gets stiff with age and loses wicking ability—use fabric softener) and chlorofiber (Blue-John's® and Thermolactyl® by Damart) are the best.[3] They absorb much less water by weight than cotton or wool and moisture does not degrade the insulating value of the fabric. Underwear listed best to worse according to water absorption are the fibers listed above (best) and in decreasing desirability, acrylics, silk, nylon, wool, cotton, and rayon. Cotton fibers can be deadly in cold, wet weather and blue jeans or cotton dungarees are the worst offenders when used as an only layer! Blue jeans are sometimes referred to as "death pants' by mountain guides. When jeans get wet, they stay wet, are difficult to dry and conduct heat away from the body and offer no insulation from the cold.

The insulation layer can be of down or synthetic fibers. While down is excellent as insulator, it is expensive and loses its insulating capabilities when wet. Down is not recommended where the danger of either outside or inside contamination with water exists. The synthetic fibers make some of the best insulation. Compared to the natural fibers (kapok, wool, cotton) these are far superior. There are two types of synthetic fibers. One is a batting (thick build up of fibers) which has protective woven material on both sides. The other is a stand lone fabric. Batting fibers include Dupont's Hollofil,® Quallofil,® Thermolite,® and Thinsulate.® Celanese makes Polarguard® and American Hoechst makes Trentron,® Pentaloft® and others.[3] Manufacturers have other brands as well. The second type of insulation is pile or fleece and this is becoming more popular. Pile and fleece have the advantage of being nonabsorbent so that water goes between the fibers, not inside, and water can be removed by wringing or swinging the garment a few times. Patagonia, Malden Mills, Columbia Sportsware and L.L. Bean (Polartec®) all make excellent fleece insulating garments. Fleece comes in various insulating capacities. Remember to choose the one right for you. Lightweight fleece (butterfleece®) won't restrict movement and fits snug against the skin but has the least insulating capacity. Midweight fleece is 40% warmer than lightweight fleece and may be good for insulation during outside aerobic activities. Heavyweight fleece is excellent but bulky. It affords superior protection especially when used under a waterproof parka in extreme conditions. Fleece is also now available as windproof fleece, sandwiching a wind-blocking membrane between fleece layers offering breathability along with wind resistance in the mid-weight fleece range.

The outer shell consists of a jacket or parka which is best if water resistant or waterproof. Remember that pants, hats and gloves also belong in this category. An insulating hat is essential in cold environments in as much as 18% of our body heat may be lost through the head. Nylon is one of the best fibers for an outer shell. The higher the denier (thickness of the fiber) the stronger the fabric. High strength nylons include fibers such as Ballistics Cloth®, Cordura®, Caprolan®, Taslan®, and others. Lighter fabrics are available if you don't need the highest strength or abrasion resistance (Supplex®, Capima®, Tactel®, Captiva®). If you take a high filament count and a super tight weave, these nylon fabrics can compete as waterproof but breathable garments (Versatech® and Super-Microft®). When total weather protection is desired, a completely windproof and waterproof outer shell or parka is required. These are designed to withstand a 3 inch per hour downpour for at least 30 minutes without getting wet. Gore-tex® was the first fabric manufactured in this category. However, now there are other waterproof breathable outer garments (Helly-tech,® Entrant,® Permia,® Waterguard,® and others).

References

1. Hudson Taylor was a missionary in China in the 1800s. He was frowned upon by other missionaries for wearing native attire and wearing his hair in the traditional Chinese pien-tze (or queue) braid.
2. REI.com website—Achieving Booted Bliss.
3. Auerbach PS, editor: *Wilderness Medicine: Management of Wilderness and Environmental Emergencies,* 3rd ed.; Gookin J, "Selections and Use of Outdoor Clothing," St. Louis, 1995, Mosby-Year Book, Inc.
4. Weiss H: *Secrets of Warmth for Comfort or Survival,* 2nd ed., Calgary, 1992, Rocky Mountain Books.

16 Personal Hygiene

Doreen Hung Mar

Bathing and Oral Hygiene
Environmental Factors
Odors
Feminine Issues
Personal Sanitation
Personal Protection

It was the best time to bathe; it was the worst time to bathe. We were headed for a bath in the river, a tributary of the Amazon. A late afternoon swim would be refreshing after two long days of trekking through the jungle and working in the clinic. Winding paths through bush led down to the gently flowing river. The opportunity to clean up was greeted with cheers, and laughter rippled over the water as soap and shampoo bubbles floated downstream.

Traipsing back to camp, however, we quickly lost the effect of washing up. Climbing up, clouds of dust from the jungle path settled onto our sweat-laden skin. From the weeds, eager insects were ready to suck the moisture from our skins. The sunset signaled feeding time for hungry mosquitoes who poised themselves to feast on our clean, exposed, repellent-free skin.

Personal hygiene is relative and dependent on the person, culture, circumstances, available resources of water, soaps and shampoos, and facilities.

While cleanliness is much more difficult to achieve in many areas of the world, a goal on a medical missions trip should be to stay as inoffensive as possible to your fellow team members, national workers, and patients.

Consideration of several factors is important for maintaining a satisfactory level of hygiene and sanitation. These factors include water availability, water purity, environmental and climatic conditions.

Bathing and Oral Hygiene

Water may be a limited resource in some areas, especially water clean enough to clean you. There is no benefit in using water that has more dirt than you do after a long hard day. Though some clean water or the use of hand sanitizers helps reduce disease transmission from soiled hands, much more is needed to maintain health.

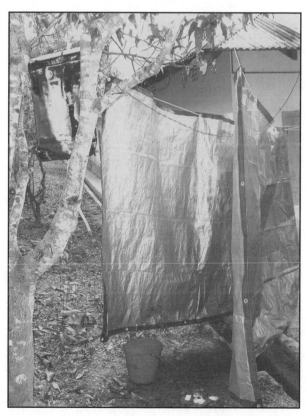

Krystina Huynh/
"Makeshift Shower—South Asia"

Even in disaster situations, people require a minimum of 5 liters of water a day for survival and this quickly increases to a daily need of 15–20 liters/day when food preparation, personal hygiene and the washing of dishes and clothing are factored in.[1]

Slightly filtered water may be used to wash, but remember to protect areas where microbes may enter and cause infection—that is, close your mouth and eyes while washing. This may sound like advice to the brink of paranoia, but in reality, entry of organisms via these portals is possible and could cause serious health problems. You should also avoid contact with water sources like ponds, lakes, streams, or rivers that may harbor waterborne diseases such as Schistosomiasis, Leptospirosis, and other potential infestations—investigate disease potential before diving or stepping into polluted waters.

Alternative bathing options in remote areas include the "bucket bath" or a portable shower. A private shower stall can be created by hanging tarps strategically. A bucket of clean, perhaps even heated water, a tin cup for dipping, and a bar of soap are all that is needed for a good bath. Another possibility is a portable shower which is a heavy-duty plastic bag with a shower nozzle. These can be purchased through camping supply stores and are light weight and easy to transport. The bag can be filled with water and laid out in the sun during the day to provide a warm shower in the evening.

Any water that enters the mouth should be purified. Only a very small amount is necessary for brushing your teeth to maintain good oral hygiene, especially in conjunction with fluorinated toothpaste. Be sure to floss. Between brushing, you can keep the mucous membranes moist with adequate hydration and sugar-free candies or gum. In very dry or cold weather conditions, high altitudes, or in the case of chronic mouth breathing, throat lozenges or candies and saline nasal sprays will also help keep membranes moist.

Environmental Factors

The environment impacts your ability to maintain a certain level of comfort and cleanliness. Hot and humid weather creates a desire to wash frequently. Trapped moisture could contribute to fungal skin infections and miliaria (heat rash). Use of powders, light but modest clothing, and frequent breaks (if possible) where one can cool off might help prevent skin problems from occurring.

Dry, hot, desert-like conditions help evaporate sweat quickly, but also can leave caked-on dirt and dust that contribute to clogged skin pores and cause uncomfortable skin conditions. Frequent cleansing of particularly sensitive areas assists in preventing infections and rashes.

Cold climates often imply accompanying dry air and, therefore, can lead to dry and chapped skin. Itching from lack of moisture may result in chaffing and might progress to bleeding and possible infections where the skin is cracked. Don't forget to pack moisturizers and to use them frequently. If there is a small area of cracked skin, such as on a fingertip, that is particularly tender and not infected, you may consider sealing it with thick creams, paraffin, Dermabond,® or a super glue brand, after cleaning. This method helps reduce the tenderness while the skin heals by protecting the exposed and sensitive nerve endings.

In very dry conditions the nasal mucosa can become irritated. Normal saline nose spray can alleviate this problem.

Odors

There is no substitute for frequent washing with deodorant soaps and for application of deodorants and powders to prevent offensive body and foot odors. Good foot health is critical on these trips for comfort, endurance, and general well being. Be sure to bring appropriate, comfortable, and broken-in shoes for any trip. Marketed by the travel industry, silver-threaded socks claim to inhibit bacterial and fungal growth and, therefore, odors, even with extended wear without washing! The Fox River Mills brand of X-Static® socks and liners use a silver-coated nylon fiber. With any given product, the silver content may range from 5–19%, depending on the sock or liner. The silver acts as an antimicrobial agent and transfers heat away from the foot. It is a permanent component of the thread, and is still effective with repeated washing. These socks are attractive enough for the business wear setting and tough enough for fairly rugged trekking. For more information, you may contact your nearby sports store or Jenni Dow at 651-426-2891 or www.foxsox.com.

Note: If possible, use biodegradable soaps, shampoos, and detergents for washing clothes. Dispose of these waters away from your drinking water source.

Feminine Issues

The chapter on "Women and Travel" offers more information on this topic, however, a few thoughts are worthy of consideration. The use of panty liners, plain or deodorant-scented, can help underwear and clothing last longer, stay fresher, and easier to clean afterwards.

Be sure to bring enough for the trip, plus a few extra days. Some products are extra thin, absorbent, and also have "wings."

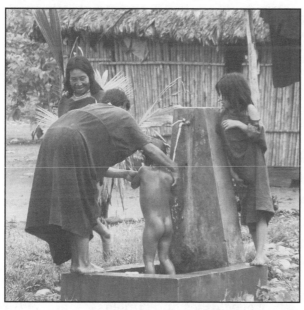

Hartmut Gross/
"Bathing in the Water Supply?"

Personal Sanitation

Environmental awareness and protection are important issues that must be considered. Indiscriminate disposal of human waste can infect water sources, harm the environment, and contribute to disease dissemination. When traveling into remote parts of the world, teams must consider the appropriate method for disposing of waste. Urination usually does not create a problem because urine evaporates rapidly and is easily washed away by rains. Avoid going close to where you are staying, especially in large groups, as the quantity does accumulate and the odor will build up. With solid waste products, however, there are several guidelines to consider.

To decrease disease transmission, keep feces away from water, fields from which food may be obtained, flies which carry disease to foods, and hands and fingers handling food and water.

Designate the location of elimination downhill, downwind, and downstream. The area for human excreta should be, preferably, about 50 meters from any drinking water source. For small holes and limited time use, the very least distance between hole and water source should be 15 meters.[2] You should distance the site of elimination from main living quarters by at least 6 meters but not more than 50 meters or one minute's walking distance from shelters, dwellings, or campsite.[2]

Small holes should be dug down approximately 15–20 cm (6–8 inches) into the soil with the use of trowels or small shovels which can be purchased from hardware or sporting supply stores. The U-dig-it® is a palm-sized stainless steel trowel with a folding handle and belt sheath ($20-27 from U-dig-it,® 3953 Brookside Lane, Boise, ID 83714; phone: 208-939-8656; E-mail: U-digit@worldnet.att.net). After defecation, the contents should be mixed with surrounding soil. The addition of a small piece of wood will also promote decomposition after the hole is covered. Beyond the use of a small hole, trench digs, latrine installation, or defecation field designations should follow the above guidelines.

One latrine should be provided for the use of a maximum of 20 people. When digging a hole is not possible, a portable unit may be necessary. There are several sources where portable toilets may be obtained, and even onetime use containers or bags are available.

1. The Coyote Bagless Toilet System,® a polyethylene box that has a separate raised toilet seat assembly, weighs nine pounds with a capacity for 55 user-days ($136 from Four Corners River Sports, P.O.Box 379, Durango, CO, 81302; phone: 800-426-7637; website: www.riversports.com).

2. Check out the River Bank System of a complete portable toilet system made of 3/16-inch thick polyethylene with waste tank and flush kit ($255, website: www.riverbankdesign.com/toilets.htm).

3. The Jon-ny Partner® is a portable toilet with an aluminum holding tank, automatic pressure release valve and a pressure nozzle attachment for a hose for fresh water flushing ($463 from Partner Steel Company, 3187 Pole Line Road, Pocatello, ID 83201; phone: 208-233-2371).

4. A rentable unit called the Bano® is a molded plastic holding tank with aluminum handles, stainless steel fasteners, and a hard plastic seat ($50 for four days from Green River Headquarters, 544 East 3900 South, Salt Lake City, UT 84107; phone: 435-564-3273; website: www.holidayexpeditions.com).

5. Single use systems are convenient and easy to carry. Information may be obtained from Restop® at their website: www.whennaturecalls.com. There are various disposable bags for liquids that contain polymers that immediately gel liquid waste. Separate bags for solid wastes are available. They contain enzymes that biodegrade feces and are environmentally safe. These containers are portable with one-way valves that help prevent spills, are sanitary, and disposable. ($8 for four Restop-1 bags for liquid wastes; $2.60 for one Restop-2 bags for both liquids and solids. Other products and packages available on their website.

There are many disposable and biodegradable products available now, including different brands of toilet paper. Otherwise, all inorganic materials should be packed-out, including toilet paper, tampons and pads, and diapers. These materials may be stored in a sealable plastic bag; consider adding a tea bag or aspirin for odor control. For personal and used medical supplies that cannot be taken out, you must consider digging a very deep hole, at least several feet or 2–3 meters deep and burying theses supplies where they cannot be easily dug up by man or animal.

Personal Protection

There are other considerations to address in practicing personal protection while overseas. Proper dress and clothing is covered in the chapter entitled "Dressing for the Job," but it should be emphasized that wearing long-sleeved shirts and long pants can significantly decrease insect bites. In addition, use proper and adequate amounts of repellent, particularly DEET, and utilize permethrin impregnated mosquito netting.

Avoid any contact with animals overseas. Very few animals, including the majority of pets are properly vaccinated for rabies, which is epidemic in some countries. Avoid blood transfusions and injections while abroad. Carry extra syringes and needles in personal luggage in case you need injectable medications and disposable equipment is not available. Extramarital sexual encounters are not only culturally inappropriate, but medically risky as well, due to the prevalence of untreated sexually transmitted diseases, including HIV, in many countries.

Bring along a complete supply plus an extra few days of your prescription medicines, copies of your prescriptions, an extra pair of eyeglasses and sunglasses, and extra batteries and supplies for hearing aids and glucose testing machines. These and any other essentials should be packed with personal, carry-on luggage.

"Cleanliness is next to godliness" is a myth. However, we do hope you show care and consideration to your teammates and to those you serve through the way you maintain personal hygiene and sanitation. May this be one of many ways you can keep yourself healthy as you seek to serve God and others throughout the world.

References
1. Medicins Sans Frontieres. *Refugee Health*, Doctors Without Borders/Medicins Sans Frontieres. London, 1997, Macmillan Education Ltd.
2. *Field Operations Guide for Disaster Assessment and Response*, U.S. Agency for International Development, Bureau for Humanitarian Response, Office of Foreign Disaster Assistance. Washington, D.C., 1998, U.S. Government Printing Office (GPO). Also available at http://www.info.usaid.gov/ofda/.

17 Women and Travel

Ann Butler

Travel health issues are different for women and men. Many of the remote areas in developing countries visited by travelers and mission workers present unique issues for women with regard to safety, hygiene, medical conditions, and pregnancy. Women who travel to these regions should acquaint themselves with available information materials about the planned destination and prepare accordingly.

Personal Safety Issues and Dress

Use common sense. Women in a new and strange environment must be extra careful. Avoid trekking out alone into an unknown area, especially at night. Familiarize yourself ahead of time with the customs and culture of your destination. Once you have arrived, the best advice is to follow the lead of the women in that culture.

This may mean having to put aside the normal independence that a woman has in the United States for the sake of the team's mission and personal safety. No one wishes to offend a country's culture or people when visiting or ministering in their land. Attention to culturally appropriate clothing and behavior will enhance your acceptance into the community you wish to serve. (See *Cultural Sensitivity* chapter for more details.) Acceptable clothing may mean wearing long skirts or dresses, sleeved shirts, and perhaps even a head scarf. Pants are acceptable in many, but not all countries, but shorts are rarely permissible except in resort areas. A good "rule of thumb" is modesty above all.

Personal Hygiene

Conditions are often primitive in the developing world, especially in rural or remote areas. This may mean that there are no modern restroom or bathroom facilities after leaving the airport, and even there, the only toilet paper may be that which you brought with you. This poses special problems for women in travel, as personal hygiene is always a concern.

When traveling to nonwestern countries, women must be mentally prepared to face the challenge of squat toilets, pit latrines, and sights and smells to which they would rather not become accustomed. Keeping a pack of tissues, alcohol hand sanitizer, and a few wet wipes on your person is an excellent plan.

One of most common questions asked about traveling abroad in remote areas concerns menstruation. Having a period while traveling can cause additional stress on women because of the added problem of hygiene and menstrual cramps. Women should be aware that the demands of travel could cause menstrual irregularities ranging from heavier to missed menses. These stresses include changes in sleeping patterns, increased activity/exercise, eating patterns, and diet. So, a woman should be prepared for the possibility of either missing her period, having an early menses, or worsening of her menstrual cramping. Of course, a missed period should be investigated with a pregnancy test if appropriate.

Because of the possibility of the stress of travel causing irregularities, it is imperative to take enough feminine hygiene products for the entire trip even if the timing of the period does not correspond. Disposable feminine hygiene products may or may not be available for purchase. Also it is important to plan to pack out your products since trash disposal receptacles may not be available in remote areas. Adding a crushed aspirin or used tea bag to a plastic bag with used feminine hygiene products will decrease odor-causing bacterial growth.

It is important to carry medications such as ibuprofen or naproxen for menstrual cramping and other premenstrual syndrome symptoms as these may not be available for purchase.

A basic hygiene pack should include the following:
- Adequate sanitary napkins/tampons
- Plastic bags for storage
- Aspirin or tea bags to add to used sanitary supplies for odor control
- Wet-wipes type hand towels
- Toilet paper—small tissue packs do well for travel
- Cotton underwear (or other appropriate fabric for hot weather/exercise, e.g. Cool Max®)
- Waterless instant hand sanitizer
- Small shovel (for remote travel)
- Optional: Lady-J urinal® or Freshette® from Sani-Fem® for prolonged periods of poor weather in remote areas.

Urinary Tract Infection

Compared to men, women are more prone to urinary tract infections (UTIs) because of anatomical reasons. The symptoms of urinary tract infections are increased urinary frequency, increased urgency, painful urination, and/or back pain. During travel additional factors such as dehydration,

inadequate toilet facilities, poor hygiene, and dietary changes can increase the risk of UTIs.

To prevent UTIs, it is important to drink adequate amounts of fluids and avoid holding urine for long periods. This may mean that in some countries the use of a pit toilet or outdoors may be necessary. Many Western women are not comfortable with the "squatting position" and may want to practice this technique a few times before traveling so that getting in and out of this position may be done without embarrassment.

To maintain hygiene in remote places, a "fanny pack" is useful to hold hand sanitizer and small tissue packs. In extremely remote travel, it might be advisable to have a prescribed antibiotic and/or urinary analgesic available just in case symptoms of UTI appear.

Older women may have the added inconvenience of stress incontinence or loss of bladder control and may wish to discuss this with a physician before traveling for possible medications and/or Kegel exercise techniques. It is advisable to carry an adequate supply of panty liners.

Vaginal Infection

Vaginitis and vaginal infections are diseases affecting the vagina, which are usually bacterial or fungal infections. During travel, women are more prone these infections for many of the same reasons as for UTIs. Two of the most common causes of vaginitis are yeast infections and bacterial vaginosis.

Yeast infections are usually caused by a fungus called *Candida albicans* and present with vaginal itching and "cottage-cheese" whitish discharge. It is not a sexually transmitted disease. It may, however, occur when a women takes an antibiotic. Traveling women taking doxycycline for malarial prevention may develop a yeast infection because of this antibiotic. Anticipation of a possible yeast infection would prompt bringing antifungal vaginal creams such as miconazole or an oral medication such as Diflucan® just in case an infection should occur.

Bacterial vaginosis is not a sexually transmitted disease either. It is caused by a change in the pH of the vaginal environment and increased growth of bacteria called *Gardnerella vaginalis*. It usually presents as a whitish to grayish discharge, vaginal itching, and/or fishy odor. Bacterial vaginosis can be treated with either metronidazole or clindamycin in oral tablet form or as a vaginal cream.

Contraception

If pregnancy is a concern, then contraception is recommended prior to and during a trip. This may be achieved either via abstinence, medications, or condoms. Menstrual control may also be an added benefit with medications. When traveling to high altitudes greater than 10,000 feet, it should be noted that there is a theoretical increased risk for deep venous thrombosis (blood clots) when taking oral contraceptives. However, hormone replacement therapy is not contraindicated at altitudes because of its physiologic doses.

It should also be noted that the medications used to prevent malaria such as doxycycline could interfere with oral contraceptives by weakening their potency.

Pregnancy

Pregnancy during travel poses another set of concerns for women. According to the American College of Obstetrics and Gynecology, the safest time for travel during pregnancy is during the second trimester (18–24 weeks). Pregnancy does not necessarily prevent travel, but advice from a physician should be sought before a trip is made.

All sexually active women should have a pregnancy test prior to extensive travel if this is a concern; this will prevent later problems. Verification by ultrasound that the pregnancy is intrauterine (pregnancy in the uterus) and not a life threatening ectopic (pregnancy in the tubes) is a must. Having an ectopic pregnancy or spontaneous abortion increases a woman's risk of

hemorrhage. Remote areas may not have adequate health care facilities to cope with such an emergency. The baby should be at least 8 weeks gestation before travel to avoid adding to the already higher risk of spontaneous abortion (25% chance with less than 8 weeks gestation).

Most airlines require a note from a physician before allowing women more than 35 weeks pregnant to fly. Pregnant women with significant anemia (less than 8.5g/dl hemoglobin) may require supplemental oxygen at higher altitudes. When traveling pregnant, it is important to realize that unexpected complications of pregnancy can occur.

Contingency plans for evacuation should be in place in case any complications do occur. Routine prenatal care should occur while traveling including prenatal vitamins and regular blood pressure checks in cases of extended trips. Prenatal vitamins may not be readily available and an adequate supply should be taken for the entire trip. Extended exposure to high altitudes should be avoided during pregnancy due to higher incidences of adverse effects.

Scuba diving is contraindicated in pregnancy. Prolonged air travel is also to be avoided because of increased risk of blood clots. If air travel is required, the pregnant traveler should request an aisle seat or a bulkhead seat to increase legroom and take exercise breaks at a minimum of once an hour.

Malaria and Pregnancy

Malaria is one of most important insect-transmitted diseases to avoid while traveling. This is especially true during pregnancy. The *falciparum* species of malaria is the most dangerous. Malaria may cross the placental barrier and infect the unborn child. Malaria also carries a higher morbidity and mortality rate in the mother and her unborn child. The disease is more severe in pregnancy, due to a weakened immune system during pregnancy. This decrease in immunity allows a higher percentage of red blood cells to be infected by parasites. Also the placenta is a preferential site for the sequestration of parasitized red blood cells.

Maternal complications of falciparum malaria include profound hypoglycemia (low blood sugar), increased anemia, kidney failure, adult respiratory distress syndrome, shock, and coma. Maternal mortality rates up to 10% can occur. Obstetrical complications of malaria include low birth weight infants, anemia, spontaneous abortion, premature births, stillbirths, and neonatal death. Malaria may cross the placental barrier and infect the unborn child.

The best advice is to avoid elective travel to malarious areas when pregnant, especially where chloroquine-resistant malaria is endemic. If travel to a malarious area is a must, it is imperative to prevent mosquito bites and taken an effective prophylactic drug. These recommendations should come from a qualified physician as some products and medications may be contraindicated in pregnancy.

Resources
1. Wendland CC, Kuhn SC: Women in the Wilderness, *Medical Missions Manual,* edited, Kuhn, W, Kuhn SC, Gross H, Augusta, GA, 2000.
2. CDC Traveler's Health Web Site at www.cdc.gov/travel
3. Anderson S: Travel Advice for Women, *The Travel and Tropical Medicine Manual,* 3rd ed., edited Jong, EC, McMullen, R, Philadelphia, PA 2003, Saunders.

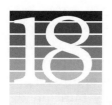# Protection from Exposure to Radiation from the Sun

Sharon C. Kuhn

Solar ultraviolet (UV) light composed of UVA I, UVA II, and UVB wavelengths enters the earth's atmosphere and can cause acute and chronic injury to the skin and eyes of exposed individuals. Of the solar radiation that reaches the earth's surface approximately 90% is UVA and 10% UVB, which is partially filtered out as it passes through the atmosphere. UVA and UVB both contribute to solar skin damage with effects ranging from acute sunburn to chronic tissue damage. UVA penetrates more deeply into the skin than UVB and has been implicated in "photoaging", causing loss of elasticity of the skin, i.e., wrinkles, and irregular pigmentation.[2] UVA also causes photoallergic and some phototoxic reactions. UVB overexposure leads to sunburn, melanogenesis, non-melanoma skin cancer (basal cell and squamous cell cancers), and also premature aging. Sun exposure is a potent cause of reactivation of herpes labialis. Ultraviolet radiation has also been shown to suppress the immune system both locally in the skin and systemically.[1] Any UVA/UVB exposure, including tanning in tanning salons or casual exposure to sunlight, contributes to the cumulative lifetime effects.[1]

Environmental Factors in UV Exposure

Several factors contribute to UV radiation exposure intensity including time of day, altitude, latitude, season, and environment. UVB peaks at midday and is intense between 10am and 3pm when the sun is high in the sky. The atmosphere absorbs and scatters UVB thus lessening its effects in the early and late hours of the day. The radiation from UVA remains constant throughout the day. UVB may increase as much as 8–10% for every 305 meter rise above sea level. UVB levels measured at an altitude of 8,500 feet (2591 meters) in Vail, CO were similar to UVB exposure hundreds of miles south in Orlando, FL.[1] Proximity to the equator (latitude) increases UV intensity significantly. The season of the year at any given latitude also affects UV exposure because of the change in the angle of the sun to the earth. Snow can reflect up to 85% of UV radiation and sand and other surfaces can also reflect the sun's rays and intensify exposure. Water is a lesser factor in reflecting the UV light, in fact UV radiation can penetrate water as much as 60 cm at midday.[1] Clouds may decrease the sun's heat, but UVA and UVB penetration may still be significant.[2]

Sunscreen and Sun Protection Factor

The sun protection factor (SPF) is calculated by dividing the dose of UV radiation needed to produce minimal erythema on skin protected by a sunscreen by the dose that produces the same degree of erythema on unprotected skin.[3] For instance, a sunscreen with an SPF of 2, blocks about 50% of UVB, an SPF of 15, blocks about 93%, and an SPF of 30, blocks about 97% of UVB, assuming it is applied properly. The SPF rating relates only to UVB protection. Other ingredients must be added to absorb UVA. Avobenzone (Parasol 1789), menthyl anthranilate, and oxybenzone absorb some UVA wavelengths. There are also physical sunblocks, zinc oxide and titanium dioxide, which block both UVB and UVA. These usually come in opaque white or colored formulations, though some newer ones are transparent.[3]

Sunscreens can minimize solar radiation skin damage, but no sunscreen protects against all UVA rays. A multitude of overstated claims led the Food and Drug Administration (FDA) to set regulations for over-the-counter (OTC) sunscreen products. As of March 1999 FDA regulations require similar labeling for all OTC sunscreen products, including sunscreen cosmetics. There is a list of allowed sunscreen active ingredients, there are label warnings and required SPF testing. Misleading terms such as "sunblock", "waterproof", "all-day protection", and "visible and/or infrared light protection" can no longer be used.[2]

Sunscreens are tested under idealized laboratory conditions where there is no wind, no excessive humidity, and no "toweling off." Therefore claims of being "water resistant" or "sweat resistant" must be taken to mean that the product will still need to be periodically reapplied.

Use of Sunscreen

Apply sunscreen half an hour before venturing outside and be careful to cover all exposed areas of skin. The nose, ears, forehead, top of head and the top of the feet are particularly vulnerable to burn. Be sure they are covered. The recommended dose of sunscreen is one ounce per application (full body).[3] Sunscreen should be reapplied every 2 hours and after swimming or heavy sweating. A light application of SPF 30 gives you only an SPF 15 protection. Because individuals tend to under-apply sunscreen

and because it is difficult to apply evenly, it is probably wise to use a product with the higher SPF of 30 to help compensate. You can estimate the amount of sunscreen necessary for travel by simply multiplying the number of days times applications per day to give you the number of ounces you will need to carry. Sunscreens and lip balm with a SPF of 15 or more are recommended for everyone over six months of age.

All sunscreens will burn the eyes if the eyes are rubbed accidentally during application. New bonding base formulas will not migrate (run down into eyes with sweat or water) after application. Sunscreens can affect your grip by causing the skin of your hands to feel slippery. The older formulations can also reduce your ability to sweat by blocking evaporation. Newer formulas work beneath the skin allowing the skin to breathe and will not affect athletic performance.[4] If you are sensitive to oxybenzone or benzephenone, then use the SPF 15 preparations that do not include them.

Protective Clothing

Clothing is critical in protection from the sun. The SPF factor of clothing depends primarily on the weave of the cloth rather that the particular fabric. A tight weave blocks the sun better than a loose weave. Dry clothing has a higher SPF than wet clothing. For example, a dry white tee shirt has an SPF of 5–9 while a wet tee shirt may have an SPF of 4 or less. Wear clothing with long sleeves and long pants to limit sun exposure. Light colors are better in hot environments. Choose a broad brimmed hat that protects not only the forehead and nose, but also the cheeks and chin and back of the neck.

Wear UV protective sunglasses. Sun may damage the eyes and can lead acutely to the formation of photokeratitis (snow blindness) or eventually to the formation of cataracts or ptyerigium.

Children and Sun Exposure

The higher the cumulative exposure to UV radiation, the greater will be the risk of non-melanoma skin cancer later in life. Children receive on average 80% of their life time exposure before age 18.[2] Use of preventive measures should begin early. Infants less than six months old should be kept out of direct sunlight and should wear clothing that covers them and a hat. Parents should use sun screen, protective hats, clothing and sunglasses, as well as sun avoidance for toddlers and older children.

Prevention Facts and Reminders

1. Limit sun exposure during the peak hours of 10 am to 3 pm.
2. Repeated exposure to the sun several days in a row causes increased UV sensitivity on the subsequent days.[2] Greater caution should be exercised each day to lessen sun exposure.
3. A suntan is a sign of skin damage and a tan does not protect the skin from further damage when exposed to solar radiation.
4. Use unscented sunscreens to avoid insects.
5. Wear protective clothing, sunglasses, and sunscreen even on cloudy days.
6. Use SPF 15, or preferably SPF 30 sunscreens liberally and reapply every 2 hours or more frequently if swimming or sweating heavily.

Treatment of Sunburn

It is best to prevent sunburn since there is no perfect treatment. If taken before exposure or prior to the appearance of erythema, aspirin or nonsteroidal antiinflammatory (NSAIDs) and topical steroid medications may slightly decrease the ensuing erythema.[3] Once the sunburn is established, treatment is symptomatic. NSAIDs or other pain relievers may be used. Cool compresses and topical anesthetics may be helpful. It is best to use non-sensitizing formulations such as those containing camphor or pramoxine rather than benzocaine and diphenhydramine. Moisturizers may also be soothing. Lotions can be refrigerated before use to provide further relief.

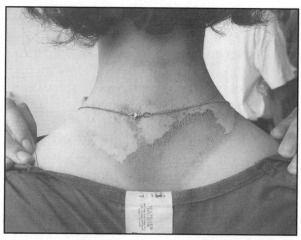

Hartmut Gross/
"Sunburned Medical Missionary"

Erythema usually begins within 4 hours of exposure and peaks at about 24 hours in a first degree sunburn. The skin may peel on days 4–7. In a second degree sunburn the skin is red and painful, and develops blisters. This can be treated as described above unless blistering is extensive, in which case medical attention should be sought. Those suffering from sunburn should drink plenty of fluids and avoid reexposure to the sun while recovering. There are many anecdotal reports suggesting a benefit to using systemic steroids in more severe sunburns; however, there are few published studies to support this.[1]

Photosensitivity Disorders

Numerous conditions can be triggered by exposure to intense sunlight and hence prevented or lessened by careful protective measures. Several commonly used medications can cause photosensitivity reactions that are either phototoxic or photoallergic. Phototoxic reactions to medication appear minutes to hours after sun exposure as an exaggerated sunburn and appear only on sun exposed skin.[2] Offending drugs may include flouroquinolones, tetracyclines, (including doxycycline), chloroquine, sulfonamides and many others. If possible, stop the suspected medication. Unfortunately, the reaction may take several weeks to resolve. Drugs can also cause photoallergic reactions. These require prior sensitization and usually present 24 hours or more following sun exposure as a pruritic, eczematous rash which will also involve non-exposed skin. Treatment requires that the offending drug be stopped.[5]

Polymorphous light eruption (PLE) is an endogenous photosensitivity disorder that appears on sun-exposed areas as a pruritic, erythematous, maculopapular, and sometimes vesicular, rash 1–2 days after sun exposure. It occurs most often in young fair-skinned women early in the summer on initial sun exposure. It will resolve on its own in 7 to 10 days.[1]

Phytophotodermatitis is another fairly common photosensitivity disorder. Many plants, such as limes and lemons containing psoralens or similar chemicals can sensitize skin. If these substances are present on the skin during sun exposure, a streaky rash may occur.

References

1. Kaplan LA, Exposure to Radiation from the Sun, *Wilderness Medicine*, 4th ed., edited Auerbach PS, St. Louis, 2001, Mosby, Inc., pp 360–384.
2. McKay M, Sun-associated Problems, *Travel Medicine*, edited Keystone JS, Kozarsky PE, Freedman DO, Nothdurft HD, Connor BA, Philadelphia, 2004, Mosby, pp 394–397.
3. Prevention and Treatment of Sunburn, *The Medical Letter*, Vol. 46 (Issue 1184):45–46, 2004.
4. Friedlander J, Lowe NJ: Exposure to Radiation from the Sun, *Wilderness Medicine: Management of Wilderness and Environmental Emergencies*, 3rd ed., editor PS Auerbach, St. Louis, Missouri, 1995, Mosby-Year Book, Inc., pp 291–311.
5. Colven R, Strother MS, Acute Skin Reactions, *The Travel and Tropical Medicine Manual*, 3rd ed., edited Jong EC, McMullen R, Philadelphia, 2003, Saunders, pp 449–458.

Resources

1. Cancer Information Service 1-800-4-CANCER
   American Cancer Society 1-800-ACS-2345
   American Academy of Dermatology
   PO Box 4014
   Schaumburg, IL 60168-4014
2. For further information concerning sunscreen and sun protection, contact:
   http://www.ftc.gov/bcp/conline/pubs/health/sun.htm

19 Motion Sickness

Jim Carroll

Physiology of Motion Sickness
Risk of Motion Sickness
Management of Motion Sickness

Motion sickness is a truly unpleasant experience of nausea and dizziness induced by movement of the body through space. The exact cause of motion sickness is unknown, but it is thought to be due to a mismatch among the four sensory systems perceiving the movement. More specifically, it seems to be caused by conflicting inputs between vision and the other systems.

Physiology of Motion Sickness

The visual system transmits signals to the occipital cortex for interpretation. The semicircular canals detect angular acceleration or deceleration of the head, such as when starting or stopping spinning, somersaulting, or turning the head. Each of the three canals lies in planes at right angles to each other. The otolith organs provide information about the position of the head relative to gravity and also detect changes in rate of linear motion. Signals arising from the components of the vestibular apparatus are transmitted to the brain stem and cerebellum. The peripheral nervous system relays information on joint position.

Motion sickness occurs most often with acceleration perpendicularly to the long axis of the body. Head movements away from the direction of overall movement are provocative. Vertical oscillatory motion at a frequency of 0.2 hertz is most likely to cause motion sickness. This is like a ship with a roll rate of 5 seconds. In fact, the term nausea is derived from the Greek word *naus*, for *ship*.[1]

Rolls at higher frequency produce less motion sickness. Adaptation tends to occur after 36–72 hours of continuous exposure.Interestingly, sitting stationary while watching a panoramic movie or flight simulator can also cause motion sickness, likely due to the conflicting visual and vestibular signals to the brain.

Nausea and vomiting are thought to be mediated by central neurotransmitters. Digestive system motility is reduced, and hyperventilation is common. Increased dopamine levels are theorized to stimulate the medulla's chemoreceptor trigger zone, stimulating the vomiting center within the reticular formation of the brain stem. The vomiting center is also stimulated by acetylcholine. The role of these chemical pathways is in part confirmed by the fact that the drugs that appear to be effective include antidopaminergics, anticholinergics, and antihistamines.

Risk of Motion Sickness

The risk for motion sickness varies with age, but almost everyone will experience motion sickness with sufficient stimulus. About one-third of the population is highly susceptible. Children under age 2 years are rarely affected. Peak susceptibility is between 4 and 10 years. Females are more susceptible than males, and oral contraceptives enhance susceptibility. The recent ingestion of foods also increases the risk. Strangely, highly conditioned individuals may be more susceptible. Individuals with migraine are thought to have a higher incidence of motion sickness. Psychological factors probably play a role.

Differential diagnosis includes vestibular disease, altitude sickness, gastroenteritis, toxin exposure, and metabolic disorders. Potential complications include hypotension and dehydration from vomiting and poor fluid intake, as well as depression and panic.

Management of Motion Sickness

Management usually amounts to the susceptible person determining what works best for his or her symptoms. Sitting near the front of the vehicle with visual fixation on the horizon often helps. If susceptible to motion sickness, one should not try to read while traveling. Head movement should be limited. Large meals should be avoided before the trip. Alcohol, smoking and disagreeable odors should be avoided. When motion sickness strikes, opening the window may help, getting "a breath of fresh air." Pressure over a point three centimeters above the distal palmar crease is said to be helpful.

Two classes of drugs may be of benefit: central cholinergic blockers or drugs that enhance dopamine-norepinephrine. The list of drugs used for motion sickness is long: scopolamine, atropine, dimenhydrinate, cyclizine, meclizine, promethazine, amphetamine, methamphetamine, and methylphenidate, to name a few.

The simplest medication to try first is dimenhydrinate (Dramamine®), 50 mg, which has an onset after one hour of administration and lasts for 6–10 hours. Meclizine (Antivert®) is a good one to try next, 25–50 mg; it has a slower onset and a longer duration of action. Obviously, either of these drugs should be taken before travel. They often cause drowsiness. Meclizine is contraindicated with respiratory problems, glaucoma, or enlarged prostate.

If the individual still gets motion sickness with either of the above medications, then the scopolamine should be considered. The patch (Transderm Scop®) delivers 1.5 mg of the drug over 3 days and is not effective until 6–8 hours after application. The patch is applied to the skin behind the ear in a hairless area. Users should wash their hands to avoid eye exposure. Tablets, 0.4 mg, may be used in lieu of the patch, taking them every 8 hours. The beneficial effect of scopolamine is said to be enhanced by 10 mg methylphenidate (Ritalin®). One should be aware that scopolamine might cause blurred vision and worsening of narrow-angle glaucoma. Essentially, over dosage looks like atropine poisoning with confusion, restlessness, and dry mouth. Scopolamine can worsen pre-existing prostate or pyloric obstruction.

If nausea and vomiting are intractable despite preventive measures, then promethazaine, 25 mg intramuscularly can be used.

Medications Commonly Used for Motion Sickness

Drugs	Dosage	Comments
Anticholinergic		
Scopolamine (Transderm Scop*)	Adults: 1 patch (1.5 mg) behind ear 4–6h before travel, change every 3 days	Not indicated in children. Contraindicated in glaucoma or difficulty urinating. May cause drowsiness, dry mouth, blurred vision. Pregnancy category C.
Antihistamines		
Dimenhydrinate (Dramamine®)	Adults: 50–100 mg PO/IM/IV q4h, max 400 mg/d Children 6-12 yrs: 25–50 mg PO/IV q4h, max 150 mg/d	May be sedating. Contraindicated in glaucoma, enlarged prostate, or pyloric obstruction. Pregnancy category B.
Meclizine (Antivert, Bonine®)	12.5–50 mg PO qid	Contraindicated in glaucoma, enlarged prostate, pyloric obstruction, or chronic respiratory problems. Pregnancy category B.
Antidopaminergic (Antiemetic)		
Metoclopramide (Reglan®)	Adults: 10-30 mg PO qid; 10 mg IV/IM q2-3h	Any may cause extrapyramidal effects. Pregnancy category B.
Prochlorperazine (Compazine®)	Adults: 10 mg PO/IM q6h; 25 mg PR q6h; 5–10 mg IV over at least 2 min Children: 0.13 mg/kg/dose	Pregnancy category C, yet considered by many as the agent of choice for prevention or relief of motion sickness in pregnancy. (Reference 5)
Promethazine (Anergan®, Phenergan®)	Adults: 12.5–50 mg PO/IM/PR q4-6h (IV not approved) Children: 0.25–0.5 mg/kg PO/IM/PR q4-6h	Pregnancy category C. May lower seizure threshold. May be sedating.
Benzodiazepines		
Clonazepam (Klonopin®) Diazepam (Valium®) Lorazepam (Ativam®)	Adults: 0.25–0.5 mg PO tid Adults: 2–7.5 mg PO qid Adults: 0.5–2 mg PO tid	All can cause dose-related drowsiness. Pregnancy category B

Medications Commonly Used for Motion Sickness (*cont.*)

Drugs	Dosage	Comments
Sympathomimetics		
Dextroamphetamine (Dexedrine®)	Adults: 5–10 mg PO qam or bid	Counteract motion sickness and have an additive effect with anticholinergic agents, as well as counteracting the sedation from other agents. Pregnancy category C.
Pemoline (Cylert®)	Adults and children: 18.75–37.5 mg PO qam	Controlled substance and may produce a positive result on drug screening. Pregnancy category B. Life threatening liver failure reported. Not indicated as first line therapy.
Methylphenidate (Ritalin®)	Adults: 10 mg tid Children > 6 yr: 5–10 mg tid	May result in insomnia if taken after 6 pm.
Other		
Ginger root (*Zingiberis rhizome, Z. officinale*)	1-9 grams of fresh or dried root PO qd	Considered safe in pregnancy. Available as capsules, powder, tea, or in candies.
Apricot or carrot juice, unroasted pumpkin or squash seeds, parsley, and peppermint tea		Many herbal remedies exist. No scientific studies exist to either support or discount any of these.
Cocculus, ignatia, ipecac, colchicum, nux vomica and tabacum		Again, no investigational studies exist. (Reference 5)

PRACTICAL TIPS FROM A MOTION SICKNESS SUFFERER

Leslie O'Neill

"...prevention is far superior to treatment once the symptoms begin."

(Dr. Jerry Lambert)

Editor's Note: These tips were tested under extreme conditions: days of riding on curvy mountain roads in buses and old open trucks and they were successful in preventing motion sickness in the author, who had to use her knowledge and medicines to help fellow travelers who were not so prepared.

1. I *religiously* took my Dramamine.® I brought along both the regular and less drowsy formulas. I took a pill one hour before we left on each trip, and then every four hours during the trip. I made it a point to keep up with the time so I did not run out of medication. I kept it in my pocket, right along with my toilet paper and anti-bacterial soap! The drowsy formula was great for that long trip over the Andes by bus, but I probably would have fallen right out of the logging truck with that formula, so I used the less-drowsy for those days.
2. I always sat in the front half of the vehicle and tried to have proper ventilation.
3. I kept salted soda crackers nearby to eat when taking medication, and for eating in between meals so my stomach did not become overly empty. I did not eat large meals on the days we traveled, but snacked on crackers, granola bars, hard candy, etc.
4. I had asked many of my friends at home to pray specifically about this potential problem, and they did! Even though I took the above "practical" measures, I know the Lord answered our prayers and was gracious to me in my weakness.

The only time I felt nauseous during all of our traveling was the night I was sitting right over the exhaust in the logging truck, and I think it was more from the smell than the motion. Once I stood up in the front of the truck and got a little "fresher" air, I began to feel better.

References

1. Gahlinger, PM: *Motion sickness. How to help your patients avoid travel travail.* Post-graduate Medicine 106: 177–184, 1999.
2. Sherman, CR: *Motion sickness: Review of causes and preventive strategies.* J Travel M; Med 8: 251–256, 2002.
3 American Botanical Council, et al.: *The Complete German Commission E Monographs: Therapeutic Guide to Herbal Medicines,* CD-ROM, editor M Blumenthal, Austin, TX, 1998, Integrative Medicine Communications.
4 Lockie A, Geddes N. *The Complete Guide to Homeopathy,* New York, 1995, Dorling Kindersley Publishing, p 222.
5 Samuel BU, Barry M: The Pregnant Traveler, *Infect Dis Clin North Am,* 12(2):325, 1998.

20 Heat Illness
Sharon C. Kuhn

Work in many developing countries involves exposure to elevated environmental temperatures, humidity, or a combination of both. Such an environment can not only reduce individual and team effectiveness through fatigue, but can be dangerous from a physiologic perspective especially if one does not understand how to adapt to such conditions. There is an abundant body of medical science to help us understand the acclimatization process and mechanisms for maintaining adequate hydration. The importance of this information can not be overemphasized. As the makers of "Camelback,®" a popular water-carrying backpack, put it, "hydrate or die."

In this chapter the emphasis will be on exertional heat illness as opposed to "classic" heat exhaustion and heat stroke. There is, however, considerable overlap in symptoms, treatment and prevention strategies in exertional and classic heat illness. Classic heat exhaustion and heat stroke are seen most often in elderly persons with multiple medical problems who are exposed to a very hot environment and who gradually develop symptoms over several days, even without physical exertion. Exertional heat illness, including heat stroke, can develop quickly in situations where individuals are performing vigorous physical work in a hot environment.

Thermoregulation

The human body is constantly producing heat as food is consumed to produce energy to maintain the metabolic processes of life. This baseline metabolic rate would cause body temperature to increase by approximately 2 degrees Fahrenheit (F) per hour if cooling mechanisms were not operative. When an individual exercises strenuously, body heat production may increase 10–20 times.[1] The body functions optimally within a fairly narrow temperature range; therefore it has numerous mechanisms to maintain this homeostasis. When external factors of heat and humidity plus internal heat production from physical exertion exceed the body's ability to cool itself, heat illnesses occur.

The basic mechanisms for heat exchange between the body and the environment are radiation, conduction, convection, and evaporation. In radiation, heat is transferred from warmer to cooler objects through electromagnetic waves. Radiant heat from the sun can be a significant factor in increasing the heat burden of the body. Conduction involves the transfer of heat from a warmer object to a cooler one through direct contact. Water conducts heat at least 25 times better that air.[1] This is why cold water immersion is the most efficient way of cooling a heat stroke victim. Convection refers to the process by which body heat is lost to air and to water vapor molecules circulating around the body. The body is cooled as the warmed molecules are moved away from the body surface by air currents. A nice breeze or a fan causes cooling through convection. The fourth method that the body uses to cool itself, and the most important as environmental temperatures rise, is evaporation. The hypothalamus is the thermoregulatory center for the body. It monitors body heat through the temperature of the blood which perfuses it and indirectly receives input from skin temperature sensors. When body temperature rises, the hypothalamus stimulates the production of sweat (a hypotonic saline solution) from the sweat glands in the skin. Blood vessels near the surface of the skin also dilate in response to heat stress to enhance the dissipation of heat. As the sweat is vaporized from the skin surface, the skin and the blood supplying it are cooled. For every one gram of sweat that is vaporized, approximately 0.6 kcals of heat are eliminated.[2] The warmer the environment, the greater the rate of perspiration. Humidity is the one major factor that limits the vaporization of sweat from the body and thus, as humidity rises, there is a decrease in the capacity for cooling.

Fluid Replacement and Thirst

For evaporation to work in cooling, the body must be hydrated well enough to produce sweat and to maintain intravascular volume in the face of marked peripheral vasodilatation. The body loses about 1.5 liters of water, or about 2% of body weight per day in maintaining normal physiologic processes. This loss is unavoidable even without added heat or stress, and must be replaced daily. Hard work in a hot environment can multiply the body's fluid losses up to 1.5 liters <u>per hour</u> or even more![1] 12%

body fluid loss produces shock and eventual death if not replenished.

A major problem for individuals working in the heat is that they do not voluntarily drink as much fluid as they lose. People usually replace only 2/3 of what is lost.[3] The body's normal thirst mechanism is either inadequate or delayed so that thirst can not be exclusively relied upon to maintain adequate hydration. This "voluntary" dehydration unintentionally increases as temperature becomes elevated and sweat losses increase. When there is a greater effort needed to obtain or carry water, people are even less likely to drink adequate amounts. Thus, "all persons in the heat should be considered dehydrated, (except immediately after a meal), unless they have recently been forced to drink more water than they desired."[3]

Certain individuals unknowingly maintain a chronic state of dehydration with chronic body water deficits of about 2 liters. Additional body fluid loss of just another 2 liters (1–2 hours in the heat) can cause a decrease in performance and an increased risk of heat illness in these individuals. In non-acclimatized individuals exposed to heat stress, there is a substantially greater loss of sodium in sweat than in the acclimatized person which further adversely impacts the thirst mechanism. With loss of sodium, the thirst may be quenched long before even minimal fluid replacement has occurred, leaving a large and potentially dangerous fluid deficit.

As acclimatization is achieved, this solute loss is less pronounced and the thirst mechanism is reset to a level more in keeping with total body fluid needs.[4] Even this degree of thirst is, however, inadequate to replace all the body's fluid losses.

Physical Fitness and Acclimatization

Each person will acclimatize to heat stress in his own way with considerable variation between individuals.[3] Nearly complete acclimatization can be achieved in 7–10 days for adults and 10–14 days for children. An hour or two per day of aerobic exercise at a relatively high intensity in the heat is sufficient to produce the desired physiologic effects of acclimatization. This process can be enhanced by improving general cardiovascular fitness under normal environmental conditions through a minimum of 20–30 minutes of aerobic exercise at least 4 times a week.[4] The benefits of acclimatization include the ability of the body to begin to sweat earlier in response to heat stress, to produce a larger volume of sweat, and to lose less salt in the sweat. Plasma volume increases both with training and with acclimatization and heart rate becomes lower with a higher stroke volume.[1] Because the cardiac output may have to increase 2–4 times to compensate for the vasodilatation resulting from heat stress, the benefits of training and acclimatization are critical.

Dressing for the Hot Environment

Heat loss through the evaporation of perspiration is the principal mechanism the body uses to prevent heat-related illness. The efficiency of evaporative heat loss depends not only on the absolute height of the ambient temperature, but is also affected by humidity, the presence or absence of wind or fans (convection) and the type of clothing. The best clothes are light colored, loosely fitting, and made of highly absorbent material. They are left in place throughout the time of heat exposure. The light color and material itself lower the amount of radiant heat from the sun which is absorbed by the body. Just wearing a light shirt can reduce the amount of heat gained from the sun significantly when compared to not wearing one.[4] The evaporation of sweat directly from the skin is more efficient for cooling than evaporation from a clinging sweat-soaked shirt, hence the recommendation for loose fitting garments. However, once wet with sweat the clothing is better for cooling than would be the case if one changed into new dry clothes. Most sweating and heat loss occurs from the head, torso and arms. The face and scalp account for 50% of sweat production. Toweling off and removing hats or protective headgear periodically will help with heat dissipation. Nonabsorbent sweat suits are dangerous to wear in hot environments since evaporation is retarded.[2]

Risk Factors for Heat Illness

There may be a delay in the onset of sweating associated with advancing age. Nevertheless, studies in middle aged marathon runners showed little to no difference in heat tolerance compared to their younger counterparts.[2] There are underlying conditions that are more common with age, including cardiac disease, diabetes, and thyroid problems that may interfere with thermoregulation and decrease the body's ability to cope with heat stress. Several classes of medications interfere with the body's ability to handle heat stress. Amphetamines, tricyclic antidepressants and thyroid hormone may increase heat production. Haloperidol decreases thirst. Drugs such as antihistamines and antidiarrheal medications decrease sweating.[3] Patients taking diuretics are already somewhat volume depleted before encountering the heat stress.

Fatal heat stroke occurs about three times more often in obese individuals compared to the thinner people.[2] Obesity stresses the heat regulatory mechanisms and fat provides insulation that prevents heat loss. Infants, children, and the elderly are at higher risk for heat illnesses. Men sweat more and at a lower temperature than do women; however, gender plays little to no role in heat-related illness if controlled for conditioning and heat acclimatization.

Predisposing Factors for Heat Illness

- Environmental temperature over 80° F
- Relatively high humidity
- Insufficient acclimatization
- Poor fitness level
- Improper hydration
- Obesity

- Extremes of age (infants, children, & elderly)
- Sustained exercise
- Febrile illness
- Certain medications (diuretics, medicines to stop diarrhea, antihistamines, some antidepressants, some psychiatric medications)
- Certain chronic diseases (vascular disease, diabetes, thyroid disorders)
- Having worked hard in a very hot environment the day before

Symptoms and Treatment of Heat-related Illnesses

Heat exhaustion occurs when an individual who is sweating profusely during exertion fails to replace fluid losses adequately. Similar problems can occur when there is a high rate of insensible water loss (for example sitting in the sun for a prolonged period when there is a nice breeze). The early symptoms of heat exhaustion are subtle and are easily overlooked. These may include: fatigue, nausea, vomiting, headache, and light-headedness which can lead to heat syncope, ataxia, tachycardia, tachypnea, and hypotension, skin pallor, and abdominal and muscle cramps. Mild confusion (trouble paying attention, trouble calculating, losing track of time) may be an early symptom which if untreated may lead to incoherent speech and even loss of consciousness and heat stroke. At first there will be profuse sweating. This may continue or the sweating may eventually cease and the skin may become cool and dry with piloerection ("goose bumps"). Initial temperature may be normal or elevated.

As soon as any symptoms of heat illness are recognized, the individual should stop work or exercise and efforts should be directed toward cooling and hydration. The individual should lie down in a cool place out of the sun, and if alert, should be given plenty of oral fluids. Water or other beverage such as a sport drink with 6% or less carbohydrate content (not alcoholic and preferably not caffeine containing) can be given at the rate of about 1–2 liters every

1–4 hours.[4] The person will need to continue to rest and drink fluids for the next 24–36 hours in order to reestablish hydration. If scales are available, 2 cups (16 ounces) of fluid should be consumed for every pound of weight lost though the dehydration. The individual should eat normally, if possible, to replace sodium losses, and should avoid any further exertion in the heat for at least 48 hours. Exertional heat illness may occur on the day following a day of high heat exposure even if the second day is cooler.

Symptoms of Heat Exhaustion[4]

- Mild confusion (trouble paying attention, trouble calculating, losing track of time)
- Fatigue
- Nausea, vomiting
- Light-headed, dizzy...may pass out (heat syncope)
- Headache
- Copious sweating
- Cool dry skin with "goose bumps" (piloerection)—late signs
- Muscle cramps, abdominal cramps
- Rapid heart rate
- Rapid breathing
- Skin pallor

Hyponatremia and Heat Illness

One other potentially serious complication that can occur in situations where heat illness is encountered is hyponatremia, or low body sodium (salt). The symptoms of hyponatremia are very similar to the symptoms of heat illness and can be life threatening. This condition has been seen in long distance competitive runners who have replaced their extensive fluid losses exclusively with plain water[1] or hypotonic fluids, e.g. quarter-strength sports drinks. It can be seen in individuals who normally drink large quantities of water, who then, in a hot environment increase this water intake even further while losing salt in their sweat and not replacing the salt loss through food or the substitution of sports drinks for water. Individuals on chronic diuretic therapy are also prone to hyponatremia prior to heat challenge. They may also have been advised to avoid salty foods and sports drinks; however, this advice may need to be tempered while working in a very hot environment.

One method of avoiding hyponatremia in these situations is to encourage the drinking of sports drinks (e.g. Gatorade® or Powerade®) for a fair portion of the fluid replacement. Having salty snacks to accompany water replacement will also help.

Fever and Hyperthermia

Persons with suspected heat illness may in fact have a gastroenteritis or other febrile illness. If the temperature fails to come down rapidly with external cooling or if the patient develops severe shivering with external cooling, an etiology other than heat stress may be present. In heat illness the body's thermal set point is not changed, therefore antipyretic drugs, such as acetaminophen, are not helpful in lowering core temperature.[1] In febrile illness, the set point is raised above 98.6°F and antipyretics are helpful. Gastroenteritis with its accompanying volume depletion can also be a predisposing factor in cases of heat exhaustion, especially in individuals working in areas where water and food sources are likely to be contaminated.

Heat Syncope

Heat syncope is most likely to occur in the first few days of exposure to heat before acclimatization takes place.[4] It is a brief loss of consciousness which can occur when an individual is exposed to a hot environment, especially if that person must stand for a prolonged period. Vasodilatation from the heat, plus gravitational pooling of blood in the lower extremities, and some degree of dehydration all contribute to the hypotension and decrease in cerebral perfusion which lead to syncope. Individuals should be advised that if they feel light-headed, nauseous, or weak, they should quickly sit down or lie down preferably in the shade or a cooler location. They should rest and drink water or a sports drink. If someone experiences syncope in a hot environment, follow the same guidelines. If the person does not immediately regain consciousness in the supine position, heat stroke or other serious illness must be considered.

Heat Cramps

Individuals engaged in strenuous exercise in the heat may develop cramps in the extremities and abdomen which can be severe. There appear to be at least two different kinds of heat cramps. Generalized muscle cramping is a common symptom of heat exhaustion. In this case the person appears ill, may have abdominal cramping, and is experiencing other symptoms such as fatigue, nausea, and vomiting.[3] The treatment is the same as for heat exhaustion: cooling, fluids, and electrolytes given orally if possible or intravenously if necessary. Another type of heat cramping has been described in which an individual who is exercising heavily in the heat develops severe cramps in the muscles that are most used, but has no other symptoms of heat exhaustion.

Cramping can occur not only during sustained exercise but even hours after such exertion is over. This type of cramping is usually associated with high sweat volumes and the consumption of large amounts of water. It responds well to stretching and the ingestion of salt containing fluids such as sport drinks. One-quarter teaspoon of salt in 1 quart of water is a tolerable replacement fluid if nothing else is available.[3]

Heat-induced Tetany and Hyperventilation

Heat-induced numbness and tingling in the extremities, carpopedal spasm and tetany have been described in patients exposed to hot environments even in the absence of significant salt and water depletion. The cramping in these individuals may occur in the abdomen, chest, and hands in addition to the legs. Hyperventilation in response to the heat appears to be a major causative factor. Rest in a cool spot and oral fluid and electrolyte replacement, and possibly rebreathing expired air are usually all that is needed for treatment.[3]

Heat Stroke

The progression from serious heat exhaustion to heat stroke with delirium and loss of consciousness can be sudden in as many as 80% of cases.[1] In heat stroke the core temperature is usually 41°C or 106°F or more; however, heat stroke may occur at lower core temperatures. The skin is usually hot and dry, but sweating may still be present. There will be severe central nervous system (CNS) dysfunction with delirium, seizures, or loss of consciousness.

Immediate cooling, preferably by cool water immersion to 39°C (102.2°F) is critical. This must be accomplished in a careful and controlled manner to avoid drowning risk. When the patient's temperature reaches 39°C, he should be removed from the cold water to prevent over cooling. If cooling by cold water immersion is not available in the field, it can be accomplished by laying the person down in a cool place, loosening or removing his clothing, sprinkling his skin with cool water and fanning him to increase evaporation. If ice is available, ice packs can be placed in the axillae and groin areas. Intravenous (IV) fluid replacement with normal saline or Ringer's lactate should be given if available at 1200 ml over the first 4 hours[1] with additional boluses as clinical symptoms warrant. Seizures can be treated with IV diazepam or phenobarbital, if medical supplies are available.

Heat stroke is a medical emergency. Action must be taken immediately to begin to cool the victim of heat stroke because the damage from heat stroke is dependent not only on the degree of the core temperature elevation, but also on the length of time that the body is exposed to the high temperature. Attention must be paid to the "ABC's" of patient care and plans for moving the patient to a quality medical facility should be made quickly if possible. It can not be overemphasized, however, that efforts to cool the patient must begin as soon as the condition is recognized. Such efforts are the key to saving the patient's life.

Other complications of exertional heat stroke include rhabdomyolysis, lactic acidosis, hypoglycemia, hyperuricemia, acute renal failure, disseminated intravascular coagulation (DIC), marked elevation of liver transaminases, and hypocalcemia. These complications are uncommon in classic nonexertional heat stroke. Ideally, these complications should be treated in a medical center, but if heat illness or heat stroke occurs in the field, cooling must be initiated prior to evacuation so that valuable time is not lost. If treated rapidly, even unconscious patients with fixed and dilated pupils have been known to recover.[1]

Prevention of Heat Illness

"An ounce of prevention is worth a pound of cure." The health care professional's primary task should be to educate those for whom he is responsible about the dangers of heat illness, ways to prevent it, and early warning signs. He should institute guidelines for prevention through regular rest breaks from strenuous work and for required fluid replacement. He should be sure that adequate supplies of pure water and palatable fluids are easily available. If possible, these should be cooled to increase compliance. Though plain water is usually adequate for fluid replacement, sports drinks are more likely to be consumed because of taste and they have the advantage of containing electrolytes which the body also loses in perspiration.

An easy way to teach individuals to gauge their hydration status is to have them pay attention to their frequency of urination and the color of the urine. Urine should be light yellow or almost clear when one is well-hydrated. Hence the athlete's "mantra" to drink until you "pee clear." By the same token, if one has worked all day in the heat and has not felt the need to urinate all day, that person is severely dehydrated. The health care professional should be aware of any medications being taken by those for whom he is responsible, and of any underlying conditions that may predispose them to heat illness.

If, in spite of all precautions, someone should become symptomatic, steps should be taken quickly to initiate cooling, rehydration, and additional treatment as indicated.

Guidelines for Prevention

1. Have team members pursue an exercise program well ahead of the trip to insure base line fitness.
2. Plan the work schedule: Start in the early morning. Break in the heat of the day. Work in the shade as much as possible. Rotate the most strenuous jobs.
3. Drink 2–4 cups of liquid before leaving for work (e.g. at breakfast).
4. Those working in the heat will need to consume approximately 3–4 quarts of fluid per day.
5. Be sure everyone has plenty of potable water or sports drink close at hand.
6. Having salty snacks available is helpful.
7. Require rest/water breaks for 5–10 minutes every hour depending on conditions.
8. Create a buddy system where people check up on each other and remind each other to drink.
9. If anyone starts to feel ill, the medical person in charge should be notified immediately. The individual should rest in a cool ventilated area and be given fluids to drink. If the situation is more serious, active cooling should be begun immediately and emergency procedures instituted.

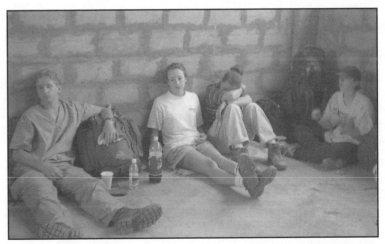

Ted Kuhn/
"Exhausted and Dehydrated Medical Team, Amazon Jungle"

References

1. Yarbrough B, Vicario S: Heat Illness, *Rosen's Emergency Medicine* 5th ed, edited Marx JA, St. Louis, 2002, Mosby, Inc. pp 1997–2006.
2. Gersoff WK, Motz HA: Environmental Factors in Athletic Performance, *Sports Injuries: Mechanisms, Prevention, Treatment*, edited Fu FH, Stone DA, Baltimore, 1994, Williams & Wilkens. pp 56–57.
3. Gaffin SL, Moran DS: Pathophysiology of Heat-Related Illnesses, *Wilderness Medicine*, 4th ed., edited Auerbach PS, St. Louis, 2001, Mosby, Inc. pp 260–263, 278–279.
4. Hubbard RW, Gaffin SL, Squire DL: Heat-Related Illnesses, *Wilderness Medicine: Management of Wilderness and Environmental Emergencies*, 3rd ed., edited Auerbach PS, St. Louis, 1995, Mosby-Year Book, Inc. pp 170–201 (Heat Exhaustion Table),.
5. Moran DS, Gaffin SL: Clinical Management of Heat-Related Illnesses, *Wilderness Medicine,* 4th ed., edited Auerbach PS, St. Louis, 2001, Mosby, Inc. p 310.

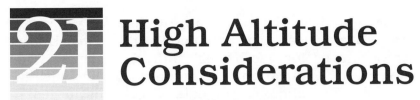

High Altitude Considerations

Cynthia Urbanowicz

Definition
Etiology
Signs and Symptoms
Prevention
Treatment of AMS
HAPE and HACE:
Serious Forms of AMS
Pearls

High altitude travelers of centuries ago attributed a certain severe and often fatal illness to "evil pestilence" and "bad humors" arising from the high mountain peaks in which they traveled. With today's ease of travel, we can leave the comfort of our homes and find ourselves standing on these same high peaks within 24 hours. High altitude travelers of long ago had one advantage over those who travel today-time. Journeys to high altitude often took months and sometimes years to reach the summit. Although these same travelers experienced signs and symptoms of acute mountain sickness (AMS), their bodies typically had time to acclimate, whereas ours often do not. It is possible to fly from Lima, Peru (sea-level) and arrive in Cusco, Peru (11, 380 feet) in only a few short hours.

Definition

High altitude is generally defined as 1,500–3,500 meters (m) or 5,000 to 11,500 ft above sea-level. Very high altitude is 3,500–5,500m or 11,500–18,000 ft. Extreme altitude would be anything over 5,500m or 18000 ft.[1] Some travelers, however, experience symptoms of AMS as low as 4,000 to 6,000 ft. This chapter will focus on very high altitude issues as this category is the

altitude at which most ministry work poses significant personal risk.

Etiology

To better understand the effects of altitude, it is necessary to review two gas laws; Boyle's law and Dalton's law. Boyle's law states, as the pressure increases, the volume decreases. Conversely, Boyle's law also states as the pressure decreases, the volume increases. Picture an ordinary balloon at sea level. If this same balloon is taken five hundred feet under the sea, it will be compressed to roughly half it's original volume. This same balloon taken to 5,000 feet in altitude will be roughly twice its original size. This is why a shampoo bottle with a bit of air trapped inside will explode all over your suitcase as you travel to high altitude!

Dalton's law addresses the partial pressures of gas. The air we breathe is a mixed gas, containing oxygen, nitrogen and carbon dioxide. Dalton's law states that the total pressure of a gas mixture equals the sum of the partial pressures that make up the mixture. This is the second major problem at altitude. The gases we breathe are simply under less pressure. At very high altitude the molecules that make up the air are farther apart, there is less pressure to help them across our capillary membranes.

In normal respiration occurring at sealevel, we inhale the mixed gases that make up our atmosphere. Our bodies and environment are wonderfully made to work in cooperation. We inhale and the gas crosses into and out of our pulmonary capillaries through the thin membrane of the alveoli, assisted by the slight "push" from the atmospheric pressure. Carbon dioxide moves briskly across the membrane to be expired while oxygen enters through the same membrane, passing into the blood for the return of freshly oxygenated blood to the heart.

At high altitude, travelers experience the gas laws at work. Inspiration occurs, but now oxygen molecules are further apart and more sluggish. Partial oxygen pressure (PaO2) in the circulating blood falls. The result is an increase in the oxygen demand; to compensate, respiration increases.

Signs and Symptoms

The internationally recognized Lake Louise Consensus defines acute mountain sickness in the setting of a recent gain in altitude, the presence of headache and at least one of the following symptoms:

- Gastrointestinal (anorexia, nausea or vomiting).
- Fatigue or weakness.
- Dizziness or light-headedness.
- Difficulty sleeping.[4]

It is important for travelers to be aware of AMS symptoms and to admit they have them. For many travelers, these trips represent a lifetime desire and their emotional and financial investments are significant. Moreover, the pressure from peers to continue on and not delay the group may be overwhelming. "Studies have shown that travelers who are on organized group treks to high-altitude locations are more likely to die of altitude illness than travelers who are by themselves. This is most likely the result of group pressure (whether perceived or real) and a fixed itinerary. The most important aspect of preventing severe altitude illness is to refrain from further ascent until all symptoms of altitude illness have disappeared."[5] Ignoring or concealing symptoms may result in a very ill individual when he can no longer hide symptoms.

Signs and symptoms of AMS are similar to other travel related illnesses and discomforts. Symptoms may be rationalized by the traveler or explained away by the well meaning friend. All illness at altitude is AMS until proven otherwise.

The Lake Louise Consensus Questionnaire has been developed as a check sheet for use by high-altitude travelers. This questionnaire contains both subjective and objective data and is a useful tool to help define a *trend* in symptoms. The worksheet may be utilized on an every hour to every eight hour basis, as the patient status dictates. Rather than looking for a specific numeric assignment, it helps patients and health professionals rate symptoms, looking for a trend. The onset of AMS can be insidious. It is recommended that every person complaining of any illness at altitude have the questionnaire initiated. A copy of the Lake Louise Questionnaire is located at the end of the chapter.

Prevention

Factors that contribute to an increased incidence of acute mountain sickness:

1. Travelers with any type of obstructive pulmonary disease.
2. Travelers with past experience of AMS symptoms.
3. Travelers who ascend at a rapid rate.
4. Travelers who exert themselves physically on arrival.
5. Travelers with anemias or any disease process that inhibits the blood's ability to carry oxygen (e.g. sickle-cell anemia).
6. Travelers with sleep apnea.
7. Travelers taking any pharmaceutical agent that depresses respiration (e.g.- sleeping pills, anti-seizure medications).

Travelers with pre-existing medical conditions that may contribute to AMS should be counseled on the dangers of high altitude travel and be medically cleared before traveling. Something closer to sea-level may be a better choice for these individuals.

"Acclimatization is the process of the body adjusting to the decreasing availability of oxygen. It is a slow process, taking place over a period of days."[2] Acclimatization requires time and slow ascent promotes better acclimatization. For maximum benefit, the first night at altitude should be spent at 10,000 feet or less.[3] This is not always practical as our modern travel methods rapidly convey us to higher altitudes.

Pre-rail and aviation travelers had the advantage of slow travel by foot, with time to acclimate to each change in altitude. Unfortunately, these same positive factors for foot travel occasionally became negative factors as the exertion and arduousness of the climb precipitated acute mountain sickness!

Normal acclimatization will result in an increase in heart rate, respiratory rate and peripheral vascular resistance. This is the normal response to an increase in the hypoxic drive. The symptoms of AMS are thought to be the body's inflammatory response to hypoxia.

A few simple steps that can reduce the incidence of AMS include:

1. Slow ascent, sleeping the first night at <10,000 feet.
2. Increase fluid intake. Dehydration is a risk factor.
3. Eat light meals high in carbohydrates
4. Restrict activity; limit physical exertion.
5. Use acetazolamide (Diamox®) preventatively.[6]
6. Avoid alcohol consumption.
7. *Never* ascend any higher if experiencing signs and symptoms of AMS.

Acetazolamide is thought to work by slightly acidifying the blood, causing an increase in respiration. In travelers with the more severe forms of AMS, a lack of increase in respiration, normal to acclimatization, has been found.[7] Common side effects include, but are not limited to increased urination and parasthesias of fingers, toes and around the lips.

The recommended dose of acetazolamide (Diamox®) is 125 mg twice a day, starting the day before travel to insure tolerance. Another acceptable dosing method is 500 mg Diamox Sequels,® once a day. The advantages of this method include greater compliance and lower incidence of side effects. Individuals with allergy to sulfonamides should not use acetazolamide.

Another pharmaceutical that may be beneficial in the prevention or treatment of AMS is dexamethasone. While dexamethasone has been proven to reduce symptoms of AMS, it has not been proven to help with acclimatization.[8] The recommended dose is 4 mg orally every 6–12 hours.

The herbal preparation, Ginkgo biloba, may reduce the severity of AMS (33%). Recent studies have reported contrary findings, some showing efficacy and another showing no benefit. Its mechanism is not understood.[9] Ginkgo biloba has not been studied as a treatment for AMS and is not recommended. The preparation causes infrequent side effects, including headache and rare episodes of bleeding. The dosage is 80–120 mg orally twice a day, starting 3 days prior to ascent. At this time, there is not sufficient evidence to support its use.

Cocoa tea (Mate de Cocoa) is often touted as a prevention and possible treatment for AMS. Evidence for or against its use is non-existent and thus the authors can not make a recommendation.

Salmeterol, a long acting inhaled beta-2-sympathomimetic has also been suggested to have a beneficial effect in the prevention of AMS. There is also insufficient literature at this time to make any recommendations about its use.

Treatment of AMS

Most significant in the treatment of AMS is the **arrest of any further ascent**. Symptoms may be treated with:

1. Rest.
2. Increased fluids if tolerated.
3. 500 mg Diamox Sequels® once a day.
4. Prochlorperazine (Compazine®) 10 mg IM for nausea, vomiting or headache. Compazine® has the added benefit of slightly acidifying the blood helping to promote acclimatization.
5. Aspirin (325 mg every 4 hours) or ibuprofen may also be given for headache.

Initiation of the Lake Louise Questionnaire is critical. Complete and regular assessment will enable providers to determine if the affected traveler is improving or deteriorating. If a poor response is noted to treatment of symptoms or overall deterioration, strongly consider a descent in altitude. A descent of as little as 2,000 ft. can significantly improve symptoms.

HAPE and HACE:

Serious Forms of AMS

High altitude pulmonary edema (HAPE) and high altitude cerebral edema (HACE) constitute the two most serious aspects of AMS. While the onset of HAPE can be quite rapid, the onset of HACE is usually much slower and insidious. Both forms are considered medical emergencies requiring immediate intervention.

HAPE is the most common serious form of AMS that occurs in high altitude travelers. High pulmonary artery pressures contribute to the onset of HAPE, theorized to be the destruction of basement cell membranes, causing fluid leak at the capillary level.[10] This is a non-cardiogenic type of pulmonary edema.

Signs and symptoms of HAPE include:
1. Cough.
2. Breathlessness at rest.
3. Weakness with slight exertion.
4. Rapid heart rate and respiration.
5. Cyanosis.
6. Audible pulmonary crackles, in a least one lobe.
7. Desaturation of oxygen with slight exertion.
8. Other symptoms of AMS may or may not be seen.

HAPE is a life-threatening medical emergency. Treatment must be immediate. Do not delay. Treatment includes:
1. Immediate and mandatory descent.
2. Limit activity as much as possible during descent.
3. Supplemental oxygen 4–6 liters per minute via nasal cannula.
4. Nifedipine 20 mg extended release orally every 8–12 hours.
5. Avoid furosemide (Lasix®).
6. Use morphine with great caution.

7. Initiate 500 mg Diamox Sequel® PO.
8. Hyperbaric therapy if available.

High altitude cerebral edema onset may occur in 1–3 days following initial ascent to high altitude. The mechanism of HACE is theorized to be an inflammatory response to hypoxia.

Signs and symptoms of HACE include:
1. Altered level of consciousness.
2. Ataxia.
3. Severe malaise.
4. Worse at night.
5. Projectile vomiting.
6. Rapid progression from coma to death.

HACE is a life-threatening medical emergency requiring immediate intervention. Do not delay! Treatment includes:

1. Immediate and mandatory descent.
2. Supplemental oxygen 4–6 liters per minute via nasal cannula.
3. 500 mg Diamox Sequel® PO.
4. Dexamethasone 8 mg IM or IV.
5. Hyperbaric therapy if available.

While descent is mandatory and immediate for both HAPE and HACE, this implies the evacuation route is known and available. When traveling to high altitude your location and altitude must be known and your escape route planned before it may be utilized. Accurate altitudes are difficult to determine without a Global Positioning Satellite (GPS). This piece of equipment will become vital in an evacuation situation. Routes out of high altitude areas may also involve an initial increase in elevation. For example, many towns and cities in Peru lie within deep bowls of mountain peaks. Roads in and out must top the rim before descent may occur. The threshold for evacuation of a traveler suspected to have the severe forms of AMS must be very low. Remember a decrease in altitude of even 2,000 ft. can mean a significant difference in the symptoms of AMS.

A potential off-label use for the ever versatile medication Viagra® (sildenafil citrate) is treatment of travelers with high altitude pulmonary edema (HAPE). Viagra®

is currently in several clinical trials for the treatment of pulmonary hypertension (not related to high altitude). At the time of this publication the results are not yet published. For several years Viagra® has been touted among climbers as an effective treatment for HAPE. This treatment has not been studied and the current evidence is anecdotal, but intriguing.

Pearls

- All illness at altitude is AMS until proven otherwise.
- Know ascent history (how high, how fast).
- Never ascend higher with signs or symptoms AMS present.
- Once evacuation is planned-don't delay.
- Know your evacuation route!!!

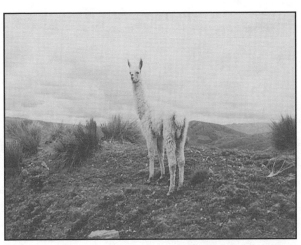

Cyndi Urbanowicz/
"Fully Acclimated"

References

1. High-altitude medicine.com
2. High-altitude medicine.com
3. Hultgren HN: *High Altitude Medicine*, Stanford, CA 1997, Hultgren Publications.
4. "The Lake Louise Consensus on the Definition and Quantification of Altitude Illness" in Sutton JR, Coates G, Houston CS (eds), Hypoxia and Mountain Medicine. Queen City Printers, Burlington, Vermont, 1992.
5. http://www.cdc.gov/travel/diseases/altitude.htm
6. High-altitude-medicine.com
7. Hultgren HN: *High Altitude Medicine*, Stanford, CA 1997, Hultgren Publications.
8. http://www.cdc.gov/travel/diseases/altitude.htm
9. High-altitude-medicine.com
10. Hultgren HN: *High Altitude Medicine*, Stanford, CA 1997, Hultgren Publications.

22 Travelers' Diarrhea

W. "Ted" Kuhn

Clinical Characteristics
Etiology
Host Factors
Acquired Immunity
Prevention
Prophylaxis
Treatment

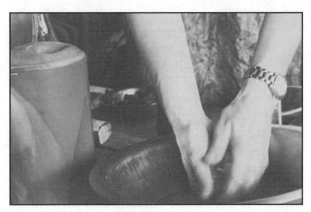

Ted Kuhn/
"Washing Hands in a Bowl"

Travelers' diarrhea (TD) is a substantial risk in the health and welfare of the traveler to the developing world. Although TD is the brunt of many jokes about travel in poor countries, the personal, economic, and health impact of TD is enormous. The exact incidence will vary from location to location, but between 20 to 90% of travelers from industrialized nations to poor nations can be expected to develop travelers' diarrhea during a one month stay. About one third of travelers with TD will be confined to bed and up to 40% will alter their itinerary due to the diarrhea. Very few travelers will need hospitalization, only 1%, but a significant number of days and resources can be wasted whether the traveler is on vacation, on business or involved in health care.

Travelers' diarrhea has been a substantial problem for the military with up to 57% of troops being affected during the first Persian Gulf conflict.[1] A similar incidence was reported in US troops deployed to Somalia. For the military, the implications are staggering, with over half the troops reporting diarrhea, a substantial percentage of troops may be unavailable for combat responsibilities when the need arises. Since the recent experience in Somalia and Persian Gulf, protocols have been implemented by the military that have dramatically decreased the incidence of diarrhea in troops.

Before strict food handling and consumption discipline was enforced on short term teams, our organization's experience was similar to the experience of the US military in Somalia and Persian Gulf. It was not unusual for teams to report an over 50% incidence of diarrhea. In a few cases, teams were unable to complete their mission and one team had to return to the US early secondary to diarrheal illness in a substantial number of team members.

When illness strikes a team, it must be remembered that not only is the person who is sick unavailable to perform duties, but another team member must be left behind to care for the ill teammate, thus making two team members unavailable for clinical responsibilities. This obviously compromises the mission of the team and is not good stewardship of human, financial, or spiritual resources.

Since enforcing safe food handling and consumption discipline on short term medi-

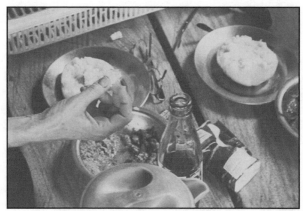

Ted Kuhn/
"Eating with Hands, West Africa"

cal teams in 1999, the incidence of travelers' diarrhea has dropped dramatically (see Chapter on "Food and Drink Safety"). Our organizational goal of 0% incidence has not yet been reached; nevertheless, diarrheal illness is distinctly uncommon on teams. Since enforcing TD precautions in 1999, even with the deployment of 40 teams with over 600 health care workers in 2005 alone, no medical team has missed a day of clinical responsibilities and no team has returned to the US early secondary to illness. The majority of medical teams now report no TD on 2 week deployments and when diarrhea does occur, it is of minor consequence affecting 1 or 2 individuals.

Prevention and early treatment have clearly been beneficial. There is a better way! Notwithstanding, this involves significant education, supervision, time and energy as well as personal and corporate discipline.

Clinical Characteristics

Definition

The classic definition of diarrhea is a stool that fits the shape of the container—in other words, a liquid stool. However, a better definition of TD would be "the passage of 3 or more loose stools in a 24 hour period associated with at least one of the following signs or symptoms: nausea, vomiting, abdominal cramping, fever, urgency, or the passage of blood or mucus in the stool[1]."

Diarrhea by Any Other Name

Not all diarrhea and abdominal discomfort in travelers is TD! Some diarrhea is caused by noninfectious etiologies, for example the implementation of a diet high in fiber in persons unused to fiber (rough milled rice or whole wheat breads), or a diet with unaccustomed spices (curry, hot peanut sauce, kimshi, picante, or "ahi") or the consumption of large amounts of fresh fruit. In some cultures, rice and beans (or lentils) are a staple, and abdominal bloating and gas are considered natural consequences. Eating 10 ripe mangoes a day, or green mango chutney will cause gastrointestinal symptoms, but this is to be expected and is not travelers' diarrhea. In South Asia there is a saying, "what goes in, comes out" and if one consumes yellow ripe mangoes or jack fruit, you can expect the passage of yellow, loose, mucoid stools.

Travelers may also develop diarrhea, cramping, and bloating when consuming milk products if they have a lactase deficiency syndrome (or have recently had diarrhea from rotavirus or *Giardia*). Water from the inside of green coconuts is often offered to those with diarrhea to replenish fluid and electrolytes. While the "coconut water" is sterile and very high in potassium, it has a high solute content and will cause an osmotic diarrhea if consumed in any significant quantity (e.g. more than just a few ounces). Better oral rehydration alternatives should be considered. We are reminded that malaria may present with diarrhea, especially in children, and mistaking *falciparum* malaria for TD may prove to be a fatal mistake[2].

Signs and Symptoms

Various studies report that the clinical course of TD varies according to geographic location and local differences in microbiologic spectrum.[2] Most often, the diarrhea begins abruptly, often on the 4–7th day of travel outside the US. There are usually 3–4 stools per day, but there may be up to 20 stools per 24 hour period. The stool is mostly watery. Blood or mucous, unusual in TD, should be considered a sign of a bacterial or parasitic etiology. There may be sufficient urgency that fecal incontinence may occur.

Vomiting is a common accompanying symptom and often occurs at the onset of the disease. Vomiting can be debilitating and lead to dehydration and electrolyte imbalance if not treated. Low grade fever lasting 2–3 days is common and high grade fever, although reported, more commonly is associated with a bacterial etiology.

The majority of TD is self-limited and uncomplicated lasting 1–2 days. Untreated, the mean duration of diarrhea is 3–5 days. Treatment substantially decreases symptoms and duration. Almost one-third of patients with TD are bedridden for 1–2 days and 40% will change their itinerary.

Complications

Complications are unusual except in those who are immunocompromised or those with chronic medical problems, especially those with diabetes, cardiac, or renal insufficiency, or those with HIV. Vomiting and diarrhea may lead to dehydration and electrolyte imbalance, and vomiting may preclude the taking of normal medications for blood pressure, diabetes or heart conditions. Oral rehydration is generally accepted as standard, but in cases where the illness is complicated by a chronic medical condition or inability to replace fluids orally, intravenous administration of fluids and medications may be prudent.

Etiology

Generally, recolonization of the bowel with "indigenous" and or "resistant" *E. coli* takes place within 3–4 days of arrival in the developing world. Although only about 60% of the time are pathogenic organisms cultured from the stool, one consistency remains, enterotoxigenic *E. coli* (ETEC) is the most commonly isolated organism responsible for TD. There is remarkable similarity in the incidence and epidemiology of ETEC in Latin America, Africa, and South Asia with a nearly 53% attack rate

among travelers. In one study, 39% of restaurant food in Mexico cultured positive for *E. coli*, and 55% of street vendor food was positive for *E. coli* and 40% of the food sold in small grocery stores was contaminated with *E. coli*. ETEC is less common in SE Asia and *Campylobacter* is one of the most common pathogens in Thailand. (*Campylobacter* in SE Asia may also be fluoroquinolone resistant).

The fact that travelers usually respond to antibiotic administration, even when a bacterial pathogen is not isolated, suggests a bacterial etiology in most undiagnosed cases of TD. Other causes of TD include *Salmonella*, *Shigella*, *Campylobacter*, and other groups of *E. coli* (EIEC, EHEC, EAEC, EPEC). These occur to a much lesser extent and more often present with bloody diarrhea or fecal leukocytes. Norovirus and rotavirus have been frequently reported as causes of large outbreaks of diarrheal illness, and the protozoan *Giardia* is also implicated. The organism *Cryptosporidium* may cause diarrheal illness in travelers and may be resistant to chlorination (but not chlorine dioxide) of water. *Cryptosporidium* should be considered in persistent diarrhea in the returned traveler who is "culture negative."

A substantial bacillary load is necessary for ETEC to induce diarrhea. Dupont demonstrated that 106 organisms were required to induce diarrhea in comparison with the relatively few organisms needed for *Shigella* (3–30) and rotavirus (3–10). "This demonstrates the marked breakdown in sanitation, as often happens in the developing world, for such high bacterial loads to be ingested.[3]"

Because substantial bacterial loads are necessary for illness to occur, simple preventive measures which may decrease the number of bacteria ingested are likely to prove invaluable. Measures such as handwashing with "clean water" or disinfecting hands with isopropyl alcohol gel prior to eating, halogenating drinking water, and eating food cooked above 158°F may substantially decrease the bacterial load consumed and thus prevent infection.

Host Factors

Travelers from "western" countries comprise the majority of those who suffer from TD and those from "northern" countries (US, UK, Europe, Canada etc.) have a higher incidence than those from "southern" countries (Central and South America). Travelers from developing nations have an incidence of diarrhea similar to that found in the host population. Increasing age is protective and the highest incidence of TD is in younger travelers. Younger travelers may have less immunity and they may have more adventurous eating habits and eat larger quantities of food (larger bacillary load). Diarrhea attack rates for children is generally as high as that in the highest risk group, young adults in the 20–29 age group).

Acquired Immunity

Protective immunity does develop after natural infection with ETEC. Importantly, there is a substantially decreased rate of attack with increasing length of stay in the host country and with increasing age. This protective immunity is demonstrated over time and may last for years after immunity develops. Since strains of ETEC vary antigenically, having traveled to another developing country and having been colonized with another ETEC strain may not provide cross immunity.

The importance of protective immunity can not be over stressed in relation to short term visitors. Those who host short term visitors and are long term occupants of the host country (and perhaps even of middle age) are likely to have developed immunity to the local *E. coli* strain. Thus they are protected from diarrhea when exposed to the bacteria.

Short term visitors, many of whom may be in the highest risk age for diarrhea (children and those ages 20–29) develop illness when exposed to the same foods normally consumed by the long term occupant. I frequently hear advice similar to this given to visitors from long term residents on the field, "This is safe to eat. I eat it all the time and I never get sick." While this is true for the middle-aged long term occupant of that country, it is true secondary to the immunity that has developed over time, not because of lack of bacterial contamination.

Equally true is that the short term visitor who has no native immunity to the host country's ETEC strain, will undoubtedly develop diarrhea after consuming the same bacterial load. While the long term occupant remains healthy, the short term visitor pays the price for the next 2 days in bed with fever, vomiting, abdominal cramping, and diarrhea for this dietary indiscretion.

Prevention

There is currently much debate about the primary prevention of TD and the usefulness of food and drink restrictions. Some feel that TD is just "part of the experience", and if you are going to get sick anyway, you might as well enjoy yourself in the meantime. One study cited less than 2% total compliance with food and drink restrictions in Swiss travelers to Thailand on a month long vacation. Most of the Swiss ate the forbidden fruit and drank potentially contaminated beverages, and if the Swiss are unable to be compliant- who can? Certainly some eating habits are highly associated with diarrhea, for example, blended fruit drinks, fruit salad, raw vegetables, ice and eating from street vendors.

There is also an association between TD and eating in restaurants- something we all do when we travel. The more flies- the greater the risk of diarrheal illness. "All inclusive" packages with prepaid food at resorts in the developing world place one at higher risk than those who choose their own meals. There seems to be a protective effect when one can choose his/her own food or prepare the food himself.[3]

One study showed no benefit in the incidence of TD between those who had been instructed in proper food and drink safety, and those who had not received this instruction. If eating in restaurants is a risk factor, and if there is little difference in risk between expensive resort (four star) dining and dining in roadside cafés,[3] then perhaps we are all doomed to spend part of our travel experience in the squat latrine.

This study notwithstanding, extensive field experience by the US military and others have demonstrated results to the contrary.

The US military in Somalia decreased the incidence of diarrhea from a 50–60% attack rate to only 4.5% over an 8 week period by strictly controlling food, monitoring water supplies and controlling fly vectors and improving field sanitation facilities, proving that prevention can and does prevent diarrhea when aggressively applied. Our own experience with medical teams also demonstrates that aggressive control of food and water makes a significant difference

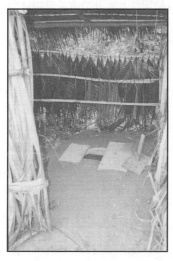

Ted Kuhn/
"Local Latrine"

in diarrheal attack rates. Our unpublished experience demonstrates results similar to the US military experience in Somalia with an attack rate of less than 4% among medical professionals on short term work assignments in the developing world.

What Works?

Perhaps most important is maintaining control over your own food and water supply. If you are able to cook and prepare your own food and the food for your team, then you can assure proper sanitary preparation of meals by applying simple safe food handling practices. In restaurants, it is preferable for one person to order the same (or similar) food for all. This not only makes ordering simple, but if food is ordered by one experienced and knowledgeable person, he/she can assure that the food is cooked well and served without raw vegetables,

salads and fruit (by simply not ordering those items).

Carbonated and hot beverages are safe and generally appreciated by team members, thus simplifying the drink order. This is what we term "active" rather than "passive" food restriction. "Passive" food restrictions involve educating people concerning what to eat and what not to eat and then relying on them to be vigilant and compliant. This probably does not work or works poorly at best.

Studies prove that it is difficult for people to remember, and compliance is a problem when eating exotic foods is considered part of the cultural experience. "Active" food restriction means that you don't serve anyone anything that they can not eat. In other words, you have maintained control over your food and water supply and everything that is served is safe. This makes mealtimes much more agreeable and takes the risk and temptation away from eating unsafe foods. As the military proved in Somalia, it works!

So what is "safe" to eat? Following a few simple rules makes all the difference. A few "do's" and "don'ts" are listed below. (Also see

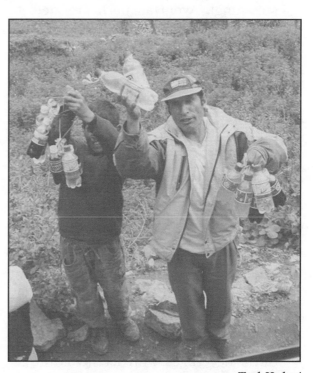

Ted Kuhn/
"Selling "Recycled" Bottled Water, South America."

chapter in this text *Food and Drink Safety* for more information)

1. Always wash your hands before preparing or consuming food (and between patients). Consider water that comes from a pipe or tube "unsafe" or contaminated. Use "safe" water for washing hands and use your own soap and your own towel if possible. If these are unavailable, use an alcohol based hand sanitizer instead of washing in potentially contaminated water with dirty soap and drying your hands on a towel laden with pathogenic bacteria.

2. If possible, use eating utensils that you have cleaned yourself (in "safe" water) or that are disposable. In a restaurant, you can ask for boiling water and soak your utensils in the water before eating. In wilderness areas, keep your utensils in a plastic container (Tupperware®) with a mixture of clean water and iodine. They will be free of bacteria by the next meal.

3. Eat only meat that has been thoroughly cooked and food that is served hot (greater than 158°F- hot to taste or steaming). Avoid all pork products to prevent trichinosis. Also, avoid eating raw fruits or raw vegetables unless the fruit is thick-skinned and you peel it yourself, e.g. bananas. Lettuce is never considered safe (even on hamburgers at McDonald's in other countries)—there are too many ridges to hide bacteria and parasites and it can not be safely cleaned.

4. Bottled water is a potential risk. (A recent study demonstrated *E. coli* contamination in 11 of 14 selected samples of bottled water in Nepal in 8 different brands[5]). Be sure the top is sealed. If uncertain of the brand, halogenate your bottled water before consuming. Boiled water and carbonated drinks in cans or bottles are safe. Be sure to clean off the tops of drink cans and bottles. Don't drink beverages with ice, avoid street vendors, and do not consume dairy products unless you know they have been pasteurized. Avoid shellfish and raw or undercooked seafood (Ceviché) even if it is "pickled".

Prophylaxis

Treatment for travelers' diarrhea has become so effective that drug prophylaxis is no longer recommended except for the immunocompromised traveler.

If you do decide to use prophylaxis, Bismuth subsalicylate (Pepto-Bismol®) has been shown to offer reasonable protection and safety. Taking 1 ounce or 2 tablets of Pepto-Bismol® 4 times daily has been shown to be effective against travelers' diarrhea but should not be taken for longer than 3 weeks. Do not use if allergic to aspirin or in children.

Several antibiotics have been shown to prevent travelers' diarrhea. Doxycycline (200 mg taken on the day before exposure, then 100 mg/day) can provide 81–86% protection. Other antibiotics shown to be effective are ciprofloxacin (Cipro®) 500 mg daily and trimethoprim-sulfamethoxazole (Septra®)160/800 mg daily.

Treatment

Oral rehydration is the cornerstone in the initial treatment of travelers' diarrhea, especially in infants, young children, and the elderly. It is a mistake to underestimate fluid losses, especially in hot environments, and fail to drink enough fluids. Canned fruit juices, sport drinks (e.g. Gatorade®), and decaffeinated sodas can be used. Oral rehydration solutions (ORS) are also excellent for fluid replacement. ORS can be purchased in commercially prepared packets, such as the World Health Organization (WHO) rehydration formula. Rehydration solutions may also be self-prepared.

Recipes
Quick ORS formula #1:
- Mix 1 teaspoon of salt and 2–3 tablespoons of sugar or honey to 1 liter of pure water.

Quick ORS formula #2
- Mix one 8-oz cup of fruit juice with 3 cups of water and 1 teaspoon of salt.

Quick ORS formula #3
- Mix 1/2 teaspoon salt, 1/4 teaspoon salt substitute (KCl), 1/2 teaspoon baking soda, and 2–3 tablespoons sugar, honey, or karo syrup to 1 liter of water.

There has been a recent controversy in the literature over the ideal composition of oral rehydration solution (ORS) and which is best in moderate and severe diarrhea. Reduced-osmolarity ORS seems to reduce the need for IV fluid administration in moderate to severe disease, but may lead to a slightly greater degree of hyponatremia.[6] Whatever the case, it would seem best to advocate a standard composition of ORS worldwide.

Table 1.
Composition of Standard and Reduced-Osmolarity WHO ORS[7]

	Standard WHO (1975)	Reduced-Osmolarity WHO (2002)
Glucose, mmol/L	111	75
Sodium, mEq/L	90	75
Potassium mEq/L	20	20
Chloride mEq/L	80	65
Citrate mmol/L	10	10
Osmolarity, mOms/L	311	245

Treatment of travelers' diarrhea may also include (bismuth subsalicylate) Pepto-Bismol,® loperamide (Imodium®), and antibiotics. If symptoms are mild, start with Pepto-Bismol.® Pepto-Bismol® is taken 1 ounce (or 2 tablets) every hour for up to 8 hours. Stop when diarrhea abates or when the total 8 ounces have been taken. If symptoms are more severe, start with an antibiotic. In Latin America, South Asia and Africa, consider ciprofloxin (Cipro®) 500 mg twice daily for 1–3 days, or TMP-SMX 160/800 (Septra®) twice daily for 3 days, or doxycycline 100 mg twice daily for 3 days, and one dose of loperamide (Imodium®) with the first dose of antibiotic. Quinolones are currently the drugs of choice for travelers' diarrhea for those over the age of 18 years.[4] They are effective against most of the causes of travelers' diarrhea except the resistant strains of *Campylobacter* in SE Asia. They may be used in younger individuals in areas of the world where resistance to the other antibiotics is significant. Azithromycin (Zithromax®) is the drug of choice in SE Asia for the antibiotic treatment of TD because of antibiotic resistance patterns to fluoroquinolones. Avoid antacids, Pepto-Bismol®, and vitamins containing iron or zinc when taking antibiotics because they may interfere with antibiotic absorption, especially the quinolones.

References
1. Peltola H, Gorbach S: Travlers' Diarrhea: Epidemiology and Clinical Aspects, *Textbook of Travel Medicine and Health*, edited by HL DuPont, R. Steffen, 2nd edition, Decker, Ontario 2001.
2. Löscher T, Connor B: Clinical Presentation and Treatment of Travelers' Diarrhea, *Travel Medicine*, edited JS Keystone, PE Kozarsky, DO Freedman, HD Nothdurft, BA Connor, Mosby 2004.
3. Brewster SJ, Taylor DN: Epidemiology of Travelers' Diarrhea, *Travel Medicine*, edited JS Keystone, PE Kozarsky, DO Freedman, HD Nothdurft, BA Connor, Mosby 2004.
4. Travelers' Diarrhea in the New Millennium: Consensus among Experts from German-speaking Countries, Steffen R, Kollaritsch H, Fleisher K, *J Travel Medicine* 2003;10: 38–45.
5. Personal communication with author from D. Shlim, August, 2003.
6. Nalin DR, et al: Clinical Concerns about Reduced-Osmolarity Oral Rehydration Solution, *JAMA*, June 2, 2004, 29(21):2632–2635.
7. Duggan C, et al: Scientific Rationale for a change in the Composition of Oral Rehydration Solution, *JAMA*, June 2, 2004, 29(21):2628–2631.

23 Malaria

Hartmut Gross and James Wilde

Anyone who plans a trip to a "Developing World" country, particularly to the tropics, should be aware of the risk of malaria. Malaria remains a major source of morbidity and mortality throughout the world, with 3 million deaths and 300 million new infections each year. It has been called the #1 life threatening infectious disease for travelers. People at particular risk for severe acute disease are young children and expatriate visitors to a malaria endemic area who experience infection for the first time. Older children and adults who are native to these endemic areas, and who are likely to have survived at least one bout of malaria previously, are at lower risk for severe disease due to a "semi-immune" state that results after the initial infection. True immunity is not produced even after repeated infections, a fact that complicates the search for a reliable vaccine.

Four Types of Human Malaria

While there are four forms of *Plasmodium* that produce malaria in humans, three are similar enough clinically that it is more practical to categorize acute disease as that due to *P. falciparum* vs. that due to the other *Plasmodia*. The other *Plasmodia* are *P. vivax*, *P. ovale*, and *P. malariae*. Although invasion of liver cells is an important component of infection from all *Plasmodia* species, *P. falciparum* and *P. malariae* produce no dormant liver stage and thus do not cause late relapse. In contrast, disease due to *P. vivax* and *P. ovale* includes a dormant liver stage that can lead to relapse 2–11 months or more after the initial infection. While parasitemia due to *P. ovale* and *P. vivax* is usually limited to young red cells (reticulocytes), and *P. malariae* tends to invade only mature cells, *P. falciparum* invades red cells of all ages. Thus, *P. falciparum* affects a far greater percentage of circulating red cells and causes a much more severe illness. *P. falciparum* is also the only human malaria parasite that produces microvascular disease, due to the adherence of *P. falciparum* parasitized red cells to the endothelial cells of capillaries of major organ systems. This can lead to particularly severe effects in the brain, kidneys, and lungs. Finally, drug resistance is substantially more common in *P. falciparum*. Because of these characteristics, disease due to *P. falciparum* tends to be much more severe than the other malaria infections and poses the greatest risk for death, particularly in the non-immune patient.

Malaria Life Cycle

In their development, *Plasmodium* are dependent upon both human and mosquito hosts to complete the life cycle. In each stage of the cycle, the organism has a different descriptive name. As there are many stages, the cycle quickly becomes a bewildering array of strange names which confuse many readers. For simplicity, the stage names have been italicized in the description which follows. The lay reader may find it easier to skip over the names and simply consider it just another step in the maturation of the organism.

Malaria is acquired after a bite from an infected anopheline mosquito. Plasmodium *sporozoites* in the salivary glands of the mosquito are injected into the human host at the time of the bite. The *sporozoites* briefly travel in the blood stream to the liver, where they invade the hepatocytes (liver cells) and multiply. Maturation to the *tissue schizont* form leads to rupture of infected hepatocytes and the release of *merozoites*, which then invade red cells. In the red cells, the parasite matures to *ring*, *trophozoite*, and finally *schizont* stages. Upon completion of the *schizont* phase of maturation, the red cell is lysed, releasing 24–32 additional *merozoites* that are then able to infect other red cells. This sequence of events in the erythrocytes constitutes the asexual reproductive cycle, and generally occurs in 48 or 72-hour intervals. In addition, differentiation of some intraerythrocytic parasites into *male and female gametocytes* also occurs. Another mosquito during a blood meal can then ingest these *gametocytes*. The *gametocytes* complete the sexual reproduction cycle in the new mosquito host, culminating in the production of *sporozoites* and continued transmission of the disease. In the absence of anopheline mosquitoes, this sexual reproductive sequence is interrupted and further spread of the disease is halted. Because hepatocyte invasion requires *sporozoites*, which come only from the bite of an infected mosquito, infection due to transfusion of infected blood results only in invasion of erythrocytes. Relapses therefore do not occur in this type of infection.

Clinical Presentation of Malaria

The familiar clinical manifestations of malaria include cyclical fevers, which coincide with the rupture of erythrocytes. This cycle occurs every 48 hours with *P. ovale* and *P. vivax*, and every 72 hours with *P. falciparum*. However, the fever tends to be more continuous in *P. falciparum* infections, with intermittent temperature "spikes." The malaria paroxysm is quite distinct. The first stage consists of severe shaking chills that may last up to several hours. In the second phase, high fever becomes prominent, and may last for several hours. Additional clinical features of this stage include headache, backache, abdominal pain, vomiting, and an altered level of consciousness. The third stage begins 2–6 hours later and is notable for the extreme diaphoresis and fatigue with resolution of fever.

The severe complications of acute malaria are due primarily to the microvascular disease typical of *P. falciparum* infections. One of the most common and devastating of these complications is cerebral malaria, which occurs in large numbers of children and other non-immune patients. Manifestations of cerebral malaria can range from subtle confusion to deep coma. Renal failure is also common, with large amounts of hemoglobin and malarial pigments in the urine leading to the clinical syndrome of "blackwater fever." Pulmonary edema is a particularly ominous development due to its high mortality rate, but this is much less common than CNS or renal involvement.

Malaria Prevention

Proper management of malaria consists of two therapeutic arms: chemoprophylaxis for prevention of disease, and chemotherapy of acute disease. Both require some knowledge of resistance patterns which have emerged around the world. Excellent prophylaxis in one country may leave one completely vulnerable in another, so the correct drug must be taken properly to provide maximal protection. In fact, resistance to chloroquine has become widespread among many isolates of *P. falciparum*. Chloroquine resistance can be assumed in all areas of the world that are endemic for malaria except Mexico, Central America, parts of the Caribbean, and in the Middle Eastern countries. Dosing and duration of the medications take into account where the medication affects the organism in its lifecycle. No currently available antimalarial drug acts on the sporozoite stage. This is part of the reason most of the medications must be continued for four weeks after departing from the malaria endemic area. Additionally, convenience and cost may be taken into account. For example, an inexpensive drug such as doxycycline must be taken daily during the trip plus an additional month. Other medications like chloroquine and mefloquine are more expensive but require only weekly administration.

In areas with chloroquine sensitive malaria, weekly chloroquine remains the drug of choice for prophylaxis. Chloroquine phosphate (brand name Aralen®) 500 mg (300 mg base) PO is given weekly beginning 1–2 weeks prior to departure and continuing for 4 weeks after return for adults. Hydroxychloroquine sulfate (brand name Plaquenil®) is an alternative to chloroquine and is sometimes better tolerated. In chloroquine-resistant areas, weekly mefloquine (brand name Lariam®) has emerged as the drug of choice with daily doxycycline 100 mg a suitable alternative. Mefloquine is dosed 250 mg PO weekly beginning 1–2 weeks prior to departure and continuing until 4 weeks after return from the malarious area. Recent studies indicate that mefloquine is safe during pregnancy and in children. Mefloquine can cause neuro-psychological side effects such as insomnia, nightmares, depression, and irritability in up to 0.5% of subjects. Frank psychosis or seizures can develop in 1 in 10,000 people during mefloquine prophylaxis, and in up to 1 in 100 when mefloquine is used to treat active disease. Until further studies are forth coming mefloquine should not be used in individuals with a history of seizures or psychiatric disorders, or with significant cardiac conduction abnormalities.

Chloroquine can infrequently cause minor adverse reactions such as dizziness, nausea, vomiting, abdominal pain, and headache. Doxycycline causes photosensitivity reactions in many people, and large numbers of women develop candidal vaginitis while taking the drug. Upset stomach and esophagitis are also common complaints because of its low pH of 2. The requirement for daily dosing makes compliance with doxycycline regimens lower. Doxycycline also should not be used in pregnant females or in children under age 8 due to possible irreversible staining of teeth. Prophylaxis with most of the antimalarial medications should be started one to two weeks prior to departure to allow time to change to a different drug should side effects occur.

Malarone®, a combination of atovaquone and proguanil, appears to be as safe and effective as mefloquine and has been licensed in the U.S. for a few years. It is typically started a day or two before entry into the malaria endemic area, taken daily while there and continued for only 7 days upon leaving the area. While convenient for short trips without the bother of trying to remember to take medication for a month after returning, it is quite expensive. It is contraindicated in pregnancy, nursing women, and in children weighing under 11 kg.

Other antimalarials in use include proguanil (alone), which is not licensed for use in the United States and is not as effective as either mefloquine or doxycycline, and primaquine, which is generally reserved for post-exposure prevention of "relapsing" malaria. Azithromycin is safe in children and in pregnant females but is not as effective as mefloquine and is very expensive. In other countries, artemesin drugs are used both for prophylaxis and treatment; however, these drugs, in spite of high safety profiles, are not yet approved for use in the US. Their short duration of action makes them ineffective when used alone, but they are very effective when used in combination with other antimalarial drugs.

Malaria Treatment

Proper treatment of acute malaria requires identification of the causative organism. This is usually accomplished through the microscopic examination of thick and thin blood smears on a glass slide. (Figure at the end of this chapter is a thin smear.) For disease due to *P. vivax, P. ovale, P. malariae* and chloroquine sensitive *P. falciparum,* a three-day regimen of oral chloroquine is recommended. None of the alternative medications offer any greater efficacy. In addition, a minimum of two weeks of primaquine is required in *P. vivax* and *P. ovale* infections in order to prevent late relapses. The dose of primaquine is 15 mg daily for two weeks if the *P. vivax* is from a temperate region. A higher dose (up to 30 mg/day for 14 days) is required to treat *P. vivax* acquired from tropical or subtropical countries. Primaquine should generally not be given to individuals with glucose-6-phosphate dehydrogenase deficiency. In more severe cases, judicious use of IV fluids, transfusions, and diuretics may be required.

Several oral medications are available for the treatment of chloroquine-resistant *P. falciparum* infections, including quinine, quinidine, mefloquine, pyrimethamine-sulfadoxine (Fansidar®), and halofantrine. The drug selected for acute disease should not be the same as that chosen for prophylaxis. Halofantrine should not be used if mefloquine resistance is suspected since resistance patterns tend to be similar. Additionally, halofantrine is not a first line drug in any country because of its adverse reaction profile. In addition, pyrimethamine-sulfadoxine should be used with caution given high rates of resistance to this agent among chloroquine-resistant organisms.

Parenteral antimalarials include quinine quinidine, and artemether. There have been no reports of resistance to quinine or quinidine among *P. falciparum* strains. Combinations of at least two of the above listed medications provide the best cure rates. Side effects may be common.

Personal protection measures are an important additional means to prevent malaria. Anopheline mosquitoes are generally active from dusk to dawn, so simply staying indoors during evening and night hours can significantly decrease the risk of acquiring the disease. Other measures include the use of insect repellants containing up to 30% DEET, permethrin-impregnated bed nets, and dressing in long sleeved shirts and trousers.

Travelers should become well acquainted with the risk of malaria and local resistance patterns before traveling to a malaria endemic area. Health information for travelers is provided through the CDC and WHO in various publications. Information can also be obtained through the Internet at www.cdc.gov and www.who.ch. The traveler should also remember that no method of malaria prophylaxis is 100% effective; yet the number one reason for failure remains noncompliance. If a non-immune traveler develops symptoms of acute malaria, medical assistance should be sought immediately. As malaria is an extremely uncommon illness in the US, and the delayed diagnosis carries a high risk of morbidity and mortality, the concerned traveler should bring to the clinician's attention the fact that malaria is a possible diagnosis. Additionally, it would be prudent to obtain consultation with a physician trained in travel medicine or tropical medicine. A list of clinics and physicians who practice travel medicine can be found in the American Society of Tropical Medicine and Hygiene website at www.astmh.org.

Drugs Recommended for Malaria Prophylaxis

Medication	Usage Regimen	Adult Dose	Pediatric Dose	Comments
Atovaquone/proguanil (Malarone®)	Begin 1–2 days before entering endemic area and throughout stay. Take for 7 additional days after leaving endemic area.	250 mg atovaquone and 100 mg proguanil HCL 1 adult tablet PO, QD	62.5 mg atovaquone and 25 mg proguanil HCL 11–20 kg: 1 tablet 21–30 kg: 2 tablets 31–40 kg: 3 tablets >40 kg: 1 adult tab every day	Primary prophylaxis in areas with chloroquine-resistant or mefloquine-resistant *P. falciparum*. Contraindicated in persons with severe renal impairment (creatinine clearance <30 mL/min). Atovaquone/proguanil should be taken with food or a milky drink. Not recommended for child <11kg; pregnant women; and women breastfeeding infants <11 kg.
Chloroquine phosphate (Aralen® and generic)	Begin one week prior to entering endemic area and continue weekly dose during stay. Take 4 additional weekly doses after leaving area.	300 mg base (500 mg salt) orally, once/week	5 mg/kg base (8.3 mg/kg salt) orally, once/week, up to maximum adult dose of 300 mg base	Primary prophylaxis only in areas with chloroquine-sensitive *Plasmodium falciparum*. May exacerbate psoriasis.
Doxycycline (Many brand names and generic)	Begin 1–2 days before entering endemic area and throughout stay. Take for 30 additional days after leaving endemic area.	100 mg orally, daily	8 years of age or older: 2 mg/kg up to adult dose of 100 mg/day	Primary prophylaxis in areas with chloroquine-resistant or mefloquine-resistant *P. falciparum*. Contraindicated in children <8 years of age and pregnant women.
Hydroxychloroquine sulfate (Plaquenil®)	Begin one week prior to entering endemic area and continue weekly dose during stay. Take 4 add'l weekly doses after leaving endemic area.	310 mg base (400 mg salt) orally, once/week	5 mg/kg base (6.5 mg/kg salt) orally, once/week up to maximum adult dose of 310 mg base	An alternative to chloroquine for primary prophylaxis only in areas with chloroquinie-sensitive *Plasmodium falciparum*. Generally better tolerated than chloroquine. May exacerbate psoriasis.

Table adapted from CDC Travelers' Health website, 2006 (reference 2) and References 4 and 9.

Drugs Recommended for Malaria Prophylaxis (cont.)

Medication	Usage Regimen	Adult Dose	Pediatric Dose	Comments
Mefloquine (Lariam® and generic)	Begin one week prior to entering endemic area and continue weekly dose during stay. Take 4 add'l weekly doses after leaving endemic area.	228 mg base (250 mg salt) orally, once/week	≤9 kg and under: 4.6 mg/kg base (5 mg/kg salt) orally, once/week 10–19 kg: ¼ tab 1/wk 20–30 kg: ¼ tab 1/wk 31–45 kg: ¾ tab 1/wk >45 kg: 1 tab 1/wk	Primary prophylaxis in areas with chloroquine-resistant *P. falciparum*. Contraindicated in persons allergic to mefloquine and in persons with active depression, a recent history of depression, generalized anxiety disorder, psychosis, schizophrenia, other major psychiatric disorderes, or seizures. Not recommended for persons with cardiac conduction abnormalities.
Primaquine	Not generally recommended for primary prophylaxis.	15–30 mg base (52.6 mg salt) orally, once/day for 7 days after departure from the malaria endemic area. Lower dose for *P. vivax* in temperate zones. Higher dose in tropical or subtropical zones (Chesson strain).	0.5 mg/kg base (0.8 mg/kg salt) up to adult dose orally, once/day for 7 days after departure from the malarious area.	Used for terminal prophylaxis to decrease the risk of relapses of *P. vivax* and *P. ovale*. Indicated for persons who have had prolonged exposure to *P. vivax* and *P. ovale* or both. Contraindicated in persons with G6PD* deficiency. Also contraindicated during pregnancy and lactation unless infant being breast-fed has a documented normal G6PD level.

Drugs Recommended for Malaria Treatment

Medication	Usage Regimen	Adult Dose	Pediatric Dose	Comments
Chloroquine phosphate (Aralen® and generic)	Dose is given daily as described.	600 mg base (1000 mg salt) orally on day one and two. Then 300 mg on day 3	10 mg/kg base (16.6 mg/kg salt) orally, up to maximum adult dose of 600 mg base. Follow with 5 mg/kg at 6, 24, and 48 hours.	Use only in areas with chloroquine-sensitive *P. falciparum*. May exacerbate psoriasis.
Mefloquine (Lariam® and generic)	Dose is given at one time or divided over one day.	228 mg base (250 mg salt) tablet. Take 3 tablets at one time and 2 more tablets 6–12 hours later	15 mg/kg as single dose followed by 10 mg/kg 6–12 hours later. Max dose is 1250 mg.	The higher dose recommended in certain areas of Thailand border. Contraindicated in persons allergic to mefloquine and in persons with active depression, a recent history of depression, generalized anxiety disorder, psychosis, schizophrenia, other major psychiatric disorders, or seizures. Not recommended for persons with cardiac conduction abnormalities.
Quinine	TID dosing required.	300 mg (salt) tablets. Take 2 tablets (650 mg) TID x 3–7 days.	Quinine sulfate 30 mg/kg/day divided three times daily.	Should be used with doxycycline, tetracycline, or clindamycin.
Atovaquone/proguanil (Malarone®)		250 mg atovaquone and 100 mg proguanil HCL (adult tablet) 4 adult tablets daily for 3 days	Children are treated using adult (250/100) or pediatric (62.5/25) tablets. Dose is given daily for 3 days. 5–8 kg: 2 peds tablets 9–10 kg: 3 peds tablets 11–20 kg: 1 adult tablet 21–30 kg: 2 adult tablets 31–40 kg: 3 adult tablets >40 kg: 4 adult tablets	

Drugs Recommended for Malaria Treatment (cont.)

Medication	Usage Regimen	Adult Dose	Pediatric Dose	Comments
Pyrimethamine-sulfadoxine (Fansidar®)	Dose is given all at one time.	500/25 mg tablets. Take 3 tablets as single dose.	500/25 mg tablets 5–10 kg: ½ tablet 11–20 kg: 1 tablet 21–30 kg: 1½ tablets 31–40 kg: 2 tablets >40 kg: 3 tablets Give dose at one time.	Caution: high rates of resistance.
Primaquine	Not generally recommended for primary prophylaxis.	15–30 mg base (52.6 mg salt) orally, once/day x 14 days. Lower dose for *P. vivax* in temperate zones. Higher dose in tropical or subtropical zones. (Chesson strain)	0.5 mg/kg base (1.0 mg/kg salt) once/day x 14 days up to adult dose.	Used for terminal prophylaxis to decrease the risk of relapses of *P. vivax* and *P. ovale*. Higher dose contraindicated in persons with G6PD* deficiency. Low dose probably tolerated. Use with caution. Also contraindicated during pregnancy and lactation unless the infant being breast-fed has a documented normal G6PD level.
Artemether/Lumefantrine (Riamet®)	Not available in US.	20/120 mg 4 tablets on day 1, followed by 4 tablets at 8 hours, then 4 tablets twice daily on days 2 and 3.	10–14 kg q dose = 1 tab 15–24 kg q dose = 2 tabs 25–34 kg q dose = 3 tabs Total of 6 doses will be given—see comments.	Two doses are given 8 hours apart on day 1. Then 2 doses are given 12 hours apart on days 2 and 3.
Doxycycline	Given with quinine	100 mg PO Bid x 7 days	4 mg/kg/day PO divided Bid x 7 days old	Not indicated in children <8 years old
Tetracycline	Given with quinine	250 mg PO Qid x 7 days	25 mg/kg/day PO divided Qid x 7 days	Not indicated in children <8 years old
Clindamycin	Given with quinine	20 mg base/kg/day PO divided Tid x 7 days	20 mg base kg/day PO divided Tid x 7 days	

Clinically suspected or diagnosed uncomplicated malaria	Possible treatment choices				
P. falciparum	A. Chloroquine (in areas where there is no chloroquine resistance)				
	B. Quinine	plus	Doxycycline or Tetracycline or Clindamycin		
	C. Atovaquone-proguanil				
	D. Mefloquine				
P. malariae	Chloroquine				
P. vivax	A. Chloroquine	plus	Primaquine		
	B. Quinine	plus	Primaquine	plus	Doxycycline or Tetracycline
	C. Mefloquine	plus	Primaquine		
P. ovale	Chloroquine	plus	Primaquine		

CDC Malaria Hotline: 770-488-7788 M–F 8am–4pm EST
770-488-7100 after hours

References

1. Gilles HM, Warrel DA, *Essential Malariology,* 3rd ed., Arnold, London, 1993.
2. http://www.cdc.gov/travel/diseases/malaria/index.htm
3. http://www.who.int/health_topics/malaria/en/
4. *Malaria* (several chapters by various authors): Travel Medicine, edited by Keystone JS, et al, Mosby, Edinburgh, 2004, pp 131–174.
5. Keystone JS: *Malaria Chemoprophylaxis in the New Millenium,* Educational Teleconference by University of Texas, Health Science Center at San Antonio, and CPE Communications, 1999.
6. Krogstad, DL, Malaria, *Tropical Infectious Diseases,* ed. Guerrant RL, Walker DU, Waller PF, Churchill Livingstone, New York, 1999, pp 736–766.
7. Malaria, *Textbook of Travel Medicine and Health,* 2nd ed., edited Dupont HL, Steffen R, Hamilton, BC Decker, Inc, 2001, pp 184-218.
8. www.astmh.org
9. Magill AJ, *Primaquine: The Past, Present and Potential,* Lecture notes from American Society of Travel Medicine and Health, 2003, Pre-meeting course.

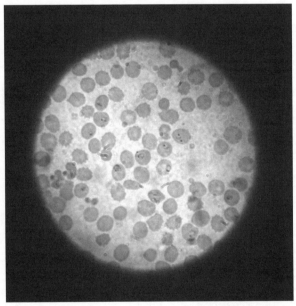

Hartmut Gross/
"Malaria; Thin Smear"

24 HIV Post-Exposure Prophylaxis

Bess Tarkington

The information listed within this chapter should help you and your team to determine an appropriate plan to address a potential occupational HIV exposure. This is a sensitive topic for multiple reasons. The emotional factor, alone, with a potential HIV exposure is significant.

HIV may be passed from one person to another when infected blood or body fluids come in contact with an uninfected person's broken skin or mucous membranes. Common ways that HIV is passed from one person to another include: sex with an HIV-infected person, the sharing of needles or injection equipment with a drug user infected with HIV, or from HIV-infected women to their babies before birth or during the birth process or through breast-feeding.

Occupational needle-stick exposure is not limited to health care workers, but to anyone working around patients, relatives or contaminated "sharps." It is important to remember that blood or body fluid splashes on intact (not broken) skin will not result in an HIV transmission. Even in a needle stick from a documented patient infected with HIV, the transmission risk of HIV is very low: 0.1%-0.3%. HIV is not airborne or food-borne and does not live long outside the body. Feces, nasal secretions, saliva, sputum, sweat, tears, urine and vomit are not considered potentially infectious unless they contain blood. Thus, the risk for transmission from these sources is low.

High risk exposures should be considered urgent medical concerns to ensure timely post-exposure management and administration of HIV Post-Exposure Prophylaxis (PEP).[2]

If Exposed

Wounds and skin sites that have been in contact with blood or body fluids should be washed with soap and water; mucous membranes should be flushed with water. No evidence exists that using antiseptics for wound care or expressing fluid by squeezing the wound further reduces the risk of blood borne pathogen transmission; however, the use of antiseptics is not contraindicated. The application of caustic agents (e.g. bleach) or the injection of antiseptics or disinfectants into the wound is not recommended.[3]

Immediately seek the advice of a health care professional knowledgeable in HIV issues who can evaluate the severity of the exposure and whether or not there is a need for a full course of post-exposure prophylaxis.

Management of an Exposure

Create a written exposure report including the following information:
- Date and time of exposure
- Risk assessment: type of fluid and type of exposure[4]
- Details including where and how the exposure occurred, and if the exposure was related to a sharp device

153

- Details of the exposure: including the type of fluid or material and the duration of contact and the condition of the skin (e.g. chapped, abraded, or intact)
- Details related to the individual or source of the exposure (e.g. this source known to be infected with HIV, an IV drug user, or a person with multiple sexual partners?)
- Obtain a laboratory evaluation of the person who was the source of the potentially infected blood or body fluid. Include testing for HIV, hepatitis B and C. Also test the person who was exposed.
- Arrange for counseling, post exposure management, and follow-up.5

Evaluating Risk

> **Low risk**: not severe, a splash exposure, solid needle, superficial injury
>
> **High risk**: severe, large bore needle, deep injury, visible blood on device, needle in patient's artery or vein.
>
> **Severity:** relates both to type of exposure and if the source is likely to be infected with HIV or if the source is unknown

We recommend that persons with a high-risk exposure initiate a three-day course of THREE antiviral medications. The quick initiation (within 2–5 hours of exposure) of the three-day course will prevent infection while allowing time for the history and laboratory profile (HIV and hepatitis B and C status) to be established and for an expert to be consulted concerning the decision whether or not to continue a full PEP regimen.

The team leader or area director will also initiate the process for the acquisition of the remainder of the four weeks of antiretroviral medication or will initiate evacuation of the exposed individual to another country where medications are available. Telephone consultation rapidly needs to be established with both a physician knowledgeable in HIV therapy and the patient's insurance carrier.

Exposures to HIV should be evaluated within hours (rather than days). The goal is to bathe the virus in anti-retroviral medications before the virus can enter or replicate within a living lymphocyte. If the source person is seronegative for HIV, baseline testing or further follow-up of the exposed person normally is not necessary.6

When a high risk HIV exposure occurs and the decision is made to continue HIV PEP, an individual's underlying medical conditions/history must also be considered (e.g. pregnancy, breast feeding, renal or hepatic disease) which may affect drug selection. At a minimum, lab monitoring for toxicity should include a complete blood count and renal and hepatic function tests.7

PEP Medication Regimens

The Centers for Disease Control recommends a basic 4-week regimen of two-drug combination or an expanded regimen of three. The author recommends the expanded three drug regimen for all post-exposure treatments if tolerated without disabling side effects. When HIV PEP is indicated, it is important to complete the recommended four-week course of medication. All antiretroviral agents have

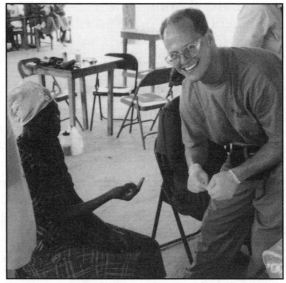

Ted Kuhn/
**"Drawing Blood in Haiti.
Remember Universal Precautions."**

been associated with side effects. It will be necessary to monitor both laboratory profiles and the individual. Side effects associated with many of the NRTIs (nucleoside reverse transcriptase inhibitors) are chiefly gastrointestinal (e.g. nausea or diarrhea). The use of PIs (protease inhibitors) has been associated with new onset diabetes mellitus, and dyslipidemia. The NNRTIs (nonnucleoside reverse transcriptase inhibitors) have been associated with severe skin reactions, including life-threatening cases of Stevens-Johnson syndrome and toxic epidermal necrolysis and hepatotoxicity.[8]

Careful evaluation of medications currently in use by the exposed person should be noted and medication adjustments should be made when needed. Further information about potential drug interactions can be found in the manufacturer's package insert.

Zidovudine (300mg) together with **Lamivudine** (150mg) comes in a combination pill (**Combivir**) to be taken twice daily. This can be taken with or without food, although with food reduces some of the GI side effects.

OR

Alternative: **Lamivudine + Stavudine** (**Lamivudine** 150mg twice a day for >/=50kg body weight or 2mg/kg of body weight if under 50kg + 40mg **Stavudine** twice a day for a person weighing >/=60kg; 30mg for a person weighing <60kg)

AND

The protease inhibitor (third drug) to add: **Nelfinivir** (1250mg twice a day with meals)
An alternative to Nelfinivir is **Indinavir** (800mg three times a day on an empty stomach) if Nelfinivir is not available or poorly tolerated.[11]

Evaluation of certain symptoms should not be delayed (e.g. rash, fever, back or abdominal pain, pain on urination or blood in the urine, or symptoms of hyperglycemia). Nausea and diarrhea are the most common side effects and may be treated with antimotility and antiemetic agents or other medications that target specific symptoms without changing the regimen. In other situations, modifying the dose interval might facilitate adherence to the regimen.[9]

Follow-up

Regardless of whether an individual receives HIV PEP, follow-up counseling, post-exposure testing, and medical evaluation should be completed. HIV-antibody testing should be performed for at least 6 months post exposure (e.g. at 6 weeks, 12 weeks, and 6 months). Although rare instances of delayed HIV seroconversion have been reported, this is an infrequent occurrence and does not warrant adding to the anxiety level of the exposed person by routinely extending the duration of post-exposure follow-up.[10]

When HIV infection is identified, the person should be referred to a specialist knowledgeable in the area of HIV treatment and counseling for medical treatment.

The emotional response to undergoing HIV PEP may be significant. Each person should be encouraged to seek counseling from an individual with knowledge and skills in this area.

Other resources available (apart from the CDC guidelines):
- PEPline: toll free: 1.888.448.4911, 24 hours/day, seven days/week
- Needle stick! Web site: ww.needlestick.mednet.ucla.edu)
- HIV Antiretroviral Pregnancy Registry www.apregistry.com/patient.htm
- FDA: www.fda.gov
- HIV/AIDS Treatment Information www.hivatis.org

References

1. Centers for Disease Control and Prevention, Updated U.S. Public Health Service Guidelines for the Management of Occupational Exposures to HBV, HCV, and HIV and Recommendations for Post exposure Prophylaxis. MMWR 2001; 50 (No. RR-11): p 7.

2. Centers for Disease Control and Prevention, Updated U.S. Public Health Service Guidelines for the Management of Occupational Exposures to HBV, HCV, and HIV and Recommendations for Post exposure Prophylaxis. MMWR 2001; 50 (No. RR-11): p 1.

3. Centers for Disease Control and Prevention, Updated U.S. Public Health Service Guidelines for the Management of Occupational Exposures to HBV, HCV, and HIV and Recommendations for Post exposure Prophylaxis. MMWR 2001; 50 (No. RR-11): p 17.

4. HIV/AIDS Care and Treatment: A Clinical Course for People Caring for Persons Living with HIV/AIDS Facilitator's Guide. Module B2. Family Health International 2004, p 380.

5. Centers for Disease Control and Prevention, Updated U.S. Public Health Service Guidelines for the Management of Occupational Exposures to HBV, HCV, and HIV and Recommendations for Post exposure Prophylaxis. MMWR 2001; 50 (No. RR-11): p 17.

6. Centers for Disease Control and Prevention, Updated U.S. Public Health Service Guidelines for the Management of Occupational Exposures to HBV, HCV, and HIV and Recommendations for Post exposure Prophylaxis. MMWR 2001; 50 (No. RR-11): p 20.

7. Centers for Disease Control and Prevention, Updated U.S. Public Health Service Guidelines for the Management of Occupational Exposures to HBV, HCV, and HIV and Recommendations for Post exposure Prophylaxis. MMWR 2001; 50 (No. RR-11): p 23.

8. Centers for Disease Control and Prevention, Updated U.S. Public Health Service Guidelines for the Management of Occupational Exposures to HBV, HCV, and HIV and Recommendations for Post exposure Prophylaxis. MMWR 2001; 50 (No. RR-11): p 27.

9. Centers for Disease Control and Prevention, Updated U.S. Public Health Service Guidelines for the Management of Occupational Exposures to HBV, HCV, and HIV and Recommendations for Post exposure Prophylaxis. MMWR 2001; 50 (No. RR-11): p 28.

10. Centers for Disease Control and Prevention, Updated U.S. Public Health Service Guidelines for the Management of Occupational Exposures to HBV, HCV, and HIV and Recommendations for Post exposure Prophylaxis. MMWR 2001; 50 (No. RR-11): p 27.

11. Center for Disease Control and Prevention. Updated U.S. Public Health Service guidelines for the management of occupational exposures to HIV and recommendations for postexposure prophylaxis. MMWR 2005;54:1-11 www.cdc.gov/mmwr/PDF/rr/rr5011.pdf

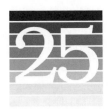

Conflict Resolution on Medical Mission Teams

David Foster

From the time of Adam and Eve conflict has been a besetting sin of the human race. Scripture records marital and familial conflicts, church conflicts, and national conflicts. On every level of interpersonal relations it is evident. Paul Tournier said it well, "Listen to all the conversations of the world, those between nations as well as those between couples. They are for the most part dialogues of the deaf. Each one speaks primarily in order to set forth his own ideas, in order to justify himself, in order to enhance himself and to accuse others. Exceedingly few exchanges of viewpoints manifest a real desire to understand the other person."1 Conflict even exists among missions teams.

Conflicts among people originate from two sources: sin and finiteness. Sin fuels many conflicts. As human beings we want our own way. We want life on our own terms. We do not naturally want to serve one another. Humans are also subject to finiteness. We have limitations. We do not have all the facts in hand. We make assumptions about what others have said or done based on inadequate information. We are plagued by both sin and finiteness and therefore continue to have conflicts.

Ken Sande in his excellent book *The Peacemaker*, says there are three ways people respond to conflict: escape, conciliate, or attack.2 The escape and attack responses both usually fall short of a godly pursuit of conflict resolution. Conciliation is the only response Christians should work toward.

Conflict on missions teams can be resolved if certain attitudinal and behavioral responses are in place. A covenant detailing roles, responsibilities, and relationships which is explained, signed, and agreed upon prior to the trip can prevent many conflicts from ever getting started. This covenant should include procedures to follow in case there is a dispute. Consequences of not following protocol should also be clearly delineated, up to and including dismissal from the team. Team leaders should model and teach servanthood. There are no conflicts that cannot be resolved with a humble, servant mind set (Phil. 2:1-16). Flexibility and humility exhibited by team members enables them to honestly deal with differences without demanding their own way.

Owning responsibility for one's own reactions and opinions is also necessary in conflict resolution. Sending "I" (owning responsibility) messages rather than "you" (blaming) messages also helps to defuse and resolve conflict. Listening to the other point of view is also an essential part of resolving disputes (Prov. 18:13, 15). The test of this listening is the verification by the speaker that the listener does indeed understand their position. Many conflicts are resolved just by this listening-clarifying-understanding process. Remembering that the ultimate goal of the mission endeavor is to glorify God, should guide both the attitudes and actions of missions participants.

Conflicts are inevitable when people gather. If those engaged in the conflict will assume the attitudes and actions mentioned above, what then is viewed as an obstacle may become an opportunity for a deeper walk with God and others.

References
1. Tournier, Paul. *To Understand Each Other.* John Knox Press, 1970.
2. Sande, Ken. *The Peacemaker.* Baker Books, Grand Rapids, 1997.

Resources
1. Lieberman, David J. *Make Peace with Anyone.* New York: St. Martin's Press, 2002.
2. Nichols, Michael P. *The Lost Art of Listening.* New York: Guilford Press, 1995.
3. Worthington, Everett L. *Forgiving and Reconciling: Bridges to Wholeness and Hope.* Downers Grove, Illinois: InterVarsity Press, 2003.

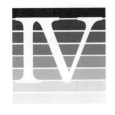

Section IV:
Medical Ministry Models in the Field

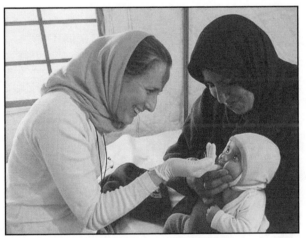

Bob Bradbury/
"Nurse with Mother and Baby"

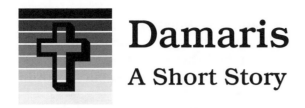

Damaris
A Short Story

W. "Ted" Kuhn

She lives only a few steps from the main path that winds through the slum of Ongata Rongi. I had walked the path several times and never noticed her home before. We were making visits to AIDS patients, who were too frail to travel the short distance to the church. Her house was made of native stone with a slanted tin roof and sagging, rotting, weathered, wooden beams. The door was quite small, only large enough for a child or small woman. My pack brushed against the top of the door frame as I stooped to pass through.

The inside was unexpectedly dark- a cheerless contrast to the bright sunshine outside. The front room was filled with smoke from an open cooking fire. The caustic fumes burned my eyes and it amazed me how anyone could live in such a small, smoke-filled, unventilated room. An opening only half the size of the front door led to an adjoining room. I pushed my body through and entered a black, crypt-like space.

I could sense the presence of another person, but my eyes, not accustomed to the dark, gave me few clues.

I switched on my flashlight. There was a wooden cot pushed to one side of the room. My knees barely touched the cot while my back pressed against the opposite wall.

I felt like I had inadvertently wondered into a small cave. Clothes were hanging from the wooden rafters. The floor was dirt and the stones were cold. There was a damp, musty smell, and the odor of cold sweat permeating air that had not circulated for days.

There was an orange blanket draped over the empty cot, yet the blanket almost imperceptibly moved. Two brown, hollow eyes stared from beneath the blanket, transfixed by the beam of light like a deer suddenly frozen in headlights. Sunken cheeks, a nearly hairless head and the bony skeleton of what appeared to have been a young woman. Legs and arms, wasted and too weak to support weight, a living portrait of death camps from times gone by. There were urine stains on the sheet. Her lips moved yet made no sound. I had met Damaris.

I opened the small shutter a crack to let in the morning sunlight. She squinted, the light painful to her dark-accustomed eyes. Her wasted body even more grotesque in the soft sunlight. She was a woman of 32. Staring into her face, I wondered, in a strange way, whether at one time she might had been pretty. Someone's lover or wife. And not as bold as I imagined the Biblical Damaris, who had enthusiastically responded to Paul's public invitation in Athens. This African Damaris had a weakened, disease-ravaged body leaving her unable to stand. Her room, a self-imposed prison cell. Yet

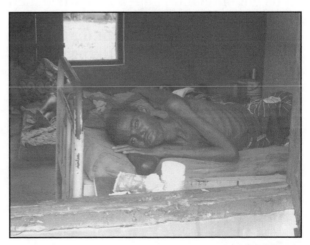

Ted Kuhn/
"Dying in Adipko"

161

like the Biblical Damaris, one of God's precious daughters.

Dying by degrees, alone in claustrophobic darkness, life going on just outside her closed window. We gave her medicine to help her swallow. She swished the white liquid in her mouth then vomited the milky substance on my friend's pants. I doubted she would do any better with the multivitamins.

There were several children ranging in ages from 4 to 12. They had been outside playing when I first entered. "Who will care for her children," I asked? "We haven't discussed it," my colleague replied. Damaris, just another unfolding tragedy among countless millions, in countless homes, in countless villages dying of AIDS in sub-Saharan Africa. In a few days or perhaps a week or two, the children playing outside will be orphans. Left alone without a mother, without food, without a home and barring the benevolence of some organization, without hope for a better future.

I had come here to meet her and her children for both the first and last time. We prayed, kneeling on the moist, dirt floor. As we prayed, she mouthed inaudible words, cracked, bleeding lips making no detectable sound. A prayer heard only by God. "We will visit if we can," we assured her. Then we walked out of her life forever, leaving the tragedy behind us like a discarded newspaper bearing yesterday's news.

AIDS attacks men and women by the very means God intended for blessing -His precious gift of relationship- a time when men and women are privileged to participate with the creator of all life, in the creation of new life. And that life in His own image. A curse instead of blessing. Separation instead of intimacy. Suffering instead of fellowship. Death instead of new birth. AIDS, an abomination to the gospel. And the sins of the parents are visited upon the children. A generation of children, innumerable millions, destined to die, robbed of the abundance of life by the ones who should have cherished them most. And those too numerous to count, often seem to count for nothing.

The future of Damaris, her children, and indeed the future of Africa is in the blood. Blood can bear life or death, blessing or curse. There is the giving of blood that saves and sustains, and defiled blood that bears death and sorrow. Sin that is covered by blood and sin that is brought on by blood. There is the blood of the covenant, and there is the blood that cries out. There is the sprinkled blood that speaks more graciously than the blood of Abel. Blood that cleanses us from guilt. And blood guiltiness. There is blood that brings us into fellowship with God and blood that separates us from the love of God. Atonement through blood. Condemnation through blood. Blood sufficient for all, or blood not sufficient at all. Sins that the blood of the Lamb can only atone and sins that the blood of lambs could never atone.

Yet, I will always remember the day I met you. There, in a far away land, in a little stone hut, along a dusty path, that leads through a slum called Ongata Rongi. Abandoned and dying of AIDS. You, alone in a small, dark room-the summation of the legacy of our generation. The Biblical namesake of a woman from Athens, known to the Apostle Paul. A woman of character and strength. A woman of faith. Damaris. Did angels bend near to listen as you prayed, your parched lips moving but making no sound? Did the Body of Christ comfort you in your time of need? And your children? And what could possibly be our testimony, when we were silent for so long? When we knew, but did not respond. When we were able, yet unwilling. Unengaged, mute witnesses to enormous tragedy? Proclaiming Christ's love, when mercy was far from us.

References
1. Kuhn W., *My Eyes, His Heart*, Winepress, October 2002.

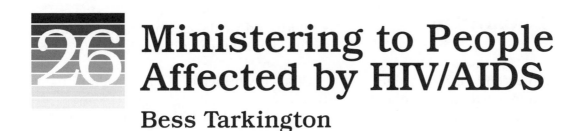

Ministering to People Affected by HIV/AIDS

Bess Tarkington

HIV/AIDS is More Than a Medical
    Condition
HIV and the Christian World View
HIV is a Disease of Relationships:
Ministering to People with HIV/AIDS

Globally more than 16 million people have died of HIV/AIDS and more than 16,000 people become newly infected each day. As the epidemic progresses and more people become ill with AIDS-related illnesses, the impact on health care systems and social safety nets increases dramatically. Many of the poorest countries already struggling with health care reforms are finding it impossible to cope with AIDS.1

HIV/AIDS Is More Than a Medical Condition

HIV/AIDS is vastly more than a medical problem. AIDS affects the whole person. Fear, anger, shame, and guilt dominate the emotions of people suffering from this infection. Socially, the person with HIV is often rejected, divorced, or abandoned, and the expense of treatment and care places enormous burdens on the person, the family, and the whole of society. Spiritually, there is hopelessness and despair.[2]

Christ died for people with HIV/AIDS too. He overcame the evil powers that lead people into activities that expose them to HIV. His grace is sufficient to bring them into eternal life, to heal their hearts and spirits, and to deliver them from bondage to evil and harmful habits. His power is sufficient to keep millions of children, young people, and adults walking in the way of life and away from those things that lead to HIV infection. He is waiting for us to take his saving and healing power to all those suffering from or at risk of contracting AIDS.[3]

"To cities filled with the homeless and impoverished, Christianity offered charity as well as hope. To cities filled with the homeless and impoverished, Christianity offered an immediate basis for attachment. To cities filled with orphans and widows, Christianity provided a new and expanded sense of family. To cities faced with epidemics, fire and earthquakes, Christianity offered effective nursing services...For what they brought was not simply an urban movement, but a new culture capable of making life in Greco-Roman cities more tolerable."[4]

Why has there been reluctance to minister to HIV/AIDS affected individuals?

1. *Fear.* Fear of death; fear of having to face unanswerable questions and seemingly unsolvable problems; fear of getting too close to persons whose life-styles are unfamiliar, unacceptable, or threatening.
2. *Prejudice.* Individuals expressing non biblical attitudes of condemnation against persons with AIDS.
3. *Tolerance of sin.* The opposite of prejudice: individuals have come to accept promiscuous sexual life-styles as normal.
4. *Misunderstanding.* Individuals seem to feel that AIDS is a medical problem and is therefore outside the domain of the church.
5. *Hopelessness.* The AIDS epidemic seems too overwhelming for any one individual or organization to address.[5]

HIV and the Christian World View

In the past, interventions to prevent HIV/AIDS have been focused on risk reduction, not primary behavior change. Prevention programs have relied on physical barriers to the virus that give only incomplete protection and are not available to vast numbers of people. This approach is accepted globally. However, faith-based messages of prevention (abstinence) are now, at last, being recognized as effective. The faith-based message understands the cultural world view and seeks to lead people to desire a selfless, compassionate and merciful worldview—with Christ's life on earth as the example.[6]

Worldview is the basis for our beliefs and our behavior. Behavior is the outward expression of the inner self. We are created for relationships: with God, with each other, with self. In our relationship with God, we love Him with our whole being and trust Him. We are obedient and we serve Him by serving others. Love for others means we consider them as a priority over ourselves. With self, our identity is this: we are bearers of the image of God. Self-acceptance is a work in progress with God being the designer/engineer. Needs of intimacy are met by God and by those He chooses for us. There is an awareness of the wholeness of life, the unity and interconnectedness of life.[7]

The existing worldview says this:
- Man is only an intelligent animal
- Man is body, mind, and feelings, with no spirit
- Man has no eternal dignity or value
- The most important person in life is ME
- What I do with my life is my own affair
- I am responsible to no one except to myself
- Other people can be used for my personal benefit[8]

HIV is a Disease of Relationships:

- With self-we don't know who we are
- With others-we seek intimacy only in a physical way, not with the whole self
- With God-we disobey his revealed pattern for life and for relationships[9]

Biblical worldview of life, love and marriage:
- We are created in God's image and have an eternal worth and destiny
- We are spiritual and physical beings
- Male and female are equal in God's sight
- God's rules for sexual behavior are to protect our health and our fulfillment
- *Agape* love is self-giving for the good of the other (Jesus is the model)
- *Filios* love considers the other better than self
- *Eros* love is God's gift to us, to be used according to God's laws and his plan
- Marriage is ordained by God and blessed by Him
- Marriage is a lifelong and growing relationship
- Marriage requires faithfulness to one another[10]

Ministering to People with HIV/AIDS

To minister to people affected by HIV/AIDS, one must first understand the origin of their beliefs, which are rooted in worldview assumptions. Typically, our worldview is transmitted to us by our culture. We seldom stop to think or reflect on it. We develop assumptions about life, the world around us, ourselves and the origin of illness.[11] Worldviews vary between cultures (thus, beliefs, values, and habits vary). And unless we understand that worldview, we cannot communicate effectively.[12]

To begin, a relationship must be developed and built. This is accomplished by listening, understanding, asking appropriate questions, guiding thoughts and discussions to a common ground where new ideas can be transmitted and decision-making can take place. LISTEN to a person's story to gain understanding and respect for the individual with whom you are developing a relationship. Develop your COMMUNICATION SKILLS. Ask indirect questions so as not to appear accusatory or self-righteous.

AFFIRM GOOD BEHAVIORS, VALUES and BELIEFS (which is ultimately leading you to a picture of their worldview). Allow for an opportunity of MUTUAL LEARNING and SHARING. Look for synthesis: putting worldviews together and finding common ground. What elements are harmful and need to be changed? Talk about them.[13]

It is important to note that in the home, parents serve as the primary educators. Developing a relationship with a parent, will in turn, encourage the education of children (by example more often than by word).

To the individual sufferer, caring for basic needs (feeding, bathing, turning) are critical. If there is family available, they can be taught and encouraged. An alternative would be to find a neighbor...or another HIV positive individual...strong and well enough to care for the one that is unable.

To children of dying parents, often the children have become the caregivers and have lost the opportunity to be children (school, play, etc.). The responsibility of caregiver has transferred to the eldest child. And this may need to continue. Support offered by neighbors and extended family will be important. It is also important to forward think—to determine how the children will be cared for when they are orphaned. The responsibility may remain with the eldest child. It is common in cultures to absorb orphaned children into the community. Is this the case in the community you are in? This notes the importance of knowing the community that you are working in.

"Memory boxes" are often put together by families/individuals affected by cancer and can also be used with AIDS patients and their families. The concept is to gather pictures, memorabilia, and other items of significance together and place them in a box/container of some kind. This may assist the family with the grieving process and over time helps them to remember and share stories of the one who has died.

HIV/AIDS is a disease of relationships. Jesus called His disciples to preach the Gospel and to minister to both spiritual and physical needs of people (Matthew 4: 18–19). We are called to love others because of the great love that God shows us (1 John 4: 7–11). We are also told that the one who loves gives of himself. Jesus came to save and not to judge. We should give and not judge others (John 3: 16). As we minister to others we must also renew ourselves, by spending time alone with the Father (2 Thessalonians 3: 13).[14]

Isaiah 61

*The Spirit of the Sovereign LORD is on me,
because the LORD has anointed me
to preach good news to the poor.
He has sent me to bind up the broken-
hearted,
to proclaim freedom for the captives
and release from darkness for the
prisoners,
to proclaim the year of the LORD's favor
and the day of vengeance of our God,
to comfort all who mourn...*

New International Version

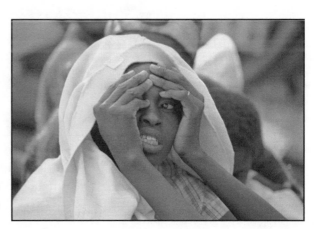

Lydia Kuhn/
"The Face of Africa"

References

1. Centers for Disease Control, Global AIDS Program: Philosophy, Updated June 15, 2002, pp 1–2.
2. Fountain, Daniel, MD, AIDS: *The 15.45 Window*, Volume 34, 1:1, 2003.
3. Fountain, Daniel, MD, AIDS: *The 15.45 Window*, Volume 34, 1:3, 2003
4. Stark, Rodney, *The Rise of Christianity*, p 161.
5. Fountain, Daniel, MD, AIDS: *The 15.45 Window*, Volume 34, 1:1, 2003
6. Fountain, Daniel, MD, *HIV, Worldview Problems and Behavior Change*, Slide 4, Global Health Missions Conference, Southeast Christian Church, November 2003.
7. Fountain, Daniel, MD, *HIV, Worldview Problems and Behavior Change*, Slide 7, Global Health Missions Conference, Southeast Christian Church, November 2003.
8. Fountain, Daniel, MD, *HIV, Worldview Problems and Behavior Change*, Slide 19, Global Health Missions Conference, Southeast Christian Church, November 2003.
9. Fountain, Daniel, MD, *HIV, Worldview Problems and Behavior Change*, Slide 12, Global Health Missions Conference, Southeast Christian Church, November 2003.
10. Fountain, Daniel, MD, *HIV, Worldview Problems and Behavior Change*, Slide 20–22, Global Health Missions Conference, Southeast Christian Church, November 2003.
11. Fountain, Daniel, MD, *HIV, Worldview Problems and Behavior Change*, Slide 31,Global Health Missions Conference, Southeast Christian Church, November 2003.
12. Fountain, Daniel, MD, *HIV, Worldview Problems and Behavior Change*, Slide 33, Global Health Missions Conference, Southeast Christian Church, November 2003.
13. Fountain, Daniel, MD, *HIV, Worldview Problems and Behavior Change*, Slide 38–40, Global Health Missions Conference, Southeast Christian Church, November 2003.
14. Rowland, Stan: *Multiplying Light and Truth through Community Health Evangelism*. GLS Publishing, Pant Nagar, Mumbai, India, 2001.

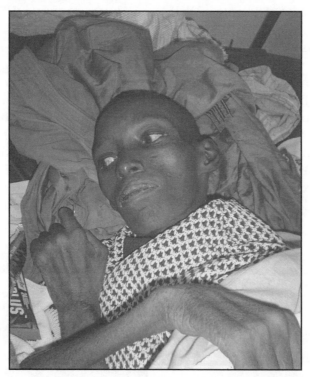

Jennifer Chapel/
**"Abandoned by Family After They
Found Out She Had HIV and TB,
East Africa."**

27 Ministering to the Needs of Street Children

Tom Stewart

Who are Street Children?
What Are the Conditions That Result in
    Street Children?
Conclusion

There are an estimated 150 million street children in the world. Much of what is known about this population is anecdotal information gleaned from the personal experience of workers in the field. There are few published studies on the demographics, sociology, psychology, and physical health of the world's street child population. Most reports are narrowly focused on one country or location.

What follows is an overview in a question and answer format. It does not deal directly with medical aspects of ministry to street children. Instead, this chapter presents a general introduction to the whole issue of homeless children and serves as a background for providing effective ministry.

Who Are Street Children?

They are the world's unwanted children. They are the "invisible" disposable children, who simply become an almost meaningless part of the landscape, usually not viewed as real people with legitimate needs. Their parents, their governments, their societies, and far too often, even the churches don't want them.

What Are the Conditions That Result in Street Children?

There are several common factors that are always found in locations where there is a significant street child problem. First, there

is always deep, persistent poverty. Second, there is severe and widespread dysfunction and breakdown of the family, often compounded by alcohol and drug abuse by parents and other adults in the child's life. Third, there is lack of effective social services for children either by the government, non-government organizations (NGOs), or by the church. A final factor, seen especially in sub-Sahara Africa, is the rampant AIDS epidemic, which has left 12–15 million children as orphans on that continent.

Since children begin life with a family (or at least a mother), how do children become street children?

Children end up on the street as a result of several common scenarios. Many children leave home as a result of threatened or actual physical and/or sexual abuse by a parent or other adult. Some homes are simply so negligent or deficient that children have little incentive to stay, even if the home is not abusive. Some are abandoned, especially by single mothers who are unable to provide for all their children (effectively abandoning some, in order to care for others). Other than in sub-Sahara Africa, most street children have at least one living parent; of course, orphaned children may also end up on the street. Street girls have often had multiple pregnancies, so some children may be homeless from birth.

Are all children on the street completely homeless?

No. Street children are a heterogeneous population. Workers tend to classify the children into two groups. The first group is described as "on" the street. These are

167

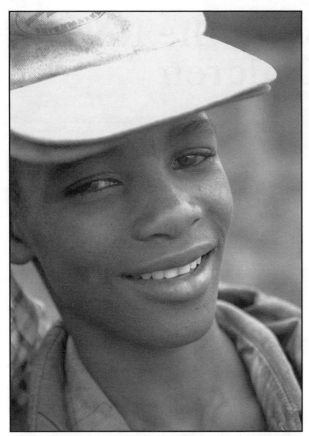

Ted Kuhn/
"Street Boy in Slums of Nairobi"

How do governments and societies respond to street children?

The attitudes, and the resulting actions, of governments and societies at large toward their street children vary widely. Some, such at the Philippines, are caring and compassionate, while others are more or less indifferent, such as countries in Eastern Europe. Still others are openly hostile and abusive toward homeless children, such as many countries in Latin America. Harassment, physical abuse, incarceration with adult criminals, and even murder of street children is not unheard of there.

What does a population of street children look like?

Although there is some variation from one geographic location to another, there are certain common demographics among most street child populations. The most obvious is that there are more boys than girls. The reasons for this appear to be complex and multiple. For example, mothers may be more protective of girls and therefore they are less likely to end up on the street. Girls, being more subject to sexual abuse and exploitation, tend to make themselves less visible than boys. They also are more likely to be victims of abduction and trafficking. The ages of children on the street typically range from about 12 through the teenage years. However, children under the age of 10 are not uncommon and even very young children are seen on the street, under the care of an older sibling.

children who retain some contact, of varying degrees, with home and a parent or other family member, while spending much, or most, of their time on the street. The second group is that of completely homeless children, described as "of" the street. These children have no contact with any parent or other relative, or any place they would describe as home. Typically the group of children "on" the street is somewhat larger percentage than those "of" the street.

Where in the world are street children found?

Significant street child populations are found in what was formerly described as "developing countries," now more commonly referred to as the "two-thirds" world. This includes most of Latin America, much of Southeast Asia, Africa, and the sub-continent of India. Mainland China has a growing street child problem, as does Russia and many eastern European countries of the former Soviet Union.

What are the substance abuse issues facing street children?

Substance abuse is a form of psychological escape for street children. Throughout the world street children routinely abuse inhalants, such as various forms of glue, which are cheap and readily available. Alcohol and other "hard" drugs are used but generally to a lesser extent.

What are the health issues facing street children?

Street children have little or no access to medical and dental care. They may not have received the usual childhood immunizations. In addition to the obvious health issues created by inhalant or other drug abuse, they face adverse weather conditions (especially in areas with cold climates), varying degrees of poor nutrition, poor dental health, traumatic injuries, chronic communicable diseases (such as tuberculosis), and the range of sexually transmitted diseases, including HIV/AIDS.

What are the psychological and developmental issues facing street children?

Street children may suffer from a host of psychological and developmental problems. Due to family dysfunction, abuse, and rejection, street children may suffer from reactive attachment disorder. They are often socially and developmentally delayed, resulting in poor interpersonal skills and inappropriate behavior. They are sexually promiscuous. Hyperactivity is not uncommon, especially in boys. Once on the street they drop out of school and many are years behind their peers academically. This results in further problems, when older children are far behind younger ones in such basic skills as reading and writing.

What are the challenges in ministering to street children?

There are special difficulties for any individual or organization wishing to work with street children. First, most of these children have never had a loving relationship with an adult. To them, adults are viewed as the source of neglect at best and abuse at worst. Establishing a relationship of compassion and thereby gaining credibility, as someone to be trusted, is the first prerequisite. Initial contacts are almost always made on the streets and hangouts where the children live. We must enter their world since they will not willingly enter ours. Second, the needs of these children are high. They suffer from deficiencies in all areas of life—spiritual, social, psychological, developmental, and academic. If these children are to become normal adults, each area must be addressed. This requires perseverance and a long-term commitment. Third, the com-

mon, if not almost universal, problem of drug abuse (especially inhalants) must be dealt with. Fourth, street children become sexually active at a young age, presenting obvious problems for those entering into a residential program.

Finally, it must be remembered that children on the streets are survivors by any means necessary. They must survive economically, which means they will do whatever is necessary to earn the money they need. This may mean menial jobs or begging, but it may also mean stealing and prostitution (by boys and girls). They must survive emotionally, which often means sexual promiscuity for girls. They may be slow to develop meaningful relationships with adults. Street children may also be highly manipulative to get what they want.

What are the challenges in medical ministry to street children?

Medical ministry to street children comes with at least all the difficulties of providing health care to homeless adults. Even if the children can be found at all and are cooperative, providing health care on the street is always severely limited due to the limitations of what diagnostic modalities can be utilized and treatments can be provided. Care provided at a "drop-in" center (a day-only non-residential facility) is somewhat better, especially if a child attends the

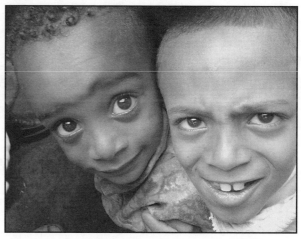

Ted Kuhn/
"Just Kids"

center daily (medications, for example, can be administered by the drop-in center staff). However, many children are quite erratic in their attendance, making effective treatment difficult due to inadequate compliance. In addition, medical records are unavailable so that, for example, it is usually not known which children have received immunizations. Truly effective care can be provided only to children who are in stable foster homes, just one of many reasons that residential care is vastly preferable to any other kind of program.

Conclusion

Ministry to street children presents us with many unique problems and possibilities. Although many work with street children in widely diverse locations around the world, very few have a global perspective on the worsening problem of homeless children. Fewer still have first hand experience with street children from different cultures. There is a great need for street child workers to share their experience and to encourage others. Together we can all learn to better help.

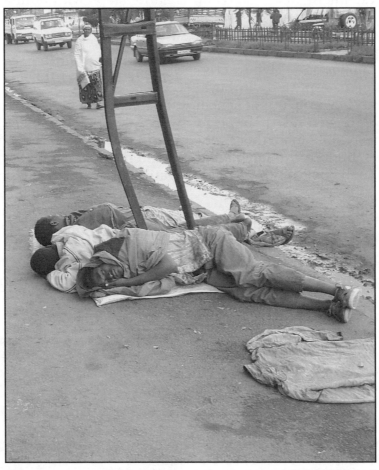

Ted Kuhn/
"Children Sleeping on the Street"

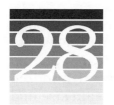

Responding to a Disaster in a Developing Country

Cynthia Urbanowicz

Preparation of Team Members: Spiritual,
 Mental and Physical
Four Phases of Disaster Relief
 Emergency/ Rescue Phase
 Relief Phase
 Recovery Phase
 Mitigation Phase

A re natural disasters increasing or are we more aware due to the ever widening communication abilities of the media? What of man-made disasters such as war? Are they also increasing and what role does media play? Developing countries with increasing populations have an increasing need for land, shelter, food sources and other natural resources. Lands located in natural flood plains, along seismic faults and in hostile areas are often unwanted and undeveloped by wealthier populations. The poor then crowd to these unwanted yet available areas.1 Land tracts are rapidly deforested in an effort to plant crops, harvest wood for cooking fires and clear areas for dwellings. Subsequently rain waters flow unchecked over eroded soil. Homes are frequently built using substandard building methods with inferior materials. Small top-heavy structures typically house numerous family members. Even a moderate flooding event or seismic activity can have a catastrophic affect on these over-populated, poorly developed areas. The result are high death tolls and immense suffering.2 The media arrives quickly to show the tragic aftermath to the world.

What should our response be as representatives of the body of Christ? We extend compassion to those affected and strive to meet their needs at the most basic physical levels *and* bring the greatest aid of all- the Gospel. Often a spiritual door is opened as victims face their own mortality. Questions arise, "How could this happen?" "Who is responsible?" "How will I go on?" In his book, *Where is God When it Hurts?* Philip Yancey explores western perceptions of pain, grief and suffering. He says, "Christian faith does not offer us a peaceful way to come to terms with death. Christ stands for Life, and his resurrection should give convincing proof that God is not satisfied with any 'cycle of life' that ends in death. He will go to any extent - he *did* go to any extent - to break that cycle." The Gospel message is not a western method of dealing with tragedy. It is the very key to life, able to cross borders, boundaries and cultures, reconciling man to God through the saving work of Christ. What of "sensitive" areas where we cannot openly share the gospel? "*But thanks be to God, who always leads us in triumphal procession in Christ and through us spreads the fragrance of the knowledge of him.*" 2 Cor 2: 15. We may share Him openly through our compassionate actions and caring mercies. This is our ultimate motivation: to share Christ in all things.

Other doors may open as disaster response teams work alongside government officials, health care workers and community leaders, allowing access and contact with areas and peoples that would happen in no other way.

Preparation of Team Members- Spiritual, Mental and Physical

Without the sound foundation of biblically based "disaster theology," disaster response workers are unprepared to deal with what meets them at the disaster site. Often unimaginable devastation, despair, hostility, aggression, abuse and apathy are all present in the same setting as hospitality, kindness and unusual openness. Victims often feel helpless, fearful and angry, yet will want to give any token of hospitality that they can manage. Taking a small cup of tea with a victim and listening can be as healing as an antibiotic. Are disaster workers prepared by their theology to answer the victim's question, "Did your god do this to me?"

Additionally, the physical and mental stress of living and working in a refugee camp can be immensely draining. Scarce food and supplies coupled with long hours of work and a high demand for services can lead to rapid burnout. Workers at disaster sites must have their own mechanism in place to debrief each day. Pastoral care and professional counseling should be available to workers, both on the field and after returning. A military unit would not be expected to last long on the front lines of battle with no support. Neither should a relief worker.

Disaster responders must have full immunizations up-to-date prior to departing for the scene. Relief workers should be aware of the need for malaria prophylaxis including appropriately treated mosquito nets for areas in which they will be working. Responders should be in excellent health. The disaster site is not an appropriate field for those with chronic medical problems that require special medicines, treatments or diets. Each worker should be able to demonstrate a reasonable degree of physical fitness, as disaster response may require hiking, heavy lifting, water crossings and long hours all in the context of extremes in hot or cold climates, including high altitude.

Responding teams must be self-sufficient, able to pump and process their own water, provide adequate nutritious food and safe, appropriate shelter for themselves. If teams arrive with a long list of their own needs and take resources from victims to satisfy those needs, they lose credibility and may cause resentment by their presence. Responding medical teams should come prepared to treat several hundred victims daily, depending on team size and configuration. Sufficient basic clinic supplies should accompany the team from its home base to the disaster site with enough to cover the clinic needs for approximately three days. This is usually adequate time to locate and obtain supplies from other NGOs (non-government organizations such as International Red Cross/ Red Crescent).

It is strongly recommended that all disaster response workers take a course that prepares them to meet the disaster field's spiritual, mental and physical demands. This chapter is not meant as a substitute for this type of training.

Four Phases of Disaster Relief

The goal of disaster relief work is to provide counseling, medical and construction assistance in the safest and most effective manner possible. Familiarity with each phase of disaster relief increases a team's ability to respond appropriately. Although the four phases of disaster relief may overlap and even recur, each phase has unique properties that define it. The four phases are:
• Emergency/ rescue
• Relief
• Recovery
• Mitigation

Emergency/ Rescue Phase

Occurring immediately post-incident (famine being the exception), this phase usually lasts several weeks. Surviving victims promptly begin to assess damage and attempt to trace loved ones. Attention is focused on locating and rescuing victims. Those who survived the initial incident may be injured or killed during precarious rescue attempts. Location of resources also becomes a crucial part of victim's response. Victims are often portrayed as helpless, shocked into inactivity. This is rarely the case. It is usually hours, days or even weeks before outside help can reach an affected area. During this period, victims frequently organize themselves, with the emergence of strong individuals who were not previously known as leaders.

Many NGOs specialize in this phase of disaster response only. The Swiss are legendary for their rescue teams with highly trained professionals, including rescue dogs. This type of rescue response requires extensive initial preparation, as well as intensive ongoing training. It is not appropriate or wise to respond during this phase unless you and your agency have this type of training *and* the appropriate support systems required for these operations. Well meaning response workers can become a hindrance as well a potential victims during ill-advised rescue attempts. The pearl of wisdom for this phase is *Rescuers Must Not Become Victims*.

It is possible, however, to begin needs assessment during this phase. Initial assessments are crucial in the logistical organization of a disaster response. Responders performing assessments during the emergency/rescue phase must have training in "scene safety." Responders must be able to discern potential hazard conditions that may not only jeopardize themselves, but also victims they wish to serve.

Responders must take an active role in their own personal protection. Each responder must have appropriate clothing and gear (Table 1).

Potential hazards include:
• Standing Water
• Moving Water
• Damaged Structures
• Power-lines
• Crowds
• Displaced Animals
• Debris Piles
• Fire
• Heat
• Disease
• Hazardous materials
• Cold
• Crime

Table 1. Personal Protection
Personal Protection
■ Over the ankle leather boots
■ Long pants
■ Long shirts
■ Eye protection
■ Hand protection
■ Head protection
Medical Providers' Body Substance Isolation
■ Gloves
■ Eye protection
■ Masks and gowns

• Terrorism
• Slope failure - landslide
• Severe weather

Relief Phase

Primarily defined by the restart and rebuilding of infra-structures (communication and medical systems, as well as governmental agencies and transportation mechanisms), the relief phase may last weeks, months or even years. Much depends on the government's response. Did the area have a disaster plan? Was it implemented? Do government resources meet the need? If resources were not adequate, were requests for international assistance made?

According to *Medecins Sans Frontieres (Doctors Without Borders)*, the top ten priorities in the relief stage are:
1. Initial assessment
2. Measles immunization
3. Water and sanitation
4. Food and nutrition
5. Shelter and site planning
6. Health care in the emergency phase
7. Control of communicable disease and epidemics
8. Public health surveillance
9. Human resources and training
10. Coordination[1]

Responding NGOs (non-government organizations) can be pivotal in this phase. The roles of NGOs vary greatly, with some groups specializing in medical response, food distribution, construction, transportation and even fund-raising. The key is communication and coordination between groups. Aggressive people groups will receive aid before those with less power to make their needs known. NGOs must take care that they do not duplicate the service of another organization while another people group goes entirely unserved.

Communication and arrangement of logistics with governments, national, regional and local is a *crucial* step in a smooth response. There is often overlap of the relief phase with the emergency/rescue phase, as time passes and successful search and rescue efforts for survivors diminish. Commonly, this occurs 10–14 days post-incident. Critical logistics (Table 2) should be arranged prior to the arrival of responders in the relief phase. Delays in transportation and procurement of necessary skills (i.e. translators, guides, and drivers) ultimately lead to detrimental delays in victims' assistance. Advance needs assessment teams can bridge this gap, making necessary contacts and arrangements.

Needs assessment teams have greater mobility than larger secondary teams. Needs assessment team composition should include a health professional, engineering, construction and professional counseling personnel. Additionally, it is essential to include persons familiar with the area to be served, referred to as "field" personnel. Field personnel are instrumental in making contacts, advising on culture and potential cultural barriers to operations. An example would be a culture in which it is forbidden for a man to touch a woman to whom he is not married. This would be problematic for male doctors treating female patients. More suitable arrangements must be made and field personnel may be the facilitators.

Recovery Phase

Recovery is defined by a move towards more permanent rebuilding of structures and infra-structures, rather than the tem-

---

> **Table 2. Advance Needs Assessments**
>
> *Logistics*
> - Official contacts made
> - Other NGOs coordinated
> - Transportation to site
> - Approximate travel time/distance/ method to site
> - Water source (at arrival point)
> - Food source (at arrival point)
> - Shelter/Lodging arrangements
> - Translators
> - Scene security

porizing measures of the relief phase. Permanent homes begin to replace tent cities. Water and sewage treatment facilities are rebuilt. Hospitals and clinics return to their role as primary health care providers as field hospitals are phased out. A great deal of overlap occurs with the relief phase. Medical facilities may be ready to resume their roles long before water treatment facilities are completed. Each disaster incident will be uniquely different from others. The restoration of systems will also be unique.

Mitigation Phase

The opportunity to *improve* systems and address preventable problems is called mitigation. Again, overlap with other stages is common. Developing countries are commonly devastated when disaster strikes as they have no disaster response plan in place, poor building methods and lack of warning systems. Areas prone to strong hurricanes, typhoons and flooding can gain great benefit from a disaster response plan. Areas in earthquake zones can also benefit from pre-planning and assessment. Warning systems common in developed countries may not exist elsewhere. Japan is the gold standard for disaster planning. Prone to strong earthquakes in heavily populated areas, the Japanese people have developed highly sophisticated response systems. Additionally, strict earthquake "proof" building codes are enforced and citizens are educated from childhood in earthquake preparedness.

These systems took the Japanese years to develop. It is unrealistic to expect this level of preparedness and prevention in a developing country, yet effort toward improvement should be made. Resources, funding and government approval will all factor into the development of these systems.

Author Judith Halpern states "Disaster Medicine is an evolving body of knowledge."[2] Halpern makes the observation regarding American disaster response, yet the same may be said of international disaster response. Each response will have unique aspects, yet will share some similar properties such as the four stages of response. As our awareness and understanding of international disasters evolves, we refine our methods of response and management. Education, planning and early intervention are crucial to disaster *prevention* and response. The question remains, "Are natural and man-made disasters on the increase or rather do we have increasing awareness?" The other question which must be asked is, "Should more resources and effort go towards disaster prevention rather than or in addition to disaster response?" Perhaps a combination of prevention and response is the answer.

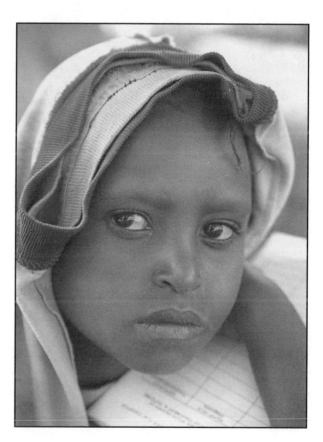

Ted Kuhn/
"Waiting in Line for Food"

References
1. Medecins Sans Frontieres: *Refugee Health- An approach to emergency situations*, London and Oxford 1997, MacMillan Education Ltd.
2. Halpern, Judith: Disaster Management and Response 2004;2:65–66, Emergency Nurses Association.

Resources
1. Wijkman, A., Timberlake, L.: *Natural Disasters—Act of God or Act of Man?* Philadelphia, PA, 1988, New Society Publishers.
2. Yancey, P: *Where is God When it Hurts?*, Grand Rapids, MI, 1990, Zondervan, p 247.

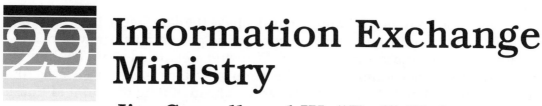

Information Exchange Ministry

Jim Carroll and W. "Ted" Kuhn

An academic team is a group of health professionals who use their role as teachers to support the church. The academic team is requested by the on-site missionary, the local church or the regional director. As with all church-sponsored medical missions, the primary goal is to see the building up of the local church. While not always the case, academic missions frequently enter the picture at a very early phase in church planting. An academic team may gain entry to a country and may begin to build relationships which will later augment church planting efforts. A related role of the academic team is to provide an opening for the long term missionary into the local community. The team's presence may also add credibility to the reputation and efforts of the missionary, as well as providing a prime opportunity for the missionary to meet with influential people in the government and society.

Other opportunities for an information exchange team occur when an established church expresses a specific community need that must be addressed from an educational standpoint. These may range from community education on the prevention of mosquito-borne diseases by appropriate use and treatment of mosquito netting, to specific continuing education for local nurses, to the introduction of some new surgical technique.

Accomplishing Change

The range of activities in which an academic team may engage are many: lecturing in areas of expertise, consultation with local health professionals, demonstration of techniques, friendship evangelism, and encouragement of seekers. Academic teams often arrive with new ideas and new practice models and may suggest change in time honored practices. Professionals, especially medical personnel, are very goal-oriented. They are accustomed to having measurable outcomes.

Short-term teams often hope to accomplish long term results in just a few days. They come with hopes of (1) doing their professional best and (2) improving the health care system. Ultimately, no one likes change and there will be variable receptivity to new ideas regardless of scientific merit. Change can be threatening and teams can be poorly received especially when viewed as 'outsiders' or 'foreigners' from another culture and another background. They should not be expected to effect permanent changes in the local system of health care in a few days or weeks! Trust and confidence has to be earned, and this is a long-term process. Eventually, perhaps after several visits, one may develop a relationship with local health care providers and can be a force for positive change. Nevertheless, short-term individuals who expect to bring quantifiable improvement on their first or second visit may be disappointed."[1]

"Notwithstanding, you may find 'champion' types (individuals from the host community or institution), i.e. those who are themselves confident and not intimidated or threatened, who are willing to learn, are strong and influential themselves and stand up to peer pressure and change. They will be the ones who can effect change in the system, ultimately after you are gone."[2] You can encourage them and assist them with further training and resources to effect change within the system. The question arises as to how to provide further educational opportunities for these 'champions.'

Routinely, it is not recommended to provide further training in the US, but rather to encourage advanced training within the educational boundaries of the host country. This means encouraging or enabling them to advance up one level within their own medical educational system. Appropriate one step training is best. Too much training results in a mismatch and dissatisfaction with resultant brain drain and counter productivity. Work primarily within their system and respect the educational structure of the host country. The perception of "outsiders" trying to "take over" may understandably be met with reluctance in the host country and runs the risk of importation of our prejudices.

Sensitivity

The cultural context always requires that the academic team member have considerable sensitivity. American academicians should not let their pride in the American medical system be an obstacle or stumbling block to the gospel. The academic aspects of the process should not become the prime focus of the trip. The personal relationships which are formed have the greatest potential for fostering the growth of the church. Getting past a friendly but formal relationship and moving on to a warm, congenial one may require more than the initial visit.

Schedules, Advanced Planning and Flexibility

Cross cultural work may be very frustrating for American academicians. One's hosts may not have the same regard for "time" and meetings and presentations may be delayed and schedules changed daily (or hourly). The team may have been given a lecture schedule ahead of time only to find that it has been altered upon arrival in the host country. Sometimes teams are given the next day's schedule only at the end of the preceding day. Lecture topics and clinical expectations can change suddenly without prior warning. There may be good reasons for the changes which we, as visitors, may not understand. For example, an important person may be visiting which will take key people away from participation. Perhaps an official is visiting and they want you to speak on a topic relevant to his/her special interest. Perhaps your primary contact is called away to another city for a meeting and those left behind to escort your team do not have the authority to make decisions about the team's schedule or lecture topics. Asians especially covet the creativity that comes from unpredictability. Life to them is more fluid and adaptable to changes around them.[3]

Western culture is more rigid and schedule oriented in contrast to most of the world which is more relational. Whatever the case, you can be assured that you will need an extra measure of grace and flexibility to have a successful outreach. You should consider praying that God will give you the patience, love and humility to weather your frustrations and anxiety. If you think you may have trouble adapting to an ever changing schedule and the uncertainty of changing presentation topics and clinical assignments, consider that this kind of outreach may not be for you.

So why plan at all, especially if we suspect our lecture topics and presentations may be changed at the last minute? Consider planning for flexibility. Planning is more than assuring that everything will be exactly as we anticipated. Planning gives us the framework, strength and resources to change quickly as the needs and requests in our host country change.[3]

As an example, one of the authors (TK) recently participated on an academic team in an Asian country. At the start, there was difficulty and delay in communicating with the host institution about their expectations and the team only received lecture topics two weeks before the scheduled departure from the US. On arrival in the host country airport, a different schedule was distributed and then again a completely new schedule the next morning. To make things more awkward, one of the lecturers was unexpectedly called back to the US for an emergency after the first day, leaving the small team with a new lecture schedule, new topics and a large knowledgeable audience.

What happened? The team had anticipated the need for flexibility and brought over 50 PowerPoint® presentations on CD from their department's repository lecture library. They had also thankfully included hundreds of clinical photos that could be pasted into new presentations. The team had access to the internet so they could search for literature on Medline from their hotel rooms each night. The result- their "planning" and flexibility resulted in a successful trip. Notwithstanding, the lectures (however professional) were not the highlight of the trip- it was the lively discussions and spontaneity stemming from the informal case presentations in the afternoons after lectures which had not been anticipated and had not been prepared ahead of time.

Common Pitfalls

In order to avoid the pitfalls of American "cultural imperialism," several issues should be kept in mind. First, be aware that the experience is better viewed as an exchange of ideas rather than our informing them of the "right way." Be sensitive to their practice styles, particularly when there is no scientific basis for one way being superior to another. Presentations should be strongly literature-based with an emphasis on well-designed studies. It may be helpful to be familiar with the medical literature on the topic in the country you are visiting. Be prepared for the audience to be quite knowledgeable and to have probing questions. A humble attitude goes a long way toward dispelling your audience's concerns about an American sense of scientific superiority.

Do not underestimate your audience! The felt needs of the physicians in the country may be quite different from what we think the needs are. Be sympathetic to their ideas first.

Teaching Methodology

Teaching techniques will change according to the host country expectations and local teaching methodology. In one setting, a PowerPoint® presentation may be so novel that it is distracting to the teaching process. In another setting, it may be expected. Group discussions and case presentations often open up more lively exchanges. In some situations, however, this type of setting might be viewed as too threatening and a cause of "loss of face." Try to be sensitive to body language and cultural cues. Be prepared for difficulties with technical equipment. The best laid plans of PowerPoint® and videos can be destroyed by lack of the needed plug adaptor or lack of electricity.

Seminars, workshops and small group discussions are all effective teaching methods which you will naturally use.[5] Interactions at the bedside during teaching rounds can evoke lively discussions and questions relating to ethics, the meaning of life and end-of-life philosophy and theology. Small group discussions may work best because change comes through role modeling and has highest "imprint value."[2] Many times participants in small groups ask penetrating questions they would feel uncomfortable asking in larger, more formal venues. In small group discussions, you can also speak freely about your experience in the practice of medicine in the US. In most countries they will be curious about the practice of medicine in America. You may also be able to weave some of your personal testimony into the discussion.

Formally, plan several lecture style presentations- at least two per team member. Everyone on the team should participate in teaching in one manner or another.[6] Prepare your presentations for an audience with a high degree of medical sophistication. It is easier to tone down a presentation that is over the audience's level of expertise, than to buff up a presentation that shoots too low.[6] Mix more advanced presentations with presentations that are practical. The goal is to help them to be able to walk out of the lecture hall and apply the information presented on patients that very afternoon. Hands-on workshops are a wonderful way to teach in the US, but this teaching methodology may be uncomfortable for participants in some countries where hands-on teaching is never done. Consult someone familiar with the training in your host country before planning workshops.

Slides are almost universally acceptable and overheads are used in most countries.[6] Overheads have the advantage of being able to be changed as the perceived level of sophistication is better understood but an overhead projector may not be available. PowerPoint® brings with it its own set of advantages and its own set of problems. In one country where the author (TK) recently taught using PowerPoint® and an LCD projector, there was a thunderstorm during the presentation and there was no available electricity for the LCD projector for several hours. The need for flexibility and grace became readily apparent. Flow charts and tables may or may not be readily understood. Here is where advance planning is helpful and investigating ahead of time the normal teaching and learning methodologies in your host country will pay off. In general jokes and puns do not translate and are best not used. Examples of practice styles and personal experience from the US are generally well appreciated and allow them to see you as a vulnerable human individual.

Most audiences will want you to speak on the "latest advances" in the topic you are presenting,[5] regardless as to whether they have mastered the "basics." Perhaps in our minds, our "professional best" is defined as cutting edge practice. Nevertheless, one should realize that it is unrealistic to expect them to be able to practice the same kind of medicine we do because of cultural, fiscal and facility constraints. Contrary to this and as a matter of pride, they will not want

medical student lectures. If you do present the "latest advances" you may be criticized for not being "practical." There is no way to avoid this controversy except by planning to address both needs. The majority of medical education is taught similarly to the US. Presentations can be structured giving the clinical presentation, differential, treatment and outcome followed by a literature review. This will be a familiar format in most countries.

Working with Translators

Many times you will be teaching using a translator. A successful relationship with your translator can make or break your presentation. Speak slowly and clearly and stop after a long phrase and after almost all sentences. Remember that for a 60 minute time slot, a 40 minute talk will more than fill the time with translation. He/she can cover for you if and when you make a cultural "faux pas." On the contrary, your translator may translate literally making you appear foolish or insensitive in front of a large crowd. Consider giving copies of your presentation to the translator ahead of time. Perhaps even consider having your PowerPoint,® your slides or overheads translated into the local language before your presentation. You will also need to brief your translator on "technical jargon," slang and special expressions before your lecture.

Handouts are generally appreciated-especially if they are bilingual. Announce at the beginning that questions are welcome after or anytime during the lecture. People can be prepared ahead of time with their questions. Many people in the audience may be hesitant to ask questions if their English is not perceived as fluent or if they have not fully understood your presentation because of language problems or problems with translation. Encourage them to write their questions and submit them in writing to your translator.[6] The good translator will "edit" the questions to avoid embarrassment and they can also be submitted anonymously to avoid embarrassment.

Gifts

Often we may be asked to bring gifts of medicines, equipment or supplies to the hospital or university where we will be teaching. They may even provide us with a "wish list" to consider bringing with us. Bearing gifts is a wonderful way of showing concern and a tangible way of upgrading their facilities and may even be good stewardship of excess equipment and supplies in the US.[4]

However, the giving of gifts may result in higher expectations for more and more gifts.[4] It is good to tie the giving of gifts with human resources, in other words, the academic teams bring the gifts with them. No teams, no gifts. This emphasizes the human element in the relationship because our interactions, our role modeling and mutual learning and encouragement lead to better health care workers, better institutions and better health for the patients in the long run. The person to person relationships that are built are also the key to sharing the greatest gift of all. Take care to remember that in the end, it is the church that is God's ultimate instrument of healing.

Notwithstanding, there are many pitfalls associated with bringing gifts. Make sure that you know whether they would be happy with used equipment or supplies, or whether they expect all new equipment. Some hospitals and administrators may be very happy with used equipment; others may be offended if you bring "second hand" equipment. Also make sure that any equipment is in working order and appropriate for the environment where it will be used (heat, humidity) and supplied with the appropriate electrical current (220 volts, 50 Hz, etc).

It may be best to make any substantial gifts of equipment (e.g. EKG machines) "official" gifts to an institution or department rather than to an individual.[4] If given to an individual, equipment may be taken home and used only by that individual and not be made available for general use. You might consider smaller gifts to individuals (e.g. glucometer) to a doctor with diabetes or to a physician who cares for patients with diabetes).

Remember that importation of durable medical supplies may be liable for import duty in many countries. Duty can sometimes be 50–100% the value of the equipment. Make sure you have an import license if needed and that you know ahead of time who will be paying the import duty- you or the beneficiary. You will need the name of the equipment, model, serial number, operating manual and approximate value to import durable medical supplies into most countries.

There is usually no "pot of money" that can be used to purchase equipment and supplies. Money must be donated just like money for other uses in mission work. It is wise to assess your monetary resources before promising to bring durable medical supplies with you. Although you may be able to get supplies and equipment at a reduced cost, you may still need to solicit a substantial amount of money for the promised equipment and unless you are willing to donate this yourself, be careful what you promise. Also remember, that purchasing equipment in the host country may be less expensive than the purchase in the US, and local vendors may provide technical support and repairs on locally purchased equipment.

Guard against medical "toys" or glamour gifts (CT scanners).[4] Always ask:

1. Is it necessary?
2. Is it helpful?
3. Is it cost effective?
4. Will they just become dependent on this (or us)?
5. Will they be able to provide the upkeep, i.e., is it affordable for them to maintain (especially parts, disposable components)[4]?

A low cost, low tech, manual machine may be much more cost effective in the long run than a fancy computerized one that can fail totally and be more difficult to fix or resupply with expensive cartridges.

Some hospitals are very possessive with their gifts and may store them or save them for a VIP and not use them for everyday medical care.[4] Hospital administrators may choose to play politics with gifts and not give the equipment to the intended department for the intended use rather giving them to another party to achieve some modicum of political favoritism. Teams can guard against this by actually having a presentation ceremony while they are there, presenting the gifts to the intended individual, department or institution. They can explain that they can assist in training or setting up the equipment or demonstrate the appropriate technique or use. This can even be tied to a meal or party for celebration, a good excuse to have fun and develop relationships and ties with one's hosts.

There are many resources within the US to obtain medical equipment for donation in other countries. Most of these are listed within this text under the chapter on *Resources for the Traveling Medical Professional*. Some donors apply restrictions on their supplies and equipment (e.g. must be used free of charge to provide care in host country). Many host countries or universities may be unwilling to donate their time and supplies free of charge. In reality, they make a living as we do, providing care to patients and charging for that service. Make sure you understand this before obtaining supplies from the donor, or traveling with equipment around the world only to find yourself in an embarrassing ethical dilemma.

The "Sweet Aroma of Christ"

We are compelled by diverse reasons to participate on an information exchange team. Hopefully, most of us are motivated to declare the good news to our peers in the medical profession in another part of the world, to provide an opportunity and platform for church planting. Others want to use and share their professional skills to improve the medical care in the host nation.[1] While these are good motivations, they may not be easily realized. In many places we are prohibited from openly declaring the gospel. To do so may be against the law of the country or against the religious mores of the people we came to serve. Sharing our faith openly may put us, our team, our long term workers or the local church at risk of persecution or reprisals.

Likewise, we need to be wise and sensitive when sharing our expertise. We must earn our right to teach and to speak.[1] The host country may not have the material resources or the social infrastructure or desire to make improvements in the health care system. Academic credentials notwithstanding, it may take several visits or even years until you are asked your opinion. And normally, it is best to wait until you are asked.

In places of the world where we cannot speak the message of the gospel, and perhaps where we can not even teach, we can demonstrate Christ himself to the people if He is truly living in us. We can model "incarnational ministry," representing Christ as best we can through the kind of persons we are and our attitude of mind, rather than in the words we say. If we are constrained by the love of Christ, we are the sweet aroma of Him to those around us- the fragrance of the likeness of Him. The treasure we hold in our earthen vessels will be revealed. We have this treasure in jars of clay; to show that this all-surpassing power and love is from God and not from us and He will draw men unto Himself through us.[1]

Summary

As with all medical outreaches, pointing toward the church is the ultimate goal. Teaching is best done by mimicry and patterning and role modeling is the key.[2] Observing the personal and patient care interactions of a committed Christian health care worker living his/her faith can be truly inspiring and transformational. Your manner, approach, interactions with the sick, the dying and the poor, the thoroughness with which you provide compassionate care is an apologetic for the gospel. In actuality they are not seeing you, but Christ in you through the transforming work of the Holy Spirit.

References

1. Tsang, Reginald in msips.org faq #30, 2004, MSI FAQ.
2. Tsang, Reginald in msips.org faq #51, 2004, MSI FAQ.
3. Tsang, Reginald in msips.org faq #34, 2004, MSI FAQ.
4. Tsang, Reginald in msips.org faq #28, 2004, MSI FAQ.
5. Tsang, Reginald in msips.org faq #26, 2004, MSI FAQ.
6. Tsang, Reginald in msips.org faq #20, 2004, MSI FAQ.

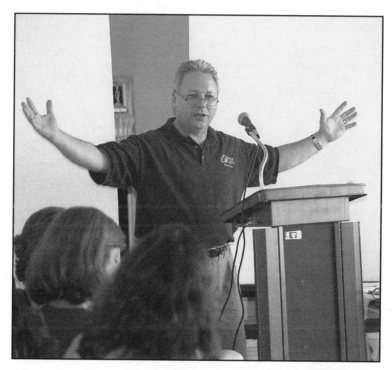

Ted Kuhn/
"David Foster Teaching"

Student Outreach Ministry
Jim Carroll and Hartmut Gross

The goals of student outreach in the context of medical missions ministries differ somewhat from the typical approach to medical missions. Whereas the usual focus is the building up of the local church, the incorporation of students into the process adds the important aspect of teaching and fostering student growth and mentoring the next generation of medical missionaries. Perhaps the main teaching point for the student is that medical missions help the local church grow and flourish. They must realize that a medical team's purpose is to see this intent through as they do their work, and then prepare to step out of the way.

To achieve the goals of student outreach, learners must be mentored in several ways. The first educational stimulus comes with the anticipation of the adverse environmental and medical conditions. Seminars with necessary content to help prepare these novices for the novel situations should be conducted. As appropriate for the planned trip, information about altitude sickness, cold injury, heat illness, infectious diseases, tropical medicine, and local culture must be covered. Especially rewarding is the enthusiasm with which students study and learn this material. This dedication is not entirely surprising, since their lives and well-being will depend on the information. With good pre-field training, the students will be able to "hit the ground running" once they arrive at the destination, ready and knowledgeable, even though not yet experienced. During a typical two weeks period of travel, medical students will have learned more about environmental emergencies and tropical diseases than most physicians learn during their residency or medical practice.

Having experienced these conditions and diseases first hand, the learners will retain this information more permanently.

Students should embrace the idea of working with others in a team setting and must strive to learn and be productive in varied, difficult settings. These environments will be quite different from what they are accustomed. This includes watching, applying and later helping others to learn, as well as looking out for their colleagues, while still being overseen by mentors themselves (e.g. water purification). Handling personal sacrifice at times for the sake of the team is a skill which some must learn (e.g. helping pack up the laboratory while the rest of the team begins a walk through the village). Many individuals experience "culture shock" in a different country, and working in a group may be helpful in adjusting to these feelings.

Teaching in general medical areas is another important goal. The foreign mission field provides a setting where much of the "business" aspect of modern medical practice is stripped away, leaving the core areas of history and physical examination to be explored in more depth and at the most basic level. This is especially true when using nonmedical translators, when one must ask simple questions and be sure that the answer one receives, after several layers of interpretation, is to original query. One must learn to draw upon one's own resourcefulness. There is no specialty lab or x-ray availability. There are no consultants and return visits for reevaluation are not an option. Medical decisions must be made on the spot; this skill and confidence must be learned with time and experience and under sage tutelage. The use of a portable labora-

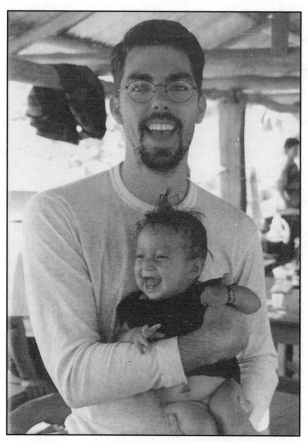

Rick Norton/
"Medical Student and Child"

tory provides a way to learn basic laboratory medicine. Honing the simple skills of phlebotomy and wound care in less than ideal situations helps develop a sense of independence as a health practitioner.

In order to accomplish these goals, the same principles as used for medical teaching in the United States are applied. During clinics the student sees the patient first and then with the preceptor, discussing the case and establishing a diagnosis and treatment. Mentoring relationships will quickly form between student and preceptor. Additional case discussions will occur in the evening and around meals, so that all may daily share and learn from each individual's learning experience.

In addition to general medicine, the students will be exposed to aspects of medicine not encountered in the US. They will see diseases not seen by most US health practitioners: dengue, malaria, measles, leishmaniasis, severe malnutrition, and parasitic infestations, to name a few. It is truly eye-opening to realize through first hand experience, that malaria and tuberculosis are still among the most deadly, common illnesses in the world. Students should be taught to deal with emergencies that may develop in wilderness situations. They must learn to take care of their own health in unsanitary conditions by managing water needs, knowing what to eat and what not to eat to avoid becoming sick themselves.

Debriefing sessions are an important part of the learning process in medical missions. Often, there is considerable and surprising emotional impact in seeing profoundly ill patients in settings with very limited resources. Sometimes the response may be to withdraw from the experience or to harden one's heart for self-protection. Medical teams work in places where pain and death are an everyday reality, and where relief or cures are not anticipated by the indigenous people. The most simple of interventions (e.g. temporary alleviation of pain with Tylenol®) are met with the most profound gratitude. This can be exhilarating, and at the same time deeply disturbing. Debriefing sessions, both during and after the trip, help the student integrate the experience and learn from it, fully.

Growth in the knowledge of the Scripture must be fostered, particularly as it relates to the task at hand. The student should learn to see how the Word of God relates to the work he or she will do and how God cares for His people in different cultural contexts. It is hoped that students will become engendered to involve themselves in medical missions on a longer term basis. In many ways the events of these missions may lead the student to conclude that this is what she or he wishes to do for a life's work.

Trip logistics and the accomplishment of the goals and methods require considerable planning of the venture. From the standpoint of the trip leaders, much thought will be given to logistics for travel, living conditions, and food preparation. This usually entails extra personnel being assigned to the trip several months in advance. For the student, the leaders should give much thought to developing the group dynamic for the trip. Additionally, much attention needs to be paid to the necessary paperwork, passports, visas, and fund raising. Students should be actively involved in all of the preparatory stages of planning the mission to gain insight into the magnitude of the project.

While several months of preparation for a two week trip may seem excessive, the time is well-spent and helps insure that all derive an uplifting and positive learning experience from the trip. As one learner succinctly phrased, "This is what we went into medicine for." Certainly, there are individuals in the developing country who will enjoy lasting physical and spiritual benefit as a result of the medical mission. Mentors will have the satisfaction of watching their pupils grow and learn. But, with their perspectives and life-styles challenged, it will be the students whose lives will be most profoundly affected, as they contemplate and plan their futures.

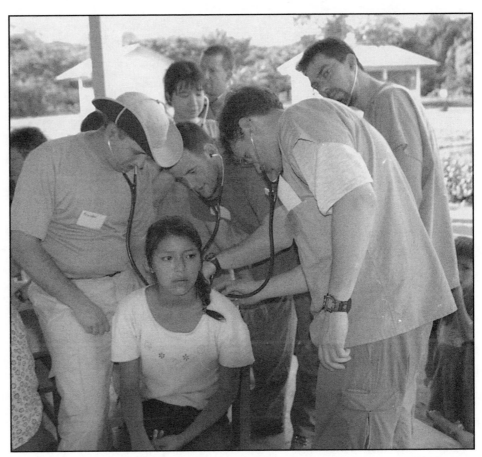

Ted Kuhn/
"Medical Students Listen to the Lungs of a TB Patient"

Reference

1. Kuhn W, International Medicine: A Unique Educational Opportunity for Emergency Medicine Residents and Faculty, *Academic Emergency Medicine*, Vol. 6, No. 7, 1999, pp 765–766.

31 Physical and Occupational Therapy in the Field

Jill Black Lattanzi, Jamie Johnson and Meghan Lee

Physical and occupational therapists are accustomed to working with patients over a significant period of time. They structure physical therapy (PT) and occupational therapy (OT) programs to meet short and long-term goals and conduct interventions to attain these goals. One might ask, what place does a physical or occupational therapist have on a short-term mission project where they might interact with a patient for twenty minutes and then never again? How valuable will their contribution be after such a short intervention?

This chapter will demonstrate the great impact that the rehabilitation professional can have with patients on the short-term mission field. It will examine the theoretical basis for short-term missions, cover cultural considerations, the establishment of sustainable practices, and the importance of joint ministry with the local church. Following a theoretical discussion is a focus on practical considerations in conducting PT and OT practice on the mission field. Considerations for PT and OT students on the field and a list of resources are provided.

Theoretical Considerations for Physical and Occupational Therapists in the Field

Physical therapists (PTs) and occupational therapists (OTs) possess tremendous potential to make vast differences in the lives of the patients in the mission field. Rehabilitative services are sparsely available in developing countries and if offered, they are limited in scope and inaccessible to the very poor. Persons who suffer strokes, spinal cord injuries, or head traumas are often medically stabilized and sent home without rehabilitative services. Children with developmental delays rarely receive PT or OT, or rehabilitative equipment such as walkers, wheelchairs, splints, and prostheses which are usually too expensive and or not available. PTs and OTs possess the knowledge, expertise and resources to make a tremendous difference in patients' functional abilities.

During the short-term mission, the PTs' and OTs' approach to the rehabilitation challenges must be different than their approach in their traditional home environment. Instead of designing a program entailing regular visits over the next month, the clinician in the field must ask the question, "what can I teach, give, or instruct the patients' family in the next 20 minutes that will make a functional difference for the long-term?"

For example, persons who have suffered a stroke often have difficulty with transfers and ambulation and yet with an appropriate assistive device and training, they may become ambulatory. A patient in rural Mexico learned to ambulate with a crutch, an Ace® wrap for the subsequent foot drop, and an arm sling. The missionary therapist taught the daughter how to assist with gait training, including training on uneven terrain. When the therapist revisited the man a year later, he was not at home because he had walked across town to visit his brother without the crutch! The daughter returned the crutch with great thanks and hope that someone else would now benefit from it (below).

Persons with arthritic knees, hips, and feet suffer immensely as many depend upon their legs as their major mode of transportation. Total joint replacements are not typically an option. The missionary therapist can make a tremendous difference simply by issuing an appropriate assistive device

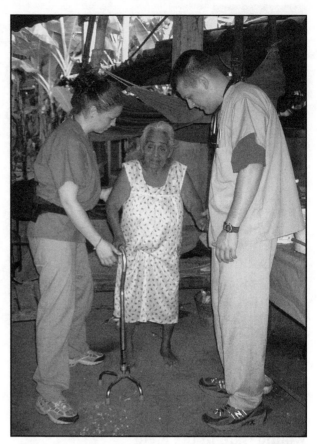

"This woman presents with degenerative arthritis of her hips and knees. She did well with the quad cane. Two student PTs conducted the assessment and intervention during the home visit."

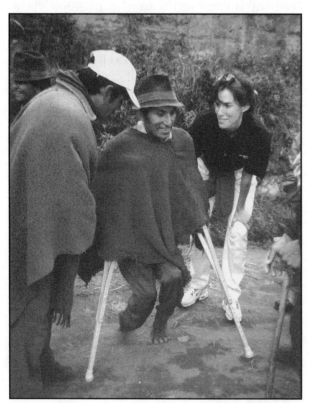

Jill Lattanzi/
"Patient was Non-ambulatory Prior to PT's Arrival"

and providing instruction in appropriate muscle building exercises (above). Children with disabilities benefit greatly from supportive splints, seating and positioning instructions, neuro-developmental activities that a parent can perform, and pediatric chairs when possible. A pediatric therapist can accomplish a great deal with a little in this environment.

The prime consideration in the provision of care is that it must be sustainable. Scenarios in the field are numerous and varied and no matter what kind of problem is encountered, the therapist should seek to insure that the interventions chosen are maintained in some way. Sustainable care constitutes care that can be continued within the context of the environment without the continued presence and intervention of the therapist. Constructing or giving a donated assistive device is an example of sustainable care. The patient is able to keep the device and continue using it in the therapist's absence. Exercise instruction is another good example of sustainable care as long as the exercises can be performed without special equipment. The competent therapist creatively adapts the exercises to the patient's resources within their environment. Theraband® is easily transported into the field, can be given to the patient, and can provide resistance to specific exercises in a myriad of ways; patients can continue exercising on their own. Fabricated splints and supports that are given to the patient are sustainable. So are any instructions to the family or patient that can be carried out without the therapist.

Ultrasound, moist heat, cold, and manual techniques are usually not sustainable and may have minimal impact on the short-term mission field. Even TENS units are not truly sustainable as they will require replacement electrodes and batteries.

Some are critical of the practice of bringing rehabilitative equipment into the country for distribution.[1] Whenever possible, materials indigenous to the area should be used to construct assistive equipment. Ideally, persons in the community would undergo training in the creation and construction of needed equipment and thus provide a sustainable service as well as create jobs for community members.

Cultural Considerations in Providing Physical and Occupational Therapy Care

The physical and occupational therapist must consider cultural differences in order to effectively interact with a patient in the field. All PT and OT interactions have the potential for cultural misunderstanding that may result in barriers to care.

The therapist will first consider his or her own cultural values and understandings. If the therapist is from the United States, he or she will most likely manifest the values of the individualistic U.S. culture (Table 1).

Table 1. Individualistic vs. Collectivistic Cultural Characteristics

Considerations for the Physical and Occupational Therapist

- Individualism/privacy vs. collectivism/group
- Time dominates vs. human interaction
- Precise time vs. loose time
- Future oriented vs. past oriented
- Doing (achieving) vs. being (personal growth)
- Competition vs. cooperation
- Human equality vs. hierarchy/rank/status
- Self-help vs. birthright inheritance
- Informality vs. formality
- Directness vs. indirectness
- Practicality/efficiency vs. idealism/theory
- Values youth vs. values elders

The common values include the importance of autonomy, independence, youth and productivity. In contrast, the rest of the world largely exhibits the values of a collectivist culture, which places a higher importance on the group rather than the individual. Thus, family and extended family and communities are considered in making major decisions. Likewise, collectivist cultures value elders and associate age with wisdom while individualistic cultures exalt youth and devalue elders. Rather than cherishing independence, the collectivist culture values interdependence.

The U.S. culture places an emphasis on time according to the clock and planning for the future. Time according to the clock is not as important in collectivist cultures and time is centered around the relationships or the activities. Collectivistic time orientation is more past or present rather than future oriented. Particularly in developing countries, the patient may be most concerned with the overwhelming cares of the present and have difficulty seeing ahead to the future. A cultural encounter between an individualist and a collectivist has the potential to clash for all of these reasons. The PT and OT professions are clearly more reflective of individualistic culture with future- orientation, an emphasis on long-term goals, and an emphasis upon independence and autonomy.

A common cultural clash with physical and occupational therapists occurs when the family of the patient insists upon assisting the patient rather than encouraging the patient's independence. Therapists often misunderstand this clash but culturally competent clinicians will recognize that an interdependence rather than independence is what is needed within the family dynamics. The therapist will find ways to incorporate the need for interdependence within the family while encouraging and expressing the potential of the patient to develop greater independence.

The PTs or OTs must also guard against the natural tendency to be ethnocentric. Ethnocentrism is the universal tendency of people to think that their ways of thinking, acting, and behaving are the only right, appropriate, and accurate ways.[2] Note that this tendency is universal—all parties in the cultural encounter tend to believe that their ways are the right ways. The PT or OT must be careful to consider interventions and ways of interaction that might be foreign. For example, a gentleman presented at a clinic in Mexico with arthritic knee pain. After learning a series of exercises to strengthen his knee musculature, he indicated that he would like to receive one of the canes that had come from the United States. The therapist easily could have given him a cane, but instead, looked closely at the cane he had. It had been constructed from polyvinylchloride (PVC) piping and was sized appropriately and fitted with a "T" cross piece for a handhold. She offered to put a crutch tip on the bottom of the cane and told him that the cane he had fashioned was actually very appropriate. She suggested that the patient could start a business of making and selling canes to those in his community who needed them. The

patient appeared to be quite pleased with the praise. A student physical therapist in the field creatively began to transform patients' walking sticks and fashion them into more appropriate canes by cutting them to the right size and fitting them with a crutch tip and axillary pads at the handhold. The PT or OT on the short-term mission field must consider the cultural encounters that will occur and be prepared to examine themselves and their choice of intervention as well as the perspective and cultural values of the patient if the interaction is to be effective.

Meeting Physical and Spiritual Needs of Patients with the Help of the Local Church

Of course, physical therapists and occupational therapists are attempting to meet the physical needs of patients, which are temporal. We know that all physical bodies degenerate with time and age and all will physically die. Our spirits, however, will live eternally. Christ is our example as He healed physical needs but exhibited primary concern for the spiritual state of people. Physical therapists and occupational therapist can follow Christ's example and strive to meet physical and spiritual needs of the patients.

The local church can be an instrument of healing, meeting the spiritual needs of the patients. In fact the physical and occupational ministry functions best in conjunction with the ministry of the local church. Often the missionary therapists will draw people with physical needs from the community, or will penetrate into the community to find those with physical disabilities. Having local church members as a part of the ministry gives credibility to the foreign therapists, as well as, allows the local body of believers to begin relationships with those served. The local believers will be the ones to follow-up with the patients spiritually long after the short-term missionaries are gone. In this way the spiritual outreach to the patients will have a greater likelihood of being sustainable.

The physical and occupational therapy mission should never conflict with the local church. The PT and OT missionaries should seek out the local church and learn of their needs and their perspective of the needs of their community. The local believers can be an excellent resource for understanding the culture and climate of the community. The church should be encouraged to see the PT and OT mission as part of their own ministry. The foreign clinicians simply provide support to the ongoing mission of the local church.

Practical Considerations for Physical and Occupational Therapists in the Field

Locating appropriate patients for physical and occupational therapy ministry can be challenging for a number of reasons. First, many times the people are not familiar with the practice of PT and OT and therefore do not understand what conditions a therapist can help. Indeed, sometimes a translation for "physical or occupational therapist" does not exist or is an unfamiliar term to the people in the community. In rural Mexico, a physical therapist is often confused with a *huesera* or "bone doctor"—a traditional healer with little formal training.

The first visit to a community may entail extensive education as to who the therapists might help. Therapists may find themselves turning away many who come with stomach pain, vision problems, or other complaints beyond the PT or OT scope of practice. The PTs or OTs might display the available assistive and adaptive equipment available and provide specific examples of treatable physical conditions, in order to facilitate understanding of the types of conditions that the therapist might assist.

Secondly, health care providers in general are not always aware of the therapist scope of practice. The therapist should not assume that because a medical practitioner does not see the need for a therapist that the need does not exist. United States medicine has become so specialized that often practitioners do not fully understand what the other is capable of doing. Practicing on the short-term mission field with a team of medical personnel provides an environment for learning more about each other's area of practice. The therapist should take advantage of this time to communicate and collaborate with fellow medical colleagues regarding the practice of physical and occupational therapies and their benefits on the field.

Lastly, the location of appropriate patients may be stymied by stereotypes and discriminatory practices of the society. Often physical disability is hidden and not readily visible to the public. Even the United States, as late as the 1920s, hid the fact that Franklin D. Roosevelt used a wheelchair after suffering polio. The Americans with Disabilities Act passed in 1994 has done much to improve accessibility and acceptance for persons with disabilities, but the U.S. society is still not completely comfortable with the differences. Other countries and other cultures possess the same tendencies to hide or de-emphasize those with physical disabilities. Disabled children and adults are out there in every society. Often they are behind closed doors, well-cared for by their loved ones, but hidden by a society uncomfortable and less accepting of the person with physical disabilities. The therapist should persist in inquiring for those in the community with physical disabilities. Sometimes trust must be gained before the community will take the therapist to those in need. The therapist should wait and pray that the Lord would lead him or her to those in need of PT or OT assistance. Those cut-off from society due to a physical disability are especially in need of experiencing the Lord's loving touch through the hands and expertise of the therapist. By taking a church member along on the visit, the church member can help make the spiritual connection and can model love and acceptance of the person as well.

The Outpatient Clinic

The outpatient clinic is simple to establish for PT and OT services. One needs an open area, preferably with shade from the heat or protection from the cold and acceptable waiting area for the patients. Typically, curtained or private areas are not required. Instead, a few chairs, a table or an exercise mat, and space are all that are needed.

The therapist can expect to see orthopedic conditions much like one would see in the United States in an outpatient ambulatory clinic. Common conditions include arthritic knees and hips, back and neck pain, foot and ankle pain, and shoulder pain and dysfunction. The therapist should quickly consider the exercises, instructions, and assistive devices or supportive equipment that would make the most sustainable difference for each patient.

In addition to orthopedic conditions, the therapist can expect to see some neurological conditions such as ambulatory or nonambulatory stroke or polio patients. Sometimes non-ambulatory patients may be brought to the clinic in a wheelbarrow, on a donkey, or carried by several family members. Children with neurological disabilities may or may not be ambulatory as their family can carry them to the clinic. Again, the therapist should consider the most functional differences he or she can make with exercises, instructions, or equipment accessible to the patient.

Community Home Visits

While the outpatient clinic is simple and the most expedient way to reach a large number of patients, the community home visits often yield very significant results. When the patient comes to the clinic, the therapist is unable to fully understand the potential barriers and obstacles the patient may encounter in their daily routine. Traveling to the home allows the therapist to understand the terrain and its challenges, the conditions of the home and potential barriers, meet the family support system, and make the most appropriate recommendations.

Obviously, when making a home visit, the therapist is more likely to encounter the people with major mobility challenges. These patients stand to benefit the greatest from the assistance of the therapist. If

therapists can take the time to get out to the home, they have the potential to make a significant difference in someone's mobility making the mutually rewarding experience more than worth the effort.

Wound Care in the Field

In addition to providing for the myriad orthopedic needs and facilitating functional independence, PTs and OTs can greatly assist in the care of wounds. The presence of decubitus and diabetic ulcers, machete wounds, burns from grenades or firearms, and pressure wounds from orthopedic malformities that create non-traditional means of weight-bearing, are just a few of the common wound findings in any country on the mission field. By debriding wound eschar and necrotic tissue to promote a proliferative granulation bed, the therapist begins the healing process. Patient education follows about the process and frequency of wound cleansing as well as how to wrap and protect the wound. The therapist should also provide the patient with a "goodie bag" of supplies, including sterile bandages, gauze, Kerlix,® and antibiotic ointments that will assist the patient for at least one week's duration of cleansing and help contribute to the sustainability of the intervention. Depending on the location of the wound, ambulatory education and appropriate assistive devices and splints may be necessary to prevent weight-bearing on an open and healing wound and to assist with function.

The high standards of wound care established in the United States must be upheld on the mission field. In the United States, a sterile environment is almost always attainable. The mission field provides challenges in this area. A typical scene is a clinic site created among the dirt floors of a rural village hut, a bench or broken chair for the patient to rest on, and hundreds of other patients crowding with anticipation nearby waiting to be seen. Despite these physical challenges, it remains essential to achieve the cleanest environment possible. This includes establishing a separate location for all sterile bandages and sharp debride-

Table 2. Wound Care Supply List for Physical Therapists on the Mission Field

- Gloves
- Sharps container
- Sterile table covering
- Kerlix® (several rolls)
- Sterile and non-sterile 4x4s (several packages)
- Sharp debridement: scalpels, tweezers, small scissors
- Wound Cleansing solution
- Saline Solution (preferably in a flush bottle)
- Hydrogen Peroxide
- Triple Antibiotic ointment
- Burn Cream
- Betadine®: bottle and swabs
- Q-tips® (2–3 packages)
- Tongue depressors (to spread ointment)
- Silvadene®
- Bucket/plastic bed pan (to soak extremities)
- Ace® bandages
- Tape (to secure bandages)

ment tools, from used scalpels and cleaning supplies (Table 2).

The clean/sterile environment must be established before the wound care procedures are performed. Hand washing and frequent changing of gloves are imperative. While it is important to strive toward high standards of cleanliness and sterilization, adaptability to the culture and environment are essential when faced with the challenges of wound care on the mission field.

Psychosocial Needs

Many patients present with a state of hopelessness as they are overshadowed by a wound that they believe will remain with them the rest of their lives. What a difference a therapist can make toward the healing of a wound, but more importantly to see how this care opens the door for the psychological, emotional, and spiritual healing of the patient as well. For example, a therapist had the opportunity to care for the wounds of an "outcast" in a tribal Amazon village. The patient's initial embarrassment to emerge from his tribal hut, much less expose his mouth that had been eaten away by a parasitic disease, became a trusting friendship as the patient saw the unconditional love displayed through the physical therapist's gentle and tender care for his wound. Through caring for this man for three days while in his village, not only did the wound tissue begin to proliferate and granulate, but also the man's heart softened to the loving truths of Christ.

On another occasion, an entire minority community was discovered in a small compound in the Philippines. Upon examination, over half of the community had skin lesions covering their entire body that had resulted from a contaminated water source. Physical therapists spent hours cleansing and applying topical antibiotic agents to wounds. Through the therapists' wound care, treatment, and education to the group, the disease was controlled. These are just a few of the many miracles that Christ has performed through physical therapists' wound care treatment and how Christ has used wound care to impact the physical and spiritual lives of patients on the mission field.

Equipment Needs

The physical and occupational therapy equipment list (Table 3 on next page) lists the recommended equipment to bring. Transporting equipment into the field is usually best accomplished by each team member carrying and checking a parcel. Four or five walkers can be duct-taped together and a packet and 6 or 7 pair of crutches can be packaged in the same manner. Large duffle bags are helpful for transporting canes, quad canes, splints, braces, and wound care materials.

Remember, all cargo should be sustainable. Leave ultrasound machines, TENS units and anything else that requires an electrical supply or batteries at home. Save

Table 3. Physical and Occupational Therapy Missions Trip Equipment List

- Folding walkers (rolling & standard)
- Crutches (wooden & aluminum, small & medium heights)
- Quad canes
- Straight canes (wooden & aluminum)
- Crutch tips & axillary pads
- Rolls of Theraband®
- Exercise pages (translated)
- Exercise mats
- Arm slings
- Miscellaneous wraps & supports

the space and utilize your time with the patient in ways that will benefit the patient the most for the long-term and in the your absence.

Students in the Field

All first year students possess enough knowledge and skill base to make great contributions in the field. After the first year of class work, a student has acquired basic examination and evaluation techniques, intervention skills, and a background in anatomy, physiology, and pathology. These tools and knowledge will allow the student to perform basic evaluations and interventions in the field. In fact, the field provides an excellent challenge as students find themselves without the assistance of technology or expensive equipment. They need to take their basic knowledge and creatively adapt PT and OT interventions to the situation to achieve the desired functional outcome.

Students gain independence, confidence, and cultural competency in the mission field. In traditional clinical affiliations, students are allowed to participate in evaluation and treatment of patients with follow-up as needed to achieve specific long and short-term goals.

In the short-term mission field, students are allowed to perform evaluations and treatment without the constraints of typical hospital or clinic settings. This freedom allows for more instruction time between therapist and students and also more time with the patient. Because follow-up care is seldom available, students must practice one of their most valuable tools: education. Providing education across cultural and communication barriers provides an excellent opportunity for students to refine their communication and education skills.

Students may consider pursuing school credit for their field experience and have successfully done so in the past. Many schools allow for independent studies or elective clinical affiliations. The criteria set forth in the American Physical Therapy Association's (APTA) Clinical Performance Instrument (CPI) to determine skills needed for performance as an entry-level therapist may be easily adapted to fit a cross-cultural setting and may serve as a guide for writing objectives to justify credit. For example, the CPI identifies the adaptation of delivery of physical therapy services to reflect respect for and sensitivity to individual differences as a very important skill for therapists and likewise would be an appropriate objective for a cross-cultural experience.[3] Another CPI criteria relates to the education of patients, family, caregivers, and other health care providers. Education is crucial for sustainable care of the patient after the student has returned home and would be another appropriate objective when preparing proposals for independent or elective study. Students may choose to write objectives relating to cultural competency, language, communication skills, evaluation techniques and interventions in the cross-cultural setting.

Conclusion

Physical and occupational therapists can make a substantial difference in the physical mobility or wound healing of a patient in the short-term. More importantly, physical and occupational therapists have the potential to minister alongside the local church and make a significant impact in a patient's spiritual healing. Caring for the patient opens doors to show the compassion and love of Christ to a patient who presents with the embarrassment, shame, or hardship of a wound or physical disability.

Acknowledging the patient as person with spiritual and emotional needs and not as a wound or disabled person is a response that is often unknown to the individual. Our attention to detail and the time spent touching a patient establishes a trust relationship that often leads to opportunities to share about Christ's tender and compassionate love for them and His care and concern about every detail in their life. May physical and occupational therapists, physical therapist assistants, occupational therapy assistants, and students answer the call to the short-term mission field and see what the Lord will do. May His name be praised!

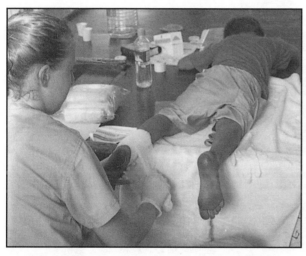

Ted Kuhn/
"PT Dressing Wound in the Field"

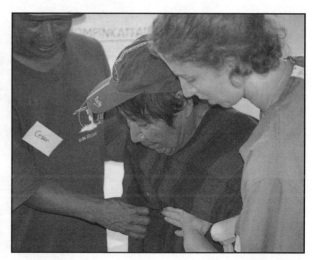

Ted Kuhn/
"Walking Again"

References

1. Purnell LD, Paulanka BJ: *Transcultural Health Care: A Culturally Competent Approach,* 2nd ed., Philadelphia, F.A. Davis, 2003.
2. Werner D: *Disabled Village Children: A Guide for Community Health Workers, Rehabilitation Workers, and Families,* 2nd ed., Palo Alto, CA, Hesperian Foundation, 1994.
3. American Physical Therapy Association CPI Instrument. Available at http://www.apta.org/Education/enrolledstudents/compBasedCPI/cpi_student.

Resources

1. Werner D: *Disabled Village Children,* Hesperian Foundation. It is available in multiple languages. The book has many illustrations and focuses upon interventions for disabled children utilizing the resources common in a rural village.
2. Leavitt R: *Cross-cultural Rehabilitation: An international perspective,* W.B. Saunders. Written by a physical therapist.
3. VHI exercise software has the ability to print out exercises in several different languages.
4. Theraband® product is available through the Hygienic Corporation and sometimes is available at no cost for PT and OT mission trips.

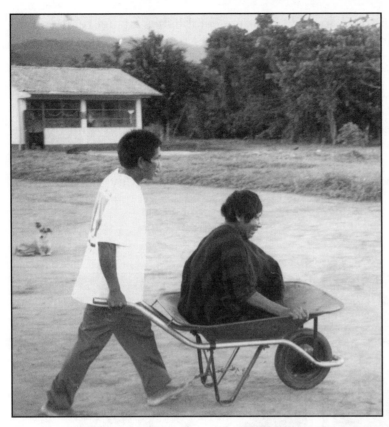

Ted Kuhn/
"From Wheelbarrow..."

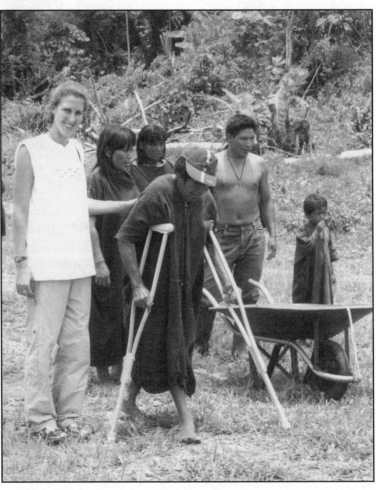

Ted Kuhn/
"to Walking"

The Village Walk: Finding Simple Solutions to Complex Problems

Hartmut Gross

Seeing someone floating by, drowning in a river you are standing beside, you instinctively reach out to rescue the individual. And a short while later, when another victim comes by, you pull him out too. And over time, as more and more victims float by, you may begin working out a sophisticated system by which you and helpers can rescue one drowning victim after the next. At some point, it may dawn on you to walk upstream and find out why all these people keep falling into the river. Perhaps there is a narrow, slippery path or a broken bridge. Recognizing a problem and carrying out a few simple measures may make a great difference and potentially even resolve the calamity. Providing medical relief work in the developing world is no different.

Upon setting up a short-term clinic in any type of setting, the medical team should quickly obtain an epidemiologic sense of what illnesses are prevalent in the community. Careful history taking and physical examinations along with some simple screens of blood, sputum, and stool will yield the diagnoses so that proper treatment may be initiated. Malaria, TB, *Cryptosporidium*, malnutrition, *Ascaris*, and hookworm, to name a few, can all be identified and the sick individuals be cured. But the next question should be, "Why are these people getting these illnesses?"—is there something we can do to prevent this?"

A leisurely team walk through the village at the end of the day does far more than relieve the stress of a busy, hectic clinic, if one keeps a sharp eye and an open mind. Children will tag along and play beside you. Several of the patients seen and treated during the clinic will be recognized and they will wave as they tend to some final evening activities before dark. The people are in their element and dressed and interacting the way they normally do from day to day. Some careful observation will answer some of the following sample questions to address the corresponding concerns:

Observations	Concerns Addressed
Protective clothing	Insect borne illness protection
Windows or screens in the home	Insect borne illness protection
Mosquito nets in use	Insect borne illness protection
Shoes	Hook worm
Houses in good repair	Poverty level assessment
Mats on the floors	Poverty level assessment
Kept up yards with flowers	Poverty level assessment
Cooking done over an open fire	Cough and eyes itching
Cooking indoors over a fire	Cough and eyes itching
People carry heavy loads	Back pain and headaches
Village well runs dry daily	Dizziness from dehydration
Running water	Basic hygiene
Bathroom area near water source	Cholera and other GI infections
Crops	Sufficient quantity and nutritious
Adverse outside influences	New illnesses, drain on resources

No preassembled check-off list of questions can be complete. However, careful observation may prompt the correct questions to identify a problem. The following are some real scenarios encountered and the simple solutions which corrected the problems.

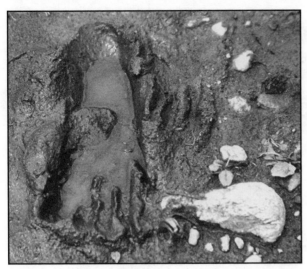

Ted Kuhn/
"Barefoot in the Jungle"

Example 1: A rural village in Honduras was found to have an epidemic of unresolved diarrhea several months after Hurricane Mitch. Stool samples confirmed a diagnosis of *Entamoeba*. The village walk revealed that there was a water tank which had been constructed a number of years earlier. There appeared to be a chlorinating device on one side clogged with branches and debris from the storm. A subsequent team with engineers was sent shortly afterward and repaired the system. Follow up showed that the diarrhea epidemic had resolved.

Example 2: An Amazon village with a cholera epidemic had many patients with severe dehydration and a number of villagers had already died. The village walk showed the pit latrines to be directly beside the village water supply. Basic education and digging of new latrines on the other side of the village stopped the development of new cases and with the treatment and resolution of the infected patients, health was restored to the community.

Example 3: In Myanmar, an outbreak of multi-drug resistant malaria was devastating several remote villages. Visiting the village demonstrated that no mosquito protection was being used. Once this was recognized, the introduction and instruction of use of permethrin-impregnated mosquito

nets dramatically reduced the incidence of new cases of malaria.

Example 4: Villages with contaminated streams as the sole water source have had teams return to drill wells. Others have had tubing run from further upstream to provide running water directly into the village. With teaching, personal hygiene that was previously barely known, has improved.

Example 5: Some problems are subtler to recognize. In the clinic, women may be noted to have stained oral mucosa and teeth. The village walk may show pots of thick liquid with the same color as the mouth staining. This regularly turns out to be a fermenting mash for making alcohol. Alcoholism may not be readily recognized and must be suspected to be identified.

Example 6: Malnourishment may have various underlying reasons. In one Amazon village, it was noted that after a one-year hiatus of a team visit, there was a marked increase in malnutrition. The society had encountered increasing contact with the outside world as a result of loggers in the area harvesting trees. Most of the village men were even working for the loggers and earning some money. How could this lead to malnutrition? The answer became evident during the village walk, looking at trash and debris lying around the village, and asking a few questions.

In many primitive Amazon cultures, it is taught from generation to generation that eating yucca root is all that is needed to survive. The other fruits and berries, while pleasant, may be foregone. Unfortunately, the starchy tuber staple is little more than that and far from sufficient dietarily. But with that little supplementation of other foods, the villagers do manage to survive. But now the loggers brought radios, flashlights, hair clips, and a myriad of other flashy, luring items. Food suddenly became a low priority. Money and food were traded for useless items, unwittingly at the expense of their own health. A long discussion was held with the village elders about the poor health of the villagers and the likely reasons for the deteriorated state. It confirmed their vague suspicions that bad influences were present. They just hadn't made the connection yet. Discussing the villagers' misguided decisions was very enlightening for the elders and the community. This intervention has helped many of the tribe's people back to better health again.

Unfortunately, other insidious influences such as tuberculosis and alcohol from the outside have also been introduced and are taking their toll. While these are far more difficult to detect on the village walk, empty bottles may be found.

Close living accommodations will be noticed. Many of the malnourished natives in this area actually develop blonde hair and can be spotted from across the village. Consider how you might try to help these people with these problems. A few questions revealed that local health workers occasionally visit to look for and treat tuberculosis patients and that food programs are available. Due to the remoteness and the social workers getting only a few hours of training, these programs have difficulty being effective. Identifying the cases for these social services and steering the resources to the most urgently needy or ill, helps greatly to facilitate the existing national programs.

Instinctively, when seeing extreme poverty, one has the urge to give money, plant food,

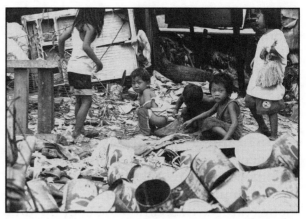

Ted Kuhn/
"Children Playing in Garbage, Slums of Manila."

and build homes for these communities. It seems counterintuitive at first, but sometimes this is the worst thing one can do, because it builds dependence upon the outside. Many villages in the past have demonstrated that they do not comprehend concepts of preparing for the future; they have after all, lived their entire lives from day to day. It is much like the story of the poultry farmer who gave his poor neighbor 5 hens and a rooster, teaching him how to care for them so they could provide eggs and more chicks. When he visited the poor man a year later and asked about the chickens, the response was, "Those 6 chickens tasted good."

Instead, these people must first realize and acknowledge that they have a problem. Next, they must determine that the problem is great enough to do something about, and worth their while and worth using some of their own resources to correct the problem. Only then is it time to begin supplying labor and supplies in graded amounts. It is better to teach the villagers to plow the fields with a donkey than to fly in a donated plow. Sadly, the plow would be used a few times, but then not be maintained because of ignorance and lack of money to buy fuel, oil or parts, and will fall into useless disrepair. This may seem very harsh. Indeed it is difficult to watch someone struggle when one knows many easier ways to accomplish tasks. But if not done by them, the villagers do not learn the skill; they do not appreciate the worth, and do not invest in building their own future.

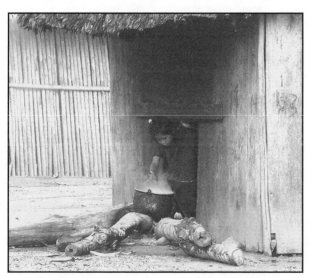

Hartmut Gross/
"Children Near Pot of Boiling Water"

It is important to remember that the people you are there to serve and help are nonetheless sovereign and you must respect the cultural differences, no matter how much you disagree with them. You cannot change everything overnight. Instead, choose to change and improve the right things at the right time. Choose a project that is easy and that you know will succeed. Don't take on more than the local community can handle, and don't make changes that cannot be kept up after you leave. Don't despair; your presence will make a difference. Future teams can expand the groundwork that you have initiated.

While walking through a village, do not forget to pause and enjoy its simplicity, the surrounding scenery, and appreciate the cultural experience. Enjoy the stroll, play with the children, catch some butterflies, kick a ball around, throw a Frisbee,® wave hello, and get to know the village and its people better.

33 Influencing Change in the Community

John Sexton

During my first medical missions trip in the summer of 1981, I had the opportunity to go to La Gonáve, Haiti, to work with a veteran missionary physician with over 20 years experience. I was thrilled to be able to work with him. We saw dozens of patients each day. One morning, he asked me what illnesses we attended that day. I did a quick summing up, and replied: "Malaria, tuberculosis and worms." He then asked which ones were preventable, and I admitted that almost all were preventable. Sadly, he said that if he had started with prevention more than 20 years before, he wouldn't need to be treating most of these illnesses today.

Short-term medical teams do gratifying work, it is one of the reasons we are drawn to them. We give back part of what God has generously given us by treating those less fortunate and we directly assist the national church with their work. Medical missions show God's love to the world and relieve suffering from health, dental and emotional problems. Additionally, the medical teams are welcomed by the community and the local church; they are invited to help prevent the illnesses and injuries that continually plague the local population. The teams are there for a short time. Many individuals will be cured, indeed some will be saved from certain death, and others will be eased from their pain and suffering, at least for a while. Yet people will continue contracting the same illnesses that were just treated. Many participants on medical trips are primary care professionals who know the importance of continued intervention to bring about improved health and are accustomed to following up on patients or to referring them to other specialists. They find they don't have this option available in this setting. Nonetheless, with some insight, sensitivity and creativity, important impacts may be made on these communities, even without the provision of typical after care to which we are accustomed.

As medical professionals, we tend to think of health and illnesses only in terms of pathophysiology. We are accustomed to looking for a medicine to treat an illness. However, impacting the health of communities, families, and individuals often can be accomplished by simple nonmedical means.

Illustrative example: A community along the American border in Mexico had a very high rate of diarrhea, and skin infections. Starting a clinic had been discussed. One observer noted that there was no running water; residents said this was a common problem in the communities along the border. Closer questioning revealed the cause for the water shortage. What was discovered, was simply that the trucks that bring water to communities could not enter because of the large holes in the roads. Merely providing shovels, wheelbarrows and other simple tools to fill in the holes greatly decreased the health problems of the community by allowing the trucks to bring in water to the community!

There are a variety of methods that can be used in assessing health and physical needs. Usually a combination of methods will be most effective. Once needs are assessed, goals can be developed and planning implemented. What follows are a few methods that a short-term team can apply to assess needs.

Going Prepared

In most rural communities in developing countries, there is a tremendous need for acute medical care, and there are often overwhelming numbers of people coming for help. Sometimes team members go without eating or getting sufficient rest, rejoicing that they are truly being used. However, each team should be encouraged to think about this issue before leaving home and examine the issue each evening during their presence in the community. It is important that team members commit to reserving time for developing solutions to the common problems they are seeing.

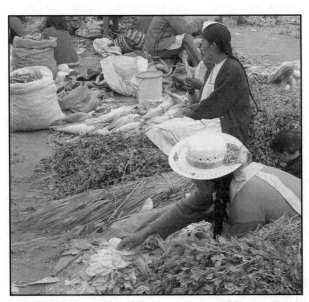

John Sexton/
"Assessing Diet in Quechua Market."

It is helpful to contact the missionaries in advance to get an idea of what problems exist and how they affecting the health of the residents in the community. Communication with previous teams can be helpful and the Internet is useful for researching diseases found in the area, locally available resources, the economy of the region, and other useful information. It may become apparent, for instance, that an orthopedic physician or a physical therapist would be invaluable for your team. Reading up on diseases, treatments, follow-up care and prevention should be done by all team members.

Illustrative example: Diabetes is very prevalent among the Belizean people. A team traveling to Belize might consider that recruiting a nurse specialized in diabetes or a nutritionist would be an asset to the team. Every member of the team should know the effects of diabetes, the impact on their area of specialty, and how to help improve patient care. In addition, bringing a large supply of commonly used and inexpensive diabetic medicines that can also be found and continued in Belize will be helpful. It is important to check with the field before bringing medicines and equipment to be sure resources are going toward what is needed.

Patient Logs

Each team should keep an accurate log of the people that they see each day and their medical problems. This is not only helpful in planning future teams, but it will also help in the recognition of common problems in the community. Each evening as a part of the routine debriefing time, the team can review the patient log looking for problems that are repeated or linked. Especially with larger teams or a busy clinic, these may not be so obvious during the clinic hours. Reviewing the individual incidences will shine light on common problems.

Illustrative example: Team members may see diarrhea and intestinal parasites among school-aged children. Individually, it may not appear epidemiologically significant. However, from the collective experience recorded in the log, it may be apparent that the incidence of diarrhea and intestinal parasites is high among children of similar age. Once recognized, it may be logical to give all the children (and adults) a dose of albendazole (Albenza®) for intestinal parasites. It may also be helpful to check the water source at the school where the children get their drinking water during school hours. In one rural Mexican community, most families used purified bottled water in the homes. However, the children drank from drinking fountains at the schools that did not have a purifying system. Discussion with teachers about bringing bottled water from home for the children reduced waterborne illnesses and improved the health and learning of their students. Alternatively, the visiting medical team could even purchase a few jugs of water to donate to the school, since the initial deposit for the bottle is often more expensive than the water itself. The initial investment may be minimal, yet produce a substantial public health intervention.

Walk Through the Community

Sometimes just walking through the community can bring both problems and solutions to light. Observant team members will see many things that are positive in the community that can be used to suggest solutions. You are encouraged to take several walks through the community during your time there. Often you will be able to see:

- How social the people are
- What their main diet is
- The health of children
- How the children are playing
- Where the water supply is and where people urinate and defecate
- Where and how the garbage is disposed
- What school and health facilities are like
- If the housing is adequate for the climate and how it impacts the health of individuals
- Churches

- Government facilities
- If there are loose animals
- What the health hazards are
- Common illnesses throughout the community that you have seen in the clinic
- The type of work the people do
- The ages of the people
- Closeness of the community to roads, rivers, and other transportation
- The economic level of the people
- Security risks

Obviously this list is incomplete. Active observation will produce other helpful information. With this information it is possible to begin making possible correlations.

- Is there a correlation between the water source, loose animals, garbage, etc. to the number of parasite cases you saw in the clinic?
- Does there seem to be a sense of community interaction, such as cooking together, washing together, groups congregating, parks or plazas, or other evidence that may relate to the community working together on a problem?
- Is the housing crowded, with multi-families, poorly ventilated, or on wet ground that may affect the health of the occupants?

Illustrative example: Participating with a medical team in two Indian villages deep in the jungle of Peru, it was noticed there was very little tuberculosis in the first village, but substantially more tuberculosis in the second village. Walking through the villages, the two were compared. The first village was isolated and initially appeared "poor," i.e., the houses were bamboo huts with thatched roofs. The second village was on a road and the community sold lumber giving them a cash crop. The houses were built with cut lumber from a sawmill, and each had a metal roof. Because of living on a road, the people were more concerned about security. The houses were enclosed and did not allow ventilation, which kept the germs in higher concentrations and infected whole families. The importance of adding ventilation to the homes to decrease tuberculosis, colds, and other airborne pathogens was shared with the village leaders, so that they could begin making these lasting changes after the team left.

Incorporate Community Health Leaders

No matter how isolated or small a community, there will be some community-recognized health leaders. It may be the medical director of a trauma center or simply the oldest woman of the village, but these people are the ones the community looks to in matters of health. Whoever this person may be, it is important to recognize his or her position, realizing that they will be in the community long after the team leaves. If it is possible to assist this leader do his or her responsibilities better, it will likely improve the health of the entire community. Working to enhance the position of these leaders and build the trust of the community may have long-term effects. Likewise, ignoring them may have detrimental effects. Simply including the leader in the team will help their credibility and influence with the community. In addition, their insight into problems, culture, resources, language, etc., can be very helpful. By ignoring the local leadership, the team may face resistance rather than support and appreciation.

Some health leaders may be physicians who can directly help the team. Even if their standards of practice are not considered to be at our level, our witness and example may improve their practice, care and compassion for the people that they are serving.

Many health workers in developing countries are lay workers. Some only teach prevention of illnesses. Some only handle malaria problems. Some only deliver babies. Many have a combination of responsibilities. Again, whatever their roles, it is important to include them. It will help them become better in their jobs by teaching, encouraging, and publicly praising them.

In the author's personal experience working two years with village health promoters in the jungle villages of Peru, the health promoters were continually placed first during our time in the villages. Although we could have done the work better ourselves and in a fraction of the time, we knew that when we left the village, the people would be relying on them. This would improve the health care of the people for years to come.

Meet Community Leaders

Simply meeting with community leaders when you first arrive in the community can enhance the chances of change occurring in the community. This meeting gives recognition of their leadership and authority that enhances your position as a guest coming into the community.

During these interactions, the leaders should be asked about the community's *strengths*, *weaknesses* and *problems*. They should be asked how they believe the community can be improved. Often these leaders will have more than information than anyone else, and will know how best to help. It is best to be a part of the solution and not the whole answer. It is important to be realistic with the community. They may say that they need a clinic with missionary doctors to staff it so it would be free. Establishing a permanent clinic will be outside of your ability. However, attempting to hear what they are saying will help bring understanding on the part of team

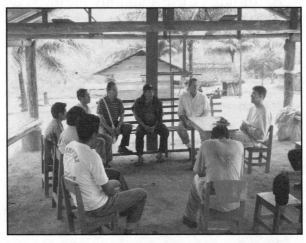

Ted Kuhn/
"Meeting with Leaders in Matoreni"

members. It is good to explore with the leaders their perception of problems in the community:

- Is there any health facility available?
- Is the cost too high?
- Is there a lack of medicines?
- Do they trust the local doctors?
- Is there a language barrier?
- Can you presently offer any help to address these issues?

Clinical Research

Sometimes doing clinical research can be an effective tool for a community. A long-term medical missionary in a rural community in Mexico knew that the school children had parasites and anemia and that these were contributing to lower school performance. She found little support for this problem locally. During a medical clinic held at the school, she asked the team to check the children for parasites and anemia, which they found in abundance. She took this information to school and community leaders to prove her point. When they examined the evidence, they initiated a plan to eliminate the problem.

Impacting Individuals for a Lasting Result

Not all chronic problems are community wide problems. There sometimes is a chronic problem that affects only one person. However, a community is made up of individuals, and each individual impacts the community. Helping him (or her) may make a lasting impact on the life of the individual as well as on their communities.

Illustrative example: In an isolated Indian village in the Peruvian jungle, an older and respected member of the community was crippled by an old knee injury and subsequent arthritis. Members of the community took turns moving this elder around the community in a wheelbarrow. A physical therapist took special interest in him and assessed his personal needs. She devised walking aids and exercises that enabled him to walk independently with pride once again. This not only impacted the man's life, but the entire community who had lovingly cared for him, corporately rejoiced with him.

Illustrative example: In rural Mexico, members of a mission construction team were introduced to a family with a nine-year-old boy with cerebral palsy who could not sit upright in a chair. Using imagination and local materials, they were able to build special chairs and furniture that allowed him to sit up with the rest of the family. A physical therapist was able to teach the parents some range of motion exercises that would decrease his spasms.

Such acts of mercy and care are a light to the community, much as the healing of the paralytic in Matthew 9. When one man was helped, the whole community responded by praising God.

Validating and Prioritizing

By making careful observations and talking with people in the community, it is necessary to validate your conclusions. Remember you are an outsider both to the community and to the culture. Conclusions should be taken to the people that are most affected. They should hear the team's impressions and have an opportunity to evaluate whether they are correct. Your impressions may be:

1. Completely accurate
2. Not exactly correct
3. Not valid
4. Valid, but not recognized by the people
5. Recognized, but not high enough priority to make changes now

Illustrative example: A medical team went to a Mexican border town to vaccinate the children, assuming that this was a need. The people said that they wanted their dogs vaccinated and not their children. Why? The government had already vaccinated the children, but there was widespread rabies in the community. The community recognized their greater need!

Bringing the information to those that are most affected is important.

Illustrative example: During a village medical trip to the Peruvian jungle, many women complained of pain to the head, neck and back. It was observed that all the women coming from the fields that evening carrying heavy baskets of food and firewood on their backs. The baskets also had a strap that went around the forehead supporting most of the weight. It was not difficult to see the cause of these head, neck and back pains! The observations were discussed with the village elders, who were all men. A change in the strap placement on the basket so the weight would be distributed to the back, and not the head and neck was recommended. They dismissed the idea. In retrospect, if the team had suggested the idea to the women, it may have been received very differently!

While validating problems, it will be necessary to assess the priorities the local people put on these problems. As outsiders, we do not view priorities as they do. We must take into account that there are many factors involved in making changes:

- Culture
- Time
- Costs
- Maintaining the changes
- Ability
- Understanding of issues
- Willingness to change
- Fears
- Resources
- Community cooperation

Setting Goals

The time comes when one or more problems that could be improved have been recognized, assessed and validated. The question of whether it is possible to assist in making a change must be answered. For short-term teams, the changes may not be fully (or even partially) realized. Whether the team suggests the changes, the community suggests them or both, the problem is the community's and its members must be in agreement with making the necessary changes. The goals set are the intended outcomes of the changes suggested and should reflect positive changes to issues identified by the team and/or the community. Some goals are large and should be broken down to smaller goals. The community may want to eradicate parasites from all the people. This is a monumental goal, and the community may become frustrated if they do not quickly reach the goal. Try to develop smaller goals that can be measurable and obtainable within a reasonable time period. Nothing succeeds like success!

Smaller steps leading up to the larger goal may include:

a. Giving a parasite treatment each year to every child
b. Have purified water for the children to drink in school
c. Teaching each family about how to avoid parasites
d. Enforcing the penning up of pigs

At the end of six months, the community can assess if they have been reaching their goals. If they haven't, the goals are still reachable. If they have succeeded, then the small goals will encourage them to reach for larger goals. If they failed, then they will not be greatly discouraged since the goal and effort was not large. They can assess and try again.

In the beginning, set small goals. Small successes will lead to larger successes. Small failures can be corrected. Start small!

Key Planning

Some key thoughts:

1. It is the community, which has the responsibility to change. Visiting teams should not take change as their responsibility, nor should they try to force change on people.
2. Teams should set reachable and measurable goals.
3. It is important to be very careful about making promises. Team members can

become eager and promise things that cannot be provided. Such promises may include future money, ongoing relationships, bringing representatives of the community to a church in the US, employment, help from other missionaries or organizations, etc. In many cultures saying "maybe" means saying "yes".

4. Sometimes people may appear to be "poor," but they may still have the needed resources. Treating someone like they are poor will offend them or cause them to see themselves as poor and think they will always need help.

5. Always be careful that the changes are within their resources.

6. Be cautious of doing all the work:
   a. There will be expectations that visitors will do all the work the next time.
   b. The community will not feel that they own it.

Summary

God has given us wonderful spiritual gifts, education, skills, abilities, resources, and vision in helping others. The Apostle Paul says in Galatians 6: 9, 10:

"Let us not become weary in doing good, for at the proper time we will reap a harvest if we do not give up. Therefore, as we have opportunity, let us do good to all people, especially to those who belong to the family of believers."

As we go to minister, we must consider how we can best help the communities, churches and ministries where we work. Considering how we can help these communities, families and individuals to decrease and prevent illnesses and poor health practices may often take extra time and seem less productive than seeing patients who come to us. However, it will often have a harvest greater than can ever be achieved during a clinic.

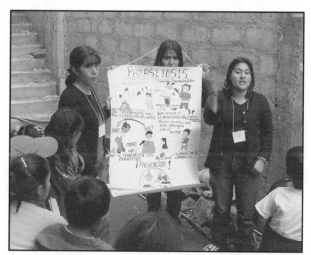

John Sexton/
"Health Teaching During Clinic"

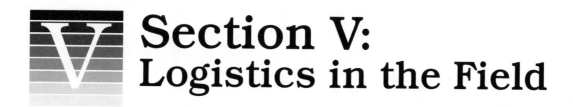

Section V: Logistics in the Field

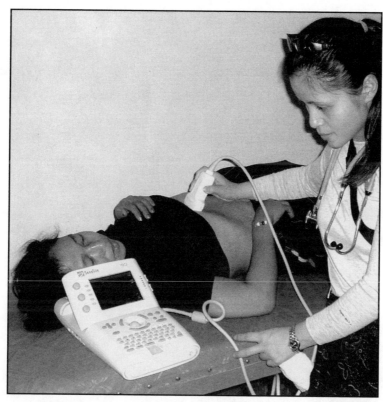

Ted Kuhn/
"The Portable Ultrasound Machine"

Logistics of Outpatient Medicine in the Developing World

Sharon C. Kuhn and W. "Ted" Kuhn

In the developing world the human needs are often great and resources are scarce. It is not unusual in an outpatient setting for a physician or medical team to be completely overwhelmed by these needs. Whether patient care is rendered in a hospital outpatient clinic, church, school building, or indeed under a tree or in an open field, it is necessary to use both human and material resources wisely in order to have a positive and lasting impact.

Some people question whether individual medical care is appropriate in the poor areas of the developing world. They argue that if the poor receive temporary relief from medical illness then they become increasingly dissatisfied with their current state. Large scale preventive health care and development projects are the necessary solution, they argue, not individually directed curative care. The situation in such places is often likened to the parable of a man drowning in a river. You jump in to save him (the curative approach), and before you know it, there is another drowning man in the river, and another and another. You spend all your time rescuing drowning people and

never have time to see why they are falling in upstream. The development model would direct your efforts upstream to prevent people from falling in. However, if you are the man drowning in the river, then rescue is indeed your highest priority even if you may fall in again. Meeting this need is a worthy and honorable goal. On the other hand, fixing the problem upstream also makes sense. The best plan may be a combination of both curative and preventative medicine. Providing quality curative medical care builds relationships and trust within the community. These relationships can be vital links during the construction of long-term preventative programs. One of the other advantages of short-term curative medical intervention is that it does relieve suffering and meets the real and perceived needs of the community without becoming institutionalized.

Putting Ideas Into Practice

Advance Preparations

1. Begin your preparations with prayer and continue to lift all the details to the Lord for his guidance.
2. Several months before the trip you will need to begin assembling the medications and supplies that you will need. These items can be acquired in many ways from your local medical community, pharmaceutical reps, and special orders from nonprofit suppliers such as King Pharmaceutical Benevolent Foundation, MAP International and International Aid. The contact information for many of these suppliers can be found in the "Resources for the Traveling Medical Professional" chapter at the end of this book.

3. Maintain regular contact with the missionary or national workers who are in charge of organizing your trip in the country you will be visiting. Find out what their expectations are for your team. Ask about the environment in which you will be working. For example, will you be seeing patients in a church building in a city or under a tree in a remote village? These types of questions will help you begin to anticipate the numbers of patients that may come and the logistical problems you may encounter.

4. Your national contact will also be able to help you find out what is available near the proposed clinic site and arrange to have many of the needed people and items present when your team arrives. For example: Will there be electricity and if so what voltage? (Take adaptors for the different types of electric plugs.) Can the receiving group provide benches or chairs and small tables for each doctor/patient/translator group? Can they provide tables for registration, the pharmacy and the laboratory? If patients will be seen in an open area or large room, then some private area will have to be found or created by makeshift curtains for use when privacy is required. Is there a suitable shaded or covered area where the patients can wait?

5. If possible, your contact should try to recruit several individuals from the receiving group to help with the clinic:
    a. Two or three people from the local community to help register the patients.
    b. Sufficient translators so that every provider, the team leader, and the triage team has a translator.
    c. A doctor, nurse, or other health care worker from the culture who can help you not only see patients, but also handle the challenges of referring patients within the local health care system if needed.

Arrival at the Clinic Site

If possible, go and see the clinic site the day before you are scheduled to work. This will help you plan ahead of time some aspects of patient flow and will make the morning setup more efficient.

1. Arrive prepared. Have your medications, nursing supplies and laboratory equipment packed and ready to go the night before. Review procedures with your team and make job assignments. Take sufficient drinking water and snacks for the team and make plans for lunch ahead of time. When working in very poor areas, eating in front of hungry people is uncomfortable unless you have enough for everyone. Let your team know ahead of time if they will be expected to work all day with only breaks for drinks and snacks. If you will be eating a more substantial meal, arranging for the team to eat in shifts will allow medical care to proceed uninterrupted. This is appropriate when people are waiting long times for care or standing in the sun. If you are in a culture where people go home for lunch, many patients may leave the site and not return for several hours. In that case, the team should break as well. Your national host will advise you of these customs.

2. Evaluate the site for the most efficient way to provide for patient flow. It is not unusual for a clinic to be held in a small school, house, or church building with only one or two exits and a large central room. A building with at least two doors and some open windows and a large central area for patient care is best. Patients can register at one door and enter the exam area in a controlled manner. Then they can proceed to one of the areas where a doctor and translator are waiting within the large central room. If possible, space these groupings of chairs out so conversations can be as confidential as possible. A separate room or curtained off area will be needed for exams requiring privacy and for counseling. The pharmacy and lab will probably also be set up in this large room. In this way the doctors can have easy access to these services and the equipment will be secure. Blood specimens can be obtained

while inside. Patients who need to provide stool or urine specimens can come and go through the monitored back door. An open window to the outside is ideal for handing in urine and stool specimens from these patients and allows them to wait outside until results are ready.

3. Patients may wait for long periods to be seen and it is nice to use a shaded or protected area outside for this purpose. Patients can then be called in as health care workers become available. If possible, make sure that patients have clean water and latrines available outside as they wait. If patients wait to be seen inside the patient care area, there will be increased confusion and noise.

4. If you have a building with only one open door, there will be congestion at that door as patients are coming and going. There will be a line of patients pressing in to be seen, as well as patients bringing in laboratory specimens, and the ever-present crowd of curious onlookers. In this case, you will need to have several helpers at the door to ease patients in and out. If at all possible do not use a building with one door. In addition to the patient flow problems, it can pose a security risk.

5. Open buildings and open spaces can also be utilized for "clinics" with surprising ease. Surveyor's tape and fiberglass rods (used for electric fencing) will mark off open areas. The surveyor's tape can be wrapped around the fiberglass rods or trees or stakes. People will generally not violate the marked off area. You can mark off the registration and patient care areas as well as the lab and pharmacy. Tarps come in handy for creating privacy. With a little imagination and planning, this can work quite well.

How Many Patients Can Be Seen?

In a full day of clinic providers will see on average 20 patients each. This may seem like a low number, but remember when working through a translator, patient care will be slowed substantially. In some cases, one may

be working through two translators, which makes patient care even more challenging. When there are not enough translators, no matter what the size of the medical team, progress will be slow. Generally there is a need for one translator for every patient care provider, the team leader and ideally two or three more to help with triage/registration, and perhaps the laboratory, pharmacy or nursing care. If the team leader is a physician, do not include him when deciding how many patients will be seen. If there are medical students or nurses acting as provider extenders, a physician will be overseeing them and not seeing patients himself. Children are usually seen more quickly. If a laboratory is available and more complex care can be given, the pace will slow, especially if a physician must read some of the laboratory tests. Plan to see fewer than the expected number of patients on the first day as your team with the translators learns the system and how to work together. Leave enough room in the schedule to see the inevitable emergency patient or V.I.P.

Triage Scenarios

There are at least four types of situations (scenarios) that can greet a medical team as they arrive at the clinic site. How these are handled will depend on the number of potential patients and their behavior, the size of the team, the size of the facility and the number of translators. The national leader and the team leader should try to anticipate ahead of time which scenario is most likely, based on their understanding of the area and be proactive in their planning. For example, if a huge crowd is expected after a general announcement, "tickets" allowing one to be seen at the clinic could be given out selectively ahead of time. The leaders and the team need to discuss possible scenarios and agree on a plan of action should the unexpected occur.

Scenario 1: The team will comfortably be able to meet the needs of the assembled people with the resources available.

Scenario 2: You will be able to meet the needs of all the patients, but resources will

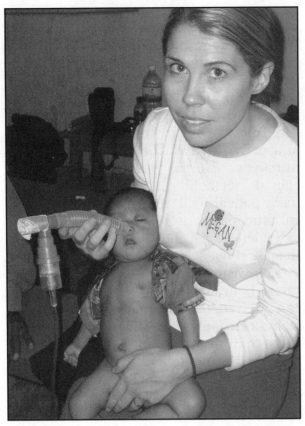

Krystina Huynh/
"Giving Aerosolized Medications Using Bicycle Pump Nebulizer."

be stretched and personnel will be pushed to their limits.

Scenario 3: Clearly, the team will not be able to meet the needs of the assembled crowd because there are several hundred people waiting by the time the team arrives. In some countries, patients will wait for their turn quietly in line for long periods. With a cooperative crowd and an effective triage system, the sickest patients in this large assembly and as many others as possible may be cared for in the time available. This plan can be made acceptable to the community when the details are discussed with and agreed upon by community leaders and if it is carefully explained to those hoping to be seen. However, at the end of the day, there will be people with unmet needs. This creates frustration and sometimes anger in both the community and the team. Driving your team to the point of exhaustion to see "just a few more patients" may only compound the problem and make care during

subsequent days more difficult. In heavily populated, needy areas, it is beneficial to plan to hold clinic in the same location for several days.

Scenario 4: The numbers of people are large; however, unlike the patient people in Scenario 3, in this situation everyone pushes forward forming an unruly crowd that is very difficult to triage. If triage is impossible or unacceptable, there is a potential for an unsatisfactory outcome or even violence. An attempt to create order should be made through the community leaders. If this fails, it may be safest to leave before the crowd gets out of hand. Explain to the community leaders that you are sorry but that it is impossible to provide any medical care under the circumstances. Let the responsibility rest with them for the chaotic conditions. Otherwise, you will struggle all day and at the end of a long and stressful day, people will be angry and your legacy in that community will be a negative one. This whole situation becomes less likely if the nationals in charge have planned ahead. They could let the word go out in the days before your arrival that the doctors will only be able to see a limited number of people in order to give each patient a good thorough exam. They may keep "advertising" to a minimum, and just have their church members invite needy friends and neighbors. If triage will be done, it helps to tell the community how patients will be chosen, e.g. "first come first serve" or "sicker ones first."

The first scenario is delightful, but it is the most unusual. When presented with the stresses of the second or third scenario, remember that the team cannot work at this intensity day after day. Plan for enforced rest breaks and refreshments during the workday, and a half or full day off after every second or third day of intense patient care. When there are more patients present than can be seen, it is best to have a medically oriented member of the local community assist with triage as he/she may understand culturally sensitive concerns that might otherwise cause unnecessary conflict. Some triage decisions will be made on "political" grounds instead of medical priorities. It is best to accept this as the cost of doing business in that community if it does not occur too frequently. It is virtually impossible for outsiders to understand all the cultural undercurrents, so let a trusted local member of the community guide these decisions. Triage fewer patients than the team can actually see. To turn away patients in the evening that have been triaged in the morning can cause considerable conflict within the team and within the community. To wait patiently all day only to be told in the evening you cannot be seen is a tough pill to swallow! At triage be sure that the total number of family members to be seen is clarified and that each one is given a chart. It is not uncommon for one member of the family to bring other family members or children with them expecting care for everyone with only one ticket. In a family oriented society, not to care for the other family members may be unacceptable. Planning for this and other "emergencies" at the start of the day is the best way to assure smooth patient flow throughout the day. After triage is complete, the rest of the crowd may be dismissed home so that they do not wait for an opportunity that is unlikely to come and thus increase their disappointment.

Triage should proceed according to team resources and may be different with each team and in each community. Generally, triage patients that match the capabilities of your team members. If the team is a group of pediatricians, it may be wisest to limit your patients to the pediatric age group. Ophthalmologists may limit their patients to eye disorders, etc. Remember, traveling in an airplane does not make one an expert in another medical specialty. The best care will be given within the limits of the provider's expertise. That may mean that patients with legitimate medical concerns may not be seen. Ideally, if the team is made up of specialists, the national contact will let this be known before the team arrives so that those patients needing specialized services will come and others will not expect to be seen. If necessary, this should be explained again at the beginning of the clinic day.

It is our opinion that triage should be done by the most experienced member of the team with the help of a respected national. Often, illness is overstated or understated depending on cultural backgrounds. The astute clinician may be able to recognize subtle signs of disease that less experienced health care workers may miss. Triage can also be a trying experience. Patients may grab on to the provider's feet or hold on to his clothing or frantically push their babies in front of his face. A very calm, gentle, but firm, experienced individual is best in this job. A sense of humor also helps.

Patients can be triaged with a number system relying on cards or with numbers written directly on the patient's hand. In some countries, where cards are given out for triage, poor patients may sell these cards as a source of income. Thus you may not see the patients you triaged but an entirely different, more prosperous patient population. We generally favor permanent marking pens with numbers written on the dorsum of the right hand. This mark remains for 2–3 days, can not be sold, transferred, lost, or erased. If you are holding clinic in the same area for several days, you can use different colored markers for different days, otherwise different team members may be seeing the same patient over and over again as he returns to get medicine that can be used for other family members or sold in the market for cash.

Home Visits

Be sure to ask the local pastor or community leader if there is anyone who is too ill to be able to come to the clinic. It is a wonderful experience for all involved to send several members of the team to do a home visit. These have been some of the most precious moments teams have had. Home visits open the door not only to relieving illness and teaching home care skills to the family, but they provide a quiet opportunity for listening, sharing and praying. Church members can continue to visit and offer spiritual and emotional support after the team leaves.

Patient Referrals

Discuss with the team and national leaders ahead of time what to do for patients with complicated medical problems or those who are critically ill or dying. For patients who need further diagnosis or treatment, can community resources be accessed by the team for the patient, e.g. treatment for tuberculosis? Will the team have to pay the hospital bill for the patient who needs surgery? If a patient must be transported a long distance to receive care, and the team's vehicle is the only method available, is it possible to transport the patient (and family members) without compromising the team? Does the community expect you to provide extraordinary care or do they accept death as the natural consequence of critical illness? These questions should be addressed with the wise input of your national co-workers.

Registration

Individuals from the community may be enlisted to register the patients. It is helpful if they can legibly write the patient's name, age, and sex. Single page patient charts can be printed for this purpose or index cards (4x6) can be used. Some form of record keeping is needed for internal use in the clinic as the patient moves from triage to provider to lab and pharmacy, and if the patient needs to return the next day. The charts may also be examined by international or national officials, especially during disasters.

If nursing help is available, vital signs can be taken and recorded just after registration and any triage notes made. Patient care providers can use the charts for jotting down their notes, diagnoses, medications needed, and for requesting and recording laboratory tests. The care provider should be sure to write his name on the chart so that he can receive the results. Charts are especially helpful when several family members present together.

Supplies needed for registration and triage include: ballpoint pens, charts or index cards, indelible markers, and paper or notebooks for keeping any other records or information. Bring extra thermometers and an extra blood pressure cuff and stethoscope in case additional nursing help is available. Have caution tape or surveyor's tape to mark off the triage and registration areas if needed.

Pharmacy

Dispensing medication should be done with the same care and attention to detail as in the United States. Small coin envelopes from an office supply store work well for holding a single medication, i.e. Tylenol® or small plastic bags will do. Zippered plastic bags have the advantage of being waterproof. Write the medication name, preferably the generic name, and dosage on the envelope or plastic bag, as well as instructions. A stamp can be made in the language of the country so that the name of the medicine and the number of pills per day can be filled in easily. Some patients will need more than one medicine and often several family members are seen together. In that case you must put each one's name on his/her medicine bag.

The person acting as pharmacist can prepackage commonly used medicines such as vitamins and pain medications whenever there is a quiet moment. There should be a bottle of pure water in the pharmacy for mixing suspensions for children. Find out what size spoons, if any, people have at home so proper dispensing instructions can be given. It is very helpful if the team is able to provide measuring devices.

In most instances it is easier for the physician to come to the pharmacy to get the desired medication in case a different medicine has to be chosen due to availability or in case the dosage needs to be verified. Often the person working in the pharmacy is not a pharmacist and will need this type of assistance. The physician's translator can then describe to the patient how to take the medicines, thus alleviating the need for a translator in the pharmacy.

Supplies for the pharmacy include: ball point pens, cellophane tape, scissors and rubber bands, clean water, a large syringe or medicine cup for measuring water for suspensions, and paper or notebooks for keeping any other records or information. Pill envelopes, small and large baggies, a pill counter and a pill cutter are handy additions. Empty camera film canisters also make convenient medicine bottles, especially in humid environments. They can be prefilled and labeled long ahead of time, but they are also bulky to transport.

Laboratory

Depending on the quantity of tests being ordered, one or two persons may be able to handle everything in the lab, or there may be a need to have additional help for receiving and processing the specimens and drawing blood. Tests results need to be recorded on the patient's chart and in the lab notebook, and someone needs to be sure that the results and the patient get back to the ordering physician so that he can make the proper disposition. As noted earlier, an open window or side door near the lab location can make receiving of specimens more convenient. The patient's chart with his name, the test ordered and the physician's name can stay with the specimen while it is being processed and then be returned to the patient with the result recorded. Here again it is useful to have a number on the card as well as on the patient's hand. The patient can then return to his doctor for final instructions.

Supplies: Bring all necessary laboratory supplies and equipment for obtaining blood specimens. (See the chapter on "The Portable Medical Laboratory"). Other items include: pens, markers, a notebook, and 3 oz plastic cups for collecting urine, stool and sputum samples. In the rural areas paper cups and banana leaves (torn into pieces and used for wrapping stool specimens) make handy, biodegradable containers. Gloves are necessary for laboratory workers. Be sure to educate any nonmedical helpers on infectious disease precautions. Toothpicks make stool specimen preparation more efficient. Bring trash bags for clean up and some paper towels. Designate a "sharps" container and be sure to use it. Have plenty of hand wipes and hand sanitizer available especially if there is a shortage of clean water for hand washing. Designate the contaminated trash so that it can be disposed of properly. If in a village, tell the elders of the danger and be sure the contaminated trash is buried and burnable items are incinerated.

The End of the Day

Plan to finish patient care before the team is exhausted and before it gets dark. Because part of our witness is to be respectful of and good stewards of the area in which we have been working, when the last patient has been seen, the whole team should clean up the area. Be sure that no trash is left lying about. See to it that everything is properly disposed of. Be careful in repacking medicine and equipment so that it will be easy to find everything for setting up at the next stop. At this point, especially if the team is not staying in the area, it is fun and informative to take a walk around the neighborhood or village before leaving. It will give the team a better idea of where the patients have come from and what their challenges in living are. Some public health hazards or a possible solution to a health problem may become obvious through these observations. Any insights can be tactfully shared with national coworkers and community leaders.

Preparing to Leave

Upon preparing to leave an area following a medical mission or even during the stay, national individuals or groups may ask to be given any "leftover" medicines. Though this request may sound simple, there are several issues to consider. (See Chapter 40, "Preparing to Return Home," for further information.) The first involves the conditions under which the medicines were donated. Medicines from most benevolent organizations require that the medicine be distributed free of charge by qualified medical professionals. If this cannot be guaranteed, medicine can not be left.

Secondly, medicines are worth a significant amount of money. Much strife can be created between well-meaning individuals and groups if a medical team leaves medicines with one person or group and not another, or divides the medications up in what is seen as an "unfair" way. What was meant to be a blessing can quickly become a problem.

Sometimes a team will meet national health workers while touring a hospital or on other official business. These individuals may request medicine. Again, the problem is that one can not be sure if the medicines will be handled appropriately or whether they will be sold for a profit. Making a large donation of medicine may set an unintended precedent and create potential misunderstandings and difficulties for other teams returning to the same area who may not have the same resources.

Leaving large amounts of supplies for another team which will be coming to the same location can be problematic, but is possible under certain circumstances. First, there must be a secure place to store the medicine which will be dry, not too hot and not too cold, and where it will be under the care of a trustworthy person.

An accurate list of what has been left must be given to the team leader of the next team so that he or she will not need to bring duplicate supplies. All medicines that have been repackaged must have the medication name, dosage, and expiration date clearly marked. Finally, since much donated medicine is short-dated, any left over medication should be directed to another mission team conducting clinics within two to three months in order to use the medications effectively.

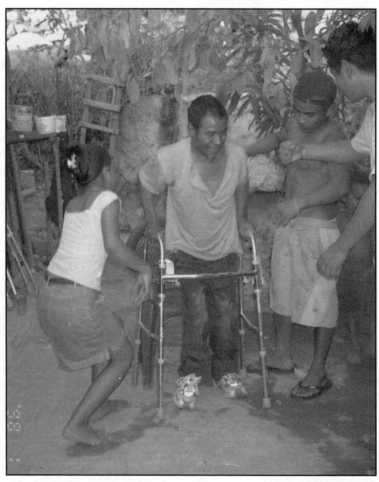

Ted Kuhn/
"Walking Again"

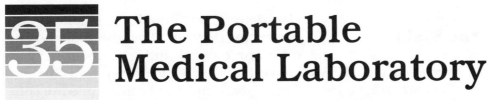

The Portable Medical Laboratory

W. "Ted" Kuhn and Hartmut Gross

Equipment and Its Usefulness
   in the Field
Additional Important Points
   to Keep in Mind
Portable Laboratory Equipment List

It is taught repeatedly in medical school that the history and physical examination of the sick patient are the cornerstones to establishing the diagnosis. In fact the patient will tell the physician the diagnosis some 60% of the time, provided he listens closely. The physical examination will yield the diagnosis an additional 30% of the time. Ancillary studies only yield a diagnosis in 10% of cases. These statistics are confirmed over and over again, provided the clinician knows what illnesses are endemic to the population being treated. However, years of experience may suddenly be rendered almost useless when working in the developing world. Illness patterns may be (and often are) very different. In fact illnesses never encountered in one's normal home practice may be the prominent maladies in a given field environment. Language barriers, use of non- (or limited) medical translators, perhaps across 2–3 languages, make history taking challenging. Fortunately, humans are humans, the world over, so exam skills are fairly uniform, but the physical findings of unusual diseases may be very perplexing. But, the help of consulting services or the luxury of sophisticated radiographic studies to make an accurate diagnosis are not available. What does one do in this dilemma?

Handing out medication based on a best guess is an option practiced by some. For example, anyone complaining of worms gets worm pills. But is that a good practice of medicine? Does it help the patient? Does it help a community? Will it make a long term difference or will the jungle close back in behind upon leaving, as though no one had ever been there? Will one return home feeling he has made a difference? Will future teams be able to draw from one's experience to continue making a positive effect in that community?

In everything we do we should strive for excellence and integrity. Nonetheless, practicing medicine in a different land with different illness makes error a real concern. While we want to do our best, the lack of support makes that goal difficult to obtain. Fortunately, we and the institutions we represent will be judged by those we are trying to serve through our accuracy and success. Yet there is one remaining resource available—the portable medical laboratory.

Carrying and using a portable medical laboratory into the developing world helps confirm the diagnosis and assists when symptoms are medically ambiguous. It also helps the medical team understand the epidemiology of diseases in the community so appropriate public health measures can be instituted. Space, weight, durability and cost are all considerations. Thus the lab needs to be small, portable, lightweight and inexpensive, basically the most "bang" for the size, weight and cost. It must be able to withstand the rigors of transport, including handling by the less than caring baggage handlers in the airports. Finally, someone must know how to use the equipment and be knowledgeable in interpreting the results of any performed tests.

Equipment and Its Usefulness in the Field

Urine dipsticks are simple, easy, and can confirm the presence of urinary tract infection (common in women in the developing world), diabetes, renal, and liver diseases. They can also be cut in half for cost savings. Devices for quick measurement of serum glucose from a single drop of blood are now universally available. They are battery operated, inexpensive, and are useful for screening for diabetes which is a real problem in some developing countries. Urine pregnancy tests help when women patients have abdominal pain, and should be used before prescribing medicines that may adversely affect the fetus during pregnancy, including some antihelminth medications. The HemaCue® machine is portable, lightweight, and accurate and runs from AA batteries. It measures hemoglobin from a finger-stick with blood placed on a cuvette. The HemaCue® machine is expensive as an initial investment but is durable, light weight, and travels well.

The centerpiece of the portable medical laboratory is the microscope. A good quality microscope with 40x, 100x, and oil immersion lens and adapted for AC or DC electricity is invaluable. A small AC/DC power inverter will allow the scope to run off a car battery and a transformer can convert 200 volt electricity to 110 volts. Since gastrointestinal complaints are common in the developing world, the ability to do a stool exam will prove useful. Stools can be examined for helminths, protozoa, and white cells using saline or Lugol's iodine. A drop of spun or unspun urine can be examined for evidence of infection or glomerulonephritis. Skin scrapings and vaginal wet preps can be examined for tinea and candida with 10% potassium hydroxide while skin scrapings can confirm scabies. With only minimal effort, stains can be used to identify patients with malaria, tuberculosis, and various bacterial infections. The Wright's or Geimsa stain can be used for malaria and other blood borne protozoa and helminths. There are rapid Geimsa stains needing less than 1 minute that are useful for malaria identification. A Kinyoun acid-fast stain for TB and a Gram's stain for bacterial pathogens can also be carried. Practice and experience is needed to learn to identify both malaria and TB. In the field artifact caused by dust or debris is easily confused with malaria parasites or tuberculosis. A plastic enclosed drying

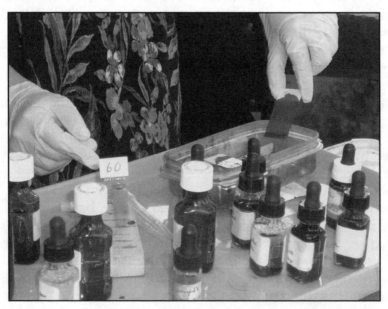

Ted Kuhn/
"Staining TB Slides with Portable Lab."

rack made from Tupperware® and tongue depressors helps keep slides clean while drying. In some countries, partially treated tuberculosis is a major problem and the initial acid-fast stain may be negative. A simple screening tool for partially treated TB is the erythrocyte sedimentation rate. Although the sedimentation rate is not specific, it is rarely, if ever, normal in patients with tuberculosis. Plastic disposable one use sedimentation rate tubes can be helpful. A word to the wise, stains often leak when exposed to varying pressure changes common with air travel and altitude. An airtight box containing the stains limits the damage and mess if the stains should leak in your suitcase or backpack.

The portable medical laboratory is an invaluable tool in the physician's armamentarium. Several equipment suppliers are listed in the "Resources for the Traveling Medical Professional" chapter. A small laboratory can be purchased for between $1,500 and $2,000, while some equipment may be borrowed from vendors for humanitarian work. When properly utilized the portable medical laboratory will vastly improve the quality and outcome of the health care provided.

Additional Important Points to Keep in Mind

- Check equipment before leaving home.
- Have some knowledge to be able to do some troubleshooting if equipment fails in the field. Consider taking spare parts, e.g. microscope bulb.
- Know the operating temperature ranges of the equipment and compare to the temperatures where you will be working.
- The laboratory always draws an interested crowd. To avoid damage to equipment and to protect onlookers from injury, plan for a safe distance of crowd control by placing barriers or ropes.
- Establish early upon arrival to a new site where the lab will be placed. A full lab may take 30 minutes to set up, which is about the time it takes for the first test requests reach the lab.

- The lab will always be the last station to close down. It makes little sense to start putting items away early. Invariably, the last test ordered in the clinic will be the test you tucked away first, under everything else. Plan on taking about 30 minutes after everyone else is finished to pack everything back into its place for safe transport.
- Plan for disposal of urine, stool, and blood samples, well away from the lab.
- Plan for disposal of used sharp implements as well as other used contaminated supplies. A pit latrine may be a good option.
- Remember to have papers documenting ownership of the equipment and the intended use. It will make bringing equipment into the country and back home much easier (see "Preparing to Return Home" chapter).

The following portable medical laboratory has been developed to accompany teams as a result of extensive field experience. Field testing included functioning of the instruments at environmental extremes including high ambient temperatures (>90 degrees F), high ambient humidity (>90%), cold (<32 degrees F) and high altitude (over 16,000 feet above sea level). Several laboratory instruments and several lab tests have proven useful and reliable over the 6 years of testing.

Portable Laboratory Equipment List

Transport
- Sturdy padded trunk or case for the equipment (e.g. Herzog® case)
- Case for microscope (e.g. Herzog® case)
- Separate waterproof case for stains (e.g. Pellikan® case)
- Some small equipment may be carry-on by team members

Electrical Devices
- Microscope with transformers (e.g. AO Microscope® (adapted for 110 volts, 220 volts, 12 volts, and solar panel)

- I-STAT® and standard (functions between 16–30⁰ C. (Na, K, Cl, BUN, Creatinine, Glucose, & Hgb)
- Capillary glucose monitor and standard (e.g. Assure®)
- Hemacue® hemaglobinometer and standard Zip-Spin® microcentrifuge (LW Scientific,® Inc—12-volt battery operated)
- Fetal Doppler® (e.g. Medasonics®)
- Ultrasound machine (SonoSite®)

Power Sources
- Batteries (all kinds)
- Solar panel (e.g. BP Solar®)
- Motorcycle batteries

Non-electric Tests
- Urine dipsticks (e.g. Uriscan®)
- Urine HCG
- Sedimentation rate
- Hepatitis A
- Hepatitis B
- HIV
- Malaria (nonspecific)

Stains and Solutions
- Gram stain
  crystal violet
  Gram's iodine solution
  decolorizer (ethanol)
  safranin counterstain
- Wright's stain
- Geimsa stain
- Kinyoun Acid Fast (cold) stain
  carbol fuchsin
  acid-alcohol

methylene blue counter stain (brilliant green)
- Hema-Quik 2®
- Stool Hema Test (Beckman Coulter®)
- Lugol's iodine
- 10% Potassium hydroxide (KOH)
- Normal saline (without preservatives)
- Phosphate buffer solution
- Irrigation water

Other Supplies
- Logbook (to record all test results)
- Plastic table cover
- Phlebotomy equipment
  Gloves
  Alcohol wipes
  Tourniquets
  Lancets
  Syringes
  2x2 gauze
  Band-Aids®
- Cups (for urine, stool & sputum)
- Toothpicks
- Microscope slides and cover slips
- Cuvettes and reagent strips for all equipment to be used
- Disposable lighter (for heat fixing slides)
- Timer (for staining techniques and sedimentation rate)
- Indelible marker (for marking specimens - and patients!)
- Reference text (with lab techniques and lots of microscope pictures)

Personal Safety
- Gloves
- TB mask

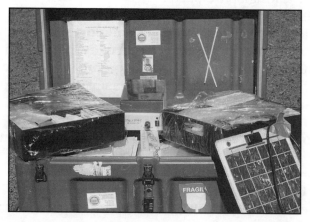

Ted Kuhn/
"Laboratory Equipment"

- Sharps containers
- Safety glasses

**Equipment Provided in the Field
Upon Request**
- Tables (level surface to set up equipment)
- Chairs
- Place to dispose of biological wastes and supplies and sharps

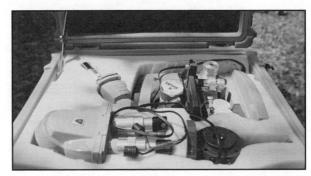

Ted Kuhn/
"Microscope in the Field"

Resources

1. Kuhn W, Fernandez E: *An Efficient, Lightweight, Durable, Portable Medical Laboratory for Diagnostic and Epidemiologic Studies in the Developing World*, submitted for publication, 2003.

36 Eyeglass Clinics

Jim Carroll, Shirley Carroll, Hartmut Gross

Eye Clinics with Non-Eye Professionals
Materials Needed
Logistics
Eye Clinics with Eye-Care Specialists
Patient Flow
Examination
Dispensary
Eyeglasses Categories

The gift of sight is held precious the world over. Eyeglasses, contact lenses, and myriad surgical procedures are so commonplace in the modern countries that they are practically taken for granted. In the developing world, however, nothing could be further from this way of thinking. Vision is clearly crucial to carry out the activities of everyday life from homemaking chores to fieldwork and from hunting to crafting. When vision dims or fails and is not corrected or restored, the affected individuals become less productive, are more likely to injure themselves and become dependent upon others willing to help them. The pride of independence and satisfaction of contributing to the community give way to the despair of being a burden. In developing nations failing vision is part of life. It is expected and accepted as inevitable and considered irreversible. Restoring vision is an unknown concept.

Eyeglass and optometry missions can serve to change that belief, restoring vision to many with something as simple as an inexpensive pair of corrective lenses. For others perhaps less tangible is the promise of slowing down the deterioration of vision through medication. Many eyes may be comforted with simple eye lubricants. Infections or trachoma may be cured or halted

before causing more injury. Other individuals may be identified who have surgically restorable eye conditions, which may be easily corrected when a surgical eye team comes in follow-up.

One of the most compelling encounters was the discovery of a young man who had sustained a gunshot wound to the face several years prior to the mission team's arrival in the Peruvian jungle. While he had survived the injury, he was blinded and had been completely dependent on others for assistance for every aspect of life. While one eye had been enucleated, the other was found to perceive light through the heavily scarred cornea. After follow-up evaluations a corneal transplant was arranged and performed. As a result, the young man has been saved from complete blindness and now has excellent vision in his eye and independently cares for himself and a family. He has also become an active and industrious contributor in his village community.

With simple training, anyone on a general medical missions team can perform initial screening for vision problems using little more than an eye chart. With that information, the decision may be made if an eye specialist needs to be brought into a community in the future. An optometrist or ophthalmologist will be needed on a missions team to provide more advanced evaluations and treatment. Even when a specialist is available, other physicians and laypersons can perform preliminary vision screening and assist with filling eyeglass prescriptions.

Preparation for the eye glass clinic should begin several months prior to the mission trip. The first task is to decide on the scope and methods to be used in the clinic. If conducted by an individual with professional training in ophthalmology or optometry, the clinic will, of course function on a more sophisticated level with the use of mydriatics, tonometer, retinoscope or ophthalmoscope.

When giving the patient their glasses, witnessing the patient's excitement of being able to see clearly is wondrous. Some of the patients will be amazed to see the leaves on the tree, having forgotten that things are not blurry. Others will rejoice to be able to read the scriptures for themselves once again. Some will be able to resume handicrafts or basket making. And others will elate to see their family and friends clearly once again. Corrective lenses are a precious tool that enables them to see more clearly and resume a forgotten or abandoned lifestyle.

Eye Clinics with Non-Eye Professionals

The following is a list of suggested supplies. This will need to be amended depending on the number of providers, the volume of patients and the services planned to be provided. Some methods for clinic logistics are also suggested.

Materials Needed

Eye Charts

Laminated, handheld Snellen (Rosenbaum) eye charts are small and practical. Be aware that illiteracy is commonplace or that the western alphabet may not be used in the host country. The tumbling E chart used for pediatric eye evaluations may prove more useful for adult exams in these situations.

Eyeglasses

Glasses should be ordered far in advance so that they will arrive already cleaned and categorized as to strengths.

Donated eyeglasses can be collected months ahead and verified via lensometer. The glasses may be ordered from one of several charitable groups who see supplying glasses for mission trips this as their ministry.

The Indiana Lions Club® has a program linked with their prison system where one can obtain labeled and verified glasses.

Eyeglasses are needed primarily in the reading glasses category. Approximately 70% of the patients' needs can be met with reading glasses or "low plus" bifocals. Some "minus" lenses are needed for an occasional myopic patient and many of them can be used for the nuclear sclerotic cataract patients. If more reading glasses are needed than can be supplied from donations, these can be ordered at low cost from Dollar Tree Stores® or similar franchises.

Several types of equipment may be used to check for the patient's prescription. The easiest to use in the authors' experience is a simple system with retinoscopy bars containing graduated lenses. Another device is called a focometer. With the latter, the patient focuses on the target and the lens correction is read from the side of the focometer. The focometer requires a fairly high level of cooperation and understanding on the part of the patient. Other devises are available, but those need more time to develop facility with their use. In order to handle large groups of patients, at least two eye charts are needed. Practice using the equipment at home before the trip.

After receiving the glasses before the trip, one should check over them to make sure the needed lenses are available. The glasses should be sorted and packed such that the loss of one or two suitcases will not represent the loss of an entire group of glasses with the same prescription.

Logistics

On the field, the team for the eyeglass clinic is usually composed of two people conducting the testing at the same time, using the two charts and two retinoscopy bars. At least one other person should be assigned to pull the prescribed glasses from the stock. This can be a time-consuming component of the project.

A translator is usually needed just for the eye clinic. While the simple instructions in another language for testing can usually be learned quickly, matters frequently arise requiring a higher level of communication (glaucoma, eye infections, injury and cataracts etc).

Choosing a suitable location for the clinic may be challenging. There must be adequate light to see the charts, but it is also desirable to avoid the team's standing in full sunlight for the entire day. Twenty feet of unimpeded space should be available for the setup of the charts. A chair should be placed just behind the 20 foot mark for the patient.

The procedure for determining the prescription should be kept as simple as possible. First, ask the patient to find out if the main need is reading glasses. Then, have the patient read the eye chart at 20 feet. If the patients under 40 years of age and can read 20/20, they do not need glasses. If the patient is over 40 and can read 20/20 for distance, it is highly likely they will need reading glasses. Find their age on the table and let them try on the corresponding "plus" or "added power" for reading.

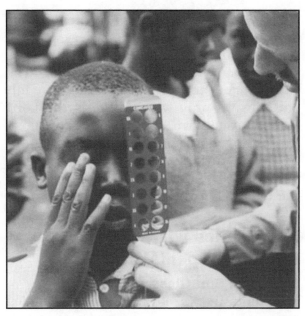

Ted Kuhn
"Vision Testing, Slums of Nairobi"

Table 1. Added Power per Age for Reading Glasses

Age	Add Power
40	+1.00 to +1.25
45	+1.25 to +1.50
50	+1.50 to +2.00
55	+2.00 to +2.25
60+	+2.50 to +3.00

Their need for plus power will usually be close to the age-predicated number. They can then be fitted with either reading glasses for that plus power or glasses that read:

- OD Plano
- OS Plano
- Add +1.00 (or whatever the power)

Plano lens have no power at the top for distance. OD means right eye, and OS means left eye. If the patient cannot read the distance chart to the 20/20 level, let them use the retinoscopy bar to see which lens corrects the vision. Find the glasses that correspond to this prescription for each eye. If the patient is over 40, they will also need additional correction to read. Their prescription should be the power for distance correction with bifocals and the "add" that corresponds to their age. If the patient is over 40 and nearsighted, in the range of -1.50 to -3.00, they can take off their glasses to read. If the patient cannot be corrected for the eye chart with the retinoscopy bar, they either have an astigmatism or a physical problem, such as a cataract or macular degeneration. You may attempt to correct for astigmatism by trying various prescriptions, but this is a difficult and trying procedure. This patient may need to be referred to the physician present, who is most knowledgeable about eye problems.

Finding the right pair of glasses for the patient after the prescription is derived is perhaps the most difficult assignment. Place all the reading glasses in one area, as these will be the ones most commonly used. Sometimes the final choice for the individual patient is decided by a combination of the correct prescription and the patient's choice of style.

Lines for glasses clinics are often intimidating in length. Even so, every patient is important, so spend as much time as is necessary with each individual. Try to discern the spiritual needs of each patient and pray with them, as the Lord leads. Patients with unmet needs or those expressing more spiritual concerns should be taken to the appropriate areas in the clinic, such as the evangelism table or to the medical area.

Eye Clinics with Eye-Care Specialists

Mydriatic Sun Glasses

Patients' pupils may be dilated and clinics are usually in an intense sun environment, so take ample pairs of mydriatic disposable sunglasses. If patient's pupils will be dilated for the examination, ample pairs of disposable sunglasses should be brought to give the patients to protect their eyes until the pupils return to normal.

Dilation Drops

Some providers opt to use a mixture of 1/3 1% Mydriacyl®, 1/3 1% Cyclogyl®, and 1/3 2.5% Neosynephrine®. This works for a rapid and effective dilation. Try to take tissues to give to the patients after the drops.

Hand Instruments for Eye Specialists

- Retinoscope with multiple rechargeable batteries
- Portable binocular indirect ophthalmoscope
- Transilluminator
- Tonopen® or Shiotz tonometer
- Retinoscopy bars

Pharmaceuticals

- 1% Mydriacyl®
- 1% Cyclogyl®
- 2.5% Neosynephrine®
- Lubricant (lots)
- Glaucoma medications
- Topical steroids
- Allergy products
- Antibiotic ointments

Most pharmaceutical companies are good about donating products. Be sure to contact them well ahead of your trip to allow time for shipping. Be sure to obtain lots of lubricants and antibiotic drops.

Patient Flow

Coordinate with the main clinic triage so that eye patients can be efficiently directed to the eye exam area. Visual acuity can be checked and recorded by a layperson. Then patients can be directed to the optometrist or ophthalmologist.

One possibility consists of having three benches set up, usually for 10 people each. Thirty patients can be seated and an assistant can be taught how to put the drops in. Once the people on the front bench are dilated, they may be examined one at a time. Once the front bench is cleared, the 2 benches behind them can move up, and the assistant calls in 10 more patients and instills the drops into their eyes. The flow will continue working in groups of 10.

The assistant may be instructed to give each patient a numbered card, to be sure they have received the drops. Making up 50 cards and taking the cards from the patients once they have been seen and then starting over, helps to keep track of how many patients have been seen. Patients see the practitioner one at a time, unless there are several providers, then they can flow through stations for retinoscopy, tonometry and ophthalmoscopy.

Examination

The exam station is usually set up in the darkest place which can be found. This is usually in a dark corner in a room. (In case of having to set up under a large shade tree outside, it is a good idea to bring a tarp and rope to help block the sun.)

The numbers of patients may be extremely large, and if there is only an individual provider, there may not be time to do everything. Some practitioners may opt to perform retinoscopy through the dilated pupil using retinoscopy bars. An external evaluation and a binocular indirect ophthalmoscopy examination may be done, based on the complaints. If the patients complain of pain, or they have hard protruding eyes that are indicative of glaucoma, then the disc should be examined. Some experienced providers may opt to make most glaucoma diagnoses from the appearance of the disc. If the patient has glaucomatous cupping, they should be treated with glaucoma medications, a year's supply if possible.

It is acknowledged that some glaucoma patients are missed by this technique. However, if there are large numbers of patients, one can help many more people using this method. Tonometry requires a greater time investment.

If there are multiple providers, then setting up assembly line type stations to do each evaluation is a good idea. Most patients have ocular surface irritations, so lubricants are typically dispensed liberally. If triage gives the patients identification cards, then patients with cataracts, glaucoma, or some problem that can be corrected by surgery, may be flagged either on the card or by making a list. That way, when a surgeon is available at the site later, those patients can be identified for the procedure.

After the examination is complete, the practitioner can write an eyeglass prescription on the patient card and identify the category of box (see below) for the people helping in the glasses dispensary. The practitioner typically will dispense all medications and instruct patients how to use them while they are still at the examination station.

Once patients are examined and given their prescription, they are sent to the dispensary. If they do not need glasses, they can be given their mydriatic sunglasses. At this time you may give them a tract introducing them to the Gospel, or if time permits, ask them about their relationship with Christ. This may of course also be done when the patients receive their prescription glasses.

Dispensary

The eyeglasses are generally boxed and categorized. It is helpful if the provider writes which category of box the dispensing assistant should look in to, in order to match with the closest prescription possible. The following is a suggested useful category guideline to use with some variation depending on the available supplies.

Eyeglasses Categories

A = +1.00 and up   SINGLE VISION
B = +2.00 to +2.75   SINGLE VISION
C = +3.00 to +3.75   SINGLE VISION
D =   0.00 to + 1.00   BIFOCALS
E = +1.00 to +1.75   BIFOCALS
F = +2.00 to +2.75   BIFOCALS
G = –0.25 to -1.75   SINGLE VISION
H = –2.00 to -2.75   SINGLE VISION
I = –1.00 to -1.75   BIFOCALS

Write the prescription on the card and the letter of the box for the assistant to look in to find that prescription. Sometimes it may be necessary to give out multiple pairs of glasses to meet the needs of certain patients. Then the assistant gives patients their mydriatic glasses, and either gives them a Gospel tract, or witnesses to them.

37 Dentistry in Primitive Settings

Annette Merlino

Education
Scope of Treatment
Logistics
Dental Equipment List

Much of the world's population does not have access to a dentist. Dental diseases is one of the most common dental disease in the world and dental infections can be deadly for those without care. Dentistry lends itself well to short-term interventions for several reasons.

- A dentist can rapidly "fix" a tooth, taking care of many dental needs in a short time.
- Gaining a sense of satisfaction.
- Freeing patients from chronic pain.
- Offering opportunities pre-, during and post-procedure to share the Gospel.

Dental services may have a significant impact on a community. Dentists may also teach other medical professionals the art of extraction, as there is such a great need, and many times, there is no dentist on a team or in the area.

The main disadvantage of dentistry is that specialized equipment is needed, making dentists less mobile than our physician colleagues.

Education

Dental education can be performed by a lay person while patients are waiting or after treatment. Bringing a plastic model of a mouth will aid in teaching brushing and flossing techniques. While Coca-Cola® is available in the most remote parts of the world, unfortunately, toothbrushes are not as readily available, nor deemed as desirable. Poor dental hygiene highlights the need for nutritional education. One may customize a presentation for each specific area.

Scope of Treatment

The dentist working in the developing world will need to decide what type of treatment to provide: restorative vs. surgical (simple extractions). While restorative dentistry has its place, if most people are in pain from abscessed teeth, simple extractions are more helpful.

Contact with community leaders to ascertain the local needs ahead of time should help in the decision of offering restorative or surgical treatment. Knowing the answers to the following questions will assist you in preparation.

- What do they perceive to be the greatest dental needs in their area?
- What is the educational level of the people you will serve?
- Do most people have healthy teeth?
- Have dentists practiced there before, and if so, what procedures did they perform?
- Is there an available local dentist?
- What type of dentistry does he or she perform? One does not want to "step on toes." For example, in the Congo, the local dentist only did extractions; therefore, the missionary dentist chose to do restorative work.
- Will you be working with children or adults or a mixed population? If you will be working with older children, you will want to offer restorations. For small children, extraction of primary teeth may be the greatest need. Plan for extractions in a mostly geriatric population. In a

233

general population, it's good to offer both restorations as well as extractions as you will probably do an equal amount of each.

- Is electricity available? Electricity will determine if restorative dentistry can be offered. You may need a transformer to convert 220V to 110V (standard U.S. voltage). Some equipment will run on either, other devices will require an external transformer. Bring a surge protector and extra fuses, especially for your compressor, as power surges can be common. If a generator will be used (perhaps provided locally), make sure that it generates sufficient amperage to run your compressor.

- Will you travel to multiple sites? Restorative dentistry requires a significant amount of time to setup and break down. You may want to limit your services to extractions if you will be traveling to different areas, especially if you will be hiking.

- Will you travel with a group? If you plan to do restorative dentistry, you will need others to pack some of your equipment and check it onto the plane.

- If you will be unable to use restorative equipment, you can still do small fillings using ART (Atraumatic Restorative Treatment). Bring some hand instruments and you can spoon out decay and fill with IRM (Intermediate Restorative Material). You can also clean teeth with hand scalers and give fluoride treatments.

Logistics

Once you determine what types of treatments you will offer, you will need to prioritize, taking the following factors into consideration: number of patients, type of need, and number of working days/hours. Look at the working space and conditions available. Assess the number of volunteers who will be able to assist.

Dental Equipment List

Quantities listed assume one dentist practicing for five days.

GENERAL EXTRACTIONS
- Forceps: 4 cowhorns, 3 upper molars, 2 upper premolar/Ant 2 lower premolar
- Elevators: 4–5 of 34 straight, 1–2 of 34S
- Syringes: 6+
- Anesthesia: 3 boxes (150 carpules), 100 long needles, 50 short needles, topical, zipper bag of Q-Tips®
- Gauze—5–7 packs
- Gloves—3 boxes

AMALGAM
- 2 high speed hand pieces
- Burs assorted
- 3–5 setups including: mirror, explorer, condenser, spoon, carver, amalgam carrier, forceps, matrix band holder
- Small spatula
- 5 mirrors and explorers
- Dappen dish, matrix bands, Dycal,® ZOE (zinc oxide eugenol) or base, mixing pad
- 100 amalgam capsules
- Amalgamator
- Cotton rolls—7 packs

COMPOSITE
- 3 setups—mirror, exp, comp. inst., spoon, forceps
- Clear matrix bands, wedges, etch, bond, brushes
- Composite—1 syringe liquid, 1 syringe reg. or 50 comps and press
- Curing light

CLEANINGS
- 5+ anterior scalers, 2+ post dental equipment setup
- Cavitron and 3–5 tips
- 3 packs gauze

STERILIZATION
- Disinfectant mix to spray
- Cold solution
- Plastic shoebox
- Pressure cooker or large pot with lid
- Hot plate
- Towels—5 hand size
- Gloves—3 boxes (100/box)
- Masks—1 box (50/box)
- Safety glasses

- Head lamp flashlight, with extra batteries

LARGE EQUIPMENT
- Air compressor unit
- Light on stand
- Transformer (as needed)
- Electric strip with surge protector
- Extension cord

MISCELLANEOUS (to give away)
- Toothbrushes and toothpaste
- Dental floss
- Instructional materials (e.g. posters, stickers, etc.)

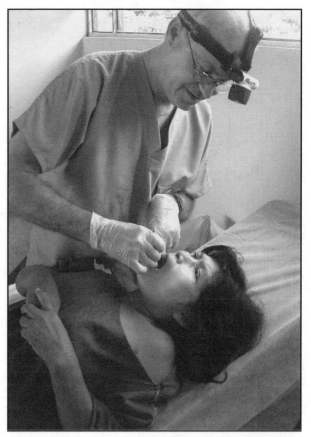

Hartmut Gross/
**"Dentist with Patient
in Rural Jungle Area."**

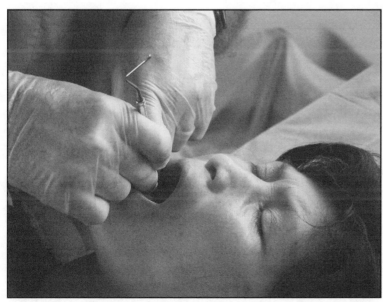

Hartmut Gross/
"First Time Patient Had Ever Seen a Dentist"

Speaking Through an Interpreter

W. "Ted" Kuhn

It was a cartoon drawing of a cat blocking the door so a dog could not enter. Above the door there was a sign,"VA Hospital." The caption read, "Don't go in there, it is full of vets." My teaching schedule at a large Asian university had suddenly been altered. I was to give a presentation I had not prepared and used a PowerPoint® presentation that I had brought with me. It was a PowerPoint® lecture someone else had developed. The first slide was the above cartoon. Thankfully, I had time to go over the slides with my interpreter prior to the presentation. After 15 minutes of trying to explain the humor in the cartoon, I gave up. Her face was expressionless and held no clue of humor or recognition. "It just does not translate," I finally admitted. We deleted the slide.

Translators (or interpreters) speak for you, just as Aaron spoke for Moses. They are special people and can make or break your ministry. Some are excellent and others will be marginal. Some will know medical terminology; others will know few if any medical or technical words. At times, children are used as interpreters, since they learn English in school. It is difficult to speak about complicated medical topics, adult, or "sensitive" issues using a child translator. Theological terms and thoughts as well as prayer are a challenge with a child translator. Prayer and discussions of scripture may also be a challenge when working with an interpreter of another faith. In some cultures a male translator will find it difficult or socially unacceptable addressing a woman and the opposite is also true. Working with a translator can be a "minefield" to the unaware. It can also

be wonderful blessing. Friendships can develop that last a lifetime. The Spirit of God can work in the heart of your translator as he interprets your prayers or as you read scripture. Nevertheless, there are some principles that are worth considering when filtering your words and thoughts through another person.

1. If you will be holding clinics or teaching in another culture, listing common words, especially medical words, or terms that you expect to use and sending them to your interpreter ahead of time allows the opportunity for study and reflection. Choosing the exact word may be critical to your ministry.

2. When lecturing overseas, speaking in a church or giving a sermon, it is very helpful to send your lecture or sermon to your interpreter several weeks ahead of time for the same reason as above. Then, before speaking, review your topic with your interpreter. "Review all technical terms and words important to your task. Also, talk about nuances, key sentences, and ideas to be covered. Discuss any explicit and implied meanings."[1]

3. Lecture handouts or presentations can be translated ahead of time and distributed in a bilingual format, so everyone can understand.

PowerPoint® presentations can be presented in a bilingual format. "If using an overhead projector, be sure to ask the interpreter or someone fluent in the language to translate and prepare these before the workshop. When using a chalk board or dry erase board, make sure you let the interpreter know which media you intend to use and what you will say. This lets the interpreter see how you handle the materials and where you will be positioned."[1]

4. Before your presentation, take time to sit down with the interpreter. Ask this person about his or her work as an interpreter. What sort of material has he worked with? Has he interpreted the kind of material you will be presenting? The more the interpreter knows, the more effective the interpretation. As you share together in conversation, the interpreter will develop a feel for how you talk and how your words flow. Also, the interpreter will gain insight about cadences."[1]

5. Does the interpreter prefer to do simultaneous, literal translation, phrase per phrase? Or does he/she prefer to let you finish an entire thought, then translate your thought using culturally appropriate terminology? "Translation is more effective and enjoyable when trainer and interpreter are a synchronized team, as together they explain, explore, show, and guide."[1]

6. Consider that a 30 to 40 minute presentation will take one hour when using a translator and plan accordingly. "When working with a translator, be sure to watch the faces and eyes of the listeners. They will help you determine whether or not the subject, idea or illustration is being grasped. Be ready to repeat or rephrase."[1]

7. Your interpreter will also translate questions from your audience back to you. The quality of the questions will give you an idea of the level of understanding in the audience. It may also be helpful to have the audience write their questions in their native language and have your interpreter translate the written questions to you. This allows for "saving face" if your lecture was poorly understood of if the question is poorly stated.

8. Interpreting for someone else can be an exhausting task. Make sure that your interpreter has plenty of rest between presentations. Also make sure you have a back-up person if one translator does not work well with you.

9. Remember, your interpreter is working as hard as you, perhaps harder. Consider that he/she needs breaks, and refreshments and lunch just as you do. It is courteous as well as expedient to ask your interpreter to accompany you to meals, to share in the benefits of the ministry and not only the work. Interpreters, like all people, are precious in the sight of God. Like Aaron and Moses, they were the most effective instrument of God's grace when they worked together.

References
1. Reekie, Robert in msips.org faq #69 2004.

The Role of Non-Medical Team Members

Doreen Hung Mar

The premise of medical missions does not preclude a non-medical person from being an integral part of a team. In fact, laypersons may make significant contributions in many different areas ranging from preparations and travel logistics, to organization and overseeing daily functions of the clinics, to ministry, to debriefing and helpful suggestions that improve the effectiveness of future teams. They can also share their experiences with other non-medical people who may "catch the vision" of medical missions.

The spiritual purpose of medical missions is to enhance, encourage, and help establish the local church's ministry to communities. Medical missions, as part of an evangelistic movement, should not be the principle goal in and of itself. Instead, they should be utilized as part of the outreach ministries of the church to bring the wonderful news of salvation for eternal healing and not just physical relief or comfort.

The non-medical person as well as the medical professional should travel and minister with the same heart and attitude as that of Christ Jesus, "taking the very nature of a servant," as exhorted by Paul in Philippians 2:5,7. Through the Holy Spirit, pray for creative gifts and insight when opportunities open where the non-medical member can make contributions that improve the success of the ministry.

Adequate preparation can impact efficiency in many ways. There are a myriad number of ways which lay people can assist, even if he/she is not traveling with the team to the host country. These range from collecting, to sorting and labeling, to packaging and packing medicines and supplies. Baggage handling is also an important issue, and a person assigned to tagging and keeping track of the bags is essential—it's hard to work without supplies if they don't arrive.

On clinic days, the non-medical team member can oversee the flow of patients from registration through triage prior to their medical evaluation, as well as monitoring the general operation of the clinic. Are the practitioners getting adequate breaks and staying well-hydrated? Do the patients who are waiting to be seen understanding and tolerating the wait-times? Are they being spiritually ministered to while waiting to be seen or while waiting for tests to get back? What more can be done to enhance their understanding or appreciation of the goals of the church? Are the patients' needs being prayed for by ministry teams?

On a medical missions trip, a person or team dedicated to ministry has a captive audience in the patients waiting to be seen by the medical personnel. An instrumentalist, like a violinist, can produce heavenly music that resonates through the deep Amazon jungle; the voice of an opera singer mesmerizes a restless audience; a storyteller, with puppet or marionette in hand, memorably entertains and educates and evangelizes to a child's spirit beyond a story simply told; skits or mime can demonstrate a message that transcends language. The message of an entertainer dedicated to showing and sharing God's love can filter through and touch the heart that sometimes even the best medicine cannot reach. No medical knowledge is needed to convey these messages.

In the trenches of medical missions work, someone with no medical experience, but with the fortitude and resolve to assist and learn, can find or be assigned numerous jobs, and even develop new skills along the way. These new areas of expertise are most often acquired in the laboratory and pharmacy that accompanies medical teams.

Finally, upon returning home, the layperson can share the vision of the eternal spiritual impact of a medical missions trip. Expressed in writing, photographs, small group presentations, speaking engagements, non-medical members can communicate how medical teams are all part of God's work to deliver His message of love and salvation for us through His Son, Jesus Christ.

Suggested Roles for Non-Medical Team Members on a Medical Missions Trip

Preparations and Logistical Help Prior to Trip

- First and foremost is prayer, enlisting intercessors and lay-borers (please forgive the pun).
- Sorting, labeling, packaging, packing of medications and supplies.
- Making Gospel bracelets or assembling ministry materials for Bible school, street evangelism.
- Procuring items like toothbrushes, floss, toothpaste, eyeglasses, glass cases, thermometers, toys, clothes, etc.
- Necessary, though mundane, tasks like cutting pharmacy labels and dipsticks, organizing lab tests and reagents.

- Copying and assembling song sheets or booklets, preparing morning devotions, evening discussion topics during debriefing sessions, internal team discussions, and organization of corporate prayer times.
- During travel, tagging all baggage, monitoring and keeping track of the number of pieces, any damaged or lost items, and if separated, tracking lost pieces to arrive at proper destination.
- Help set up meetings to orient and prepare team members to the host country and conditions to be encountered.

General Needs During Trip

- Prayer for clinic, patients and ministry—praying continuously—includes "prayer warriors" at home.
- General operation of time schedules (for travel, breaks, meals, etc.); confirmation of flights or travel arrangements.
- Water-purification—very important part of overall health of team members—need responsible person(s) to make sure clean (purified) water is available at all times. This may even entail pumping water from a river, as in trips to jungles, or simply treating all water, even bottled water, with iodine or chlorine. The water requirements also include pediatric medicine suspensions.
- Food preparation—a.k.a. a food guard, someone with almost militaristic resolve to oversee proper food preparation, cleaning of utensils and dishes, cutting of fresh fruits with the two-knife method, etc.
- Treasurer—a VIP job!!! Keeper of receipts—however difficult to obtain, however small the expense. Keeping expense records is one of the more difficult, tedious, yet most important jobs of a trip.
- Photographer, video-producer, team journalist; includes post-trip organizer and producer of trip documentation.

Needs During Clinic, Non-medical

- Prayer.
- Organization of clinic flow from registration through triage to medical provider;

certain patients may need to be escorted through this process.

- Keeping track that all personnel stay well-hydrated, especially in hot, humid environments.
- Runner—high-energy deliverer of messages, supplies, etc.
- General ministry with prayer teams for individuals, to homes (home visits), to communities.
- Distribute clothes and shoes, help sort them and fit them, especially on to little people (this job may be rewarded with lots of shy smiles); fashion sense not required.
- Play time with children—persons with endless capacity to blow bubbles or balloons (including twisting balloons for Gospel ministry); any iota of artistry, like drawing with sidewalk chalk, or making figures of clay or Play-dough;® play games (patty-cake, cat's cradle, Frisbee,® soccer, simple ball games), learn their games; present and distribute Wordless Gospel bracelets, flyers, tracts; juggler willing to teach how to juggle can use bags made of the Gospel colors.

Needs During Clinic, Medically-Related

- Language skills, interpreters/translators—even a small amount can help for simple interpretation or instructions, and also for prayer
- Dental demonstrations—tooth-brushing, flossing. If you brush and floss your teeth, you're qualified!
- Pharmacy assistant—if you can count from 1–100 and you're good with charades, you can help.
- Lab tech—potential new skills. Perform simple lab tests, e.g. pregnancy tests, urine dipsticks; learn how to draw blood—on-the-job training provided.
- Eyeglasses—learn to determine correct prescription and fit patient for eyeglasses.
- Help pump nebulizer for aerosolized treatments of lung problems.
- Consider assisting in physical or massage therapy.
- Wound care—learn to clean and dress wounds, especially burn wounds.

- Proper cleaning and disposal of blood, body fluids, wastes, needles/sharps—an undesirable but absolutely necessary job.
- Cleaning of medical instruments, and possibly body parts—also requires a servant's heart.

Ministry

- Designated person for conflict resolution and mediation.
- Prayer team.
- Evangelism team—evangelist, pastor, lay pastor, team to minister to patient(s), family, homes.
- Present or distribute evangelism materials, Bibles, tracts, flyers, Gospel bracelets and explain significance of colors.
- Audiovisual tech—run the "Jesus" film; have Bible ready to answer questions.
- Entertainment/performance—music, song, dance, stories, skits, mime, balloons, drawings, etc. that depict Biblically-oriented themes.
- Relationship building—talking with people; show interest and ask questions about their lives and life-styles (families, professions, hobbies, ways of cooking and even recipes, employment opportunities, culture, worldview, prayer needs, etc.); play with children; be a good listener; drink some tea or coffee or local nonalcoholic "social" beverage; simply "hang out."

After the Missions Trip

- Debrief, and share constructive criticism that can improve future teams.
- Write trip account—incorporate journal entries, experiences, stories from the trip that impressed you and that would encourage others to contribute or participate in a medical missions team.
- Write "thank you" notes to supporters and incorporate your trip account or a short version of it.
- Show photographs or videos, and consider sending some back to the missionaries or nationals!
- Give small group presentations or speaking engagements on how medical teams by "Word and Deed" demonstrate God's

sovereignty and His desire for peoples to be a part of His Kingdom.

- Invite and/or recruit others to join and share experiences with future medical missions teams.

- Pray about your support of medical missions, sign up for your next trip, and restart the cycle!

Share the Vision, and Ignite Spiritual Fires!

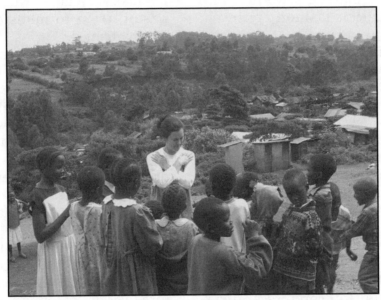

Ted Kuhn/
"Children's Ministry"

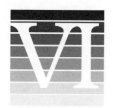

Section VI:
Returning from the Field

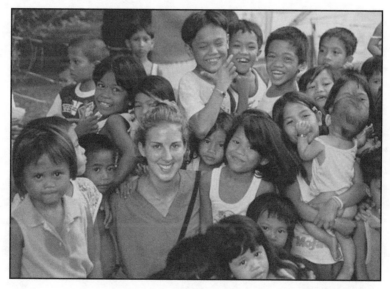

Ted Kuhn/
"New Friends"

Was It Worthwhile?
A Short Story

W. "Ted" Kuhn

It is my first day back to work after returning from Honduras. I am exhausted from the long hours of patient care in the wake of the devastation wrought by Hurricane Mitch. Although the emergency department is full of patients, my heart and mind are full of questions and a part of me is still in Central America. Was it worthwhile? Did the medical team make a difference? Would the people of the Aguan Valley have been better off if we had just sent them the money spent on airfare and support?

I remember the parable of pulling drowning people out of a river. It is often used as an argument against curative medical services. It goes something like this. I can work all day and night until I am exhausted pulling drowning people out of the river, but it is only when I discover why they are falling in upstream, and prevent them from falling in, that I can really make a difference. I have spent the last several weeks pulling drowning people out of a river and I am certainly exhausted. I even knew why they were falling in upstream and I knew how to prevent them from falling. Nevertheless, I spent these weeks as a life-guard and constructed no fence upstream. How can I justify my actions to others and defend the expense and resources spent on curative medicine in rural Honduras?

An emergency medicine resident asks me to see a patient. He presents a middle-aged woman with advanced breast cancer. She has a metastatic lesion in her back causing her constant, severe pain. She is unable to lie down or stand comfortably and recently developed weakness in her legs-the tumor expanding to her spinal cord. A "slam-dunk" for the resident- an easy patient.

Order an MRI and admit to neurosurgery for decompression. Yet, speaking with her breaks my heart. She is frail and covers her head with a bandana having lost her hair from chemotherapy. She grimaces in pain as we talk. She looks older than her years and much older than her husband-weeks of pain and suffering having taken their toll. She asks for pain relief and I give her morphine. For the moment she rests, her pain relieved. I know that soon the pain will return. We both know that in the next several days the cancer will claim her frail life. Her short future will be filled with days of discomfort as she struggles with the pain and good-byes to family and friends. I left the room but returned to check on her. She stirred and held out her hand. I extended mine. And for a moment our hands and lives touched. She wanted to thank me for the care I provided, then closed her eyes and fell back to sleep. I had thought of asking if the morphine helped, but I already knew the answer.

Ask a drowning man if he desires rescue. Ask him, even if he knows he will fall in again. What is the value of another day? Another week? A month? A year? What would his answer be? What would your answer be? Is temporary relief of pain or healing worthwhile? Indeed, it is priceless! Mercy extended in love. Even in this age of high-speed technology, physical and spiritual healing nevertheless proceed at the pace of one life touching another. Is temporary relief of suffering worthwhile? Look into the eyes of the woman dying of breast cancer. Or look into the eyes of a Honduran mother who has lost everything. And you will know the answer.

Resources
1. Kuhn W., *My Eyes, His Heart*, Winepress, 2002.

40 Preparing to Return Home

W. "Ted" Kuhn

The United States Customs Service has become increasingly strict following September 11th about re-entering the US with supplies, durable medical goods and medicines in any substantial quantity from an overseas location. Medical teams and team leaders need to be certain before they leave the US that they are in compliance with US customs policy regarding the re-importation of unused medical supplies and pharmaceuticals back into the country after the completion of a deployment.

It is a wise policy NOT to leave unused medicines and supplies in the host country after a short term medical ministry. There are numerous reasons for this:

1. Medicines and supplies can be sold on the street which would violate the agreement with many of the donor agencies that supply items to teams free of charge (or subsidized) with the understanding that these items and supplies will reach the poor without charge. This may jeopardize future relationships with donor agencies and is at least, poor stewardship.

2. There is no way to insure accountability of supplies left behind. The proceeds of supplies sold can be pocketed by one or several individuals without ability to account for the money involved. If claims are made that the supplies and medicines were sold, the individual can reply that they were given to the poor. The proceeds from supplies left behind can be substantial- often many times the yearly salary of national workers. Since there may be no records, it is one person's word against another.

3. Charges of impropriety or theft can be brought against innocent national workers or church planters if all supplies can not be accounted for. Jealousy and rivalry does exist in communities where medical teams work in the developing world. Good ministries can be discredited by well-intentioned but naive US teams. The very ministry that the team came to support, can be destroyed by careless disregard for supplies and resources.

4. If the person in the host country is not licensed to practice medicine in that country or is not medical, leaving prescription medicines that they will dispense encourages them to practice without a license and perhaps even break the law of the host country in regards to the legal practice of medicine, and it opens the possibility of accidental misuse of medication. This not only jeopardizes the national workers status in country, but the mission team's ability to return and conduct future medical ministry.

5. Rival ministries in the host country may be competing for resources. Leaving valuable supplies with one ministry encourages jealousy and suspicion between co-existing ministries.

6. Storage conditions may not be ideal and medicines and supplies may be ruined by the heat or humidity. Frequently medicine will become out of date of date before use.

7. Supplies are often needed in other countries for other ongoing or future medical outreaches and can easily be transported back to the US to be deployed with another medical team.

These and other reasons compel all of us to return to the US with unused supplies. Often you will be carrying both durable medical goods (lab, microscope) and unused pharmaceuticals in your check-through luggage upon re-entering the US. To comply with US customs requirements for returning to the US with medicines, you will need several documents:

1. The original letter from the donor agency stating that all medicines and supplies were donated free of charge (or minimal charge) and to be used for humanitarian purposes. (King pharmaceuticals provides this letter with each shipment of medicines.) SonoSite, International Aid and MAP will provide a letter at your request.
2. List of all medicines and supplies that you took *out* of the US.
3. Letter from your sending agency saying that you are a part of their international outreach and providing humanitarian services free of charge in the country you are returning from. (The Mission to the World medical department currently provides this "get-out-of-jail-free" letter to its team leaders on all medical teams.) Copy of "Organizational Letter" included in the appendix of this text.
4. List of medicines, supplies or durable medical goods that you are *returning* with back into the US. (A reasonable estimate of the amount of medicine is sufficient.)

To comply with US customs requirements for returning to the US with durable medical goods (microscope, lab equipment, I-STATs, ultrasound, surgical equipment, laptop, LCD projector, camera or anything

with a serial number) you will need to fill out a customs service Form 4455- Certificate of Registration. You will need to attach a list of all durable supplies you are returning with, description of the item and serial number. You can get the form online at- http://www.customs.gov/xp/cgov/toolbox/forms/. You will need to go to your nearest US Customs office to have your list "certified" before you leave. Once done, you can use this list repeatedly on all your trips.

All international airports will have a customs office that provides this service. In Atlanta, the customs office is across I-75 from the airport at 4341 International Parkway, exit 239—phone (404) 675-1300. US customs offices are open 8–4:30, 7 days a week. However, call before you go.

It is currently illegal to return narcotics or controlled substances into the United States. The author questioned US customs officials explicitly regarding the return into the US with small amounts of controlled substances carried in the emergency bag for use with ill or injured team members. Exceptions to this restriction are allowable under the following conditions:

1. That the individual carrying the controlled substances is a licensed medical practitioner in the US (and has his/her medical or DEA license to prove it);
2. That the amount of controlled substances carried is minimal (reasonable quantity that would be used to treat one or several sick or injured individuals).

By following these recommendations, you will be in compliance with US Customs requirements and avoid unpleasant legal entanglement in the airport upon your arrival into the US.

41 Debriefing Medical Mission Teams

David Foster

Medical mission team participants are not exempt from developing post-traumatic stress symptoms or other significant complications from incidents encountered on the missions field. Preventing such occurrences should be a primary goal of sending agencies and team leaders. Ideally, we would want all participants returning home with an eagerness for future involvement in missions work. Fortunately, there is an emerging body of literature and training is available that can assist in this process.

Exposure to stress and emotional trauma is part and parcel of short-term medical and career missions ventures. Team members may be first responders to disasters such as hurricanes, floods, and earthquakes. Often more subtle but no less difficult to deal with may be governmental corruption or incompetence which impedes providing adequate medical care. Working with previously unseen diseases or extreme levels of poverty may be uncommonly upsetting. Another, perhaps unexpected issue to work through is the long-term trauma resident missionaries have been exposed to. Their stories can be secondarily traumatizing to medical team providers. In a fallen world, difficulties occur even to God's people. This should not surprise the reader of scripture, which recounts the suffering of numerous saints and repeatedly cites suffering as the common lot of the believer (John 16:33; James 1:2; I Peter 4:12). A problem can emerge, however, when team members approach a trip in an unrealistic, romanticized fashion, which does not take into account deep differences across cultures and differences in the practice of medicine.

Literature on crisis intervention methodology, Critical Incident Stress Management, and missionary trauma provides instructive advice on how to effectively debrief and hopefully prevent posttraumatic stress from developing among missions participants. Regrettably some mission agencies have been reluctant to utilize such information. There are a myriad of reasons: fear of confronting emotionally loaded situations, fear the incident will reflect poorly on the agency, avoidance due to not wanting to deal with one's own trauma, etc.

There are several approaches to debriefing (operational debriefing; personal debriefing; and group sharing) utilized in the missions world. Typically interventions are dictated by how soon a debriefing can occur and the perceived severity of the crisis. Team members who are clear in their understanding as to role, culture, and risks before arriving on the scene will typically be less disturbed by what they experience. Premorbid level of psychological functioning is also a fairly accurate predictor of response to crises. It should also be said, however, that even veterans in missionary and medical endeavors are not exempt from the effects of trauma. Debriefing sessions should serve the functions of lessening current stress, preventing post-traumatic symptoms from developing, and where needed, referring for further pastoral and/or psychological assistance. The purpose of debriefing is not to provide counseling but to provide all participants the opportunity to relate their experience of what they have encountered.

The author has found the following format to be useful in debriefing short-term teams. It assumes daily monitoring of team members by team leaders regarding the need for one-on-one attention. It presupposes that adequate pre-trip information on culture, role, risks, and stress management has been given to participants. It utilizes a six question outline. The questions are designed to begin with facts, move to feelings and return to facts. They are to be presented at the end of a trip, normally the last evening before departure or after a particularly difficult day in a non-threatening atmosphere. Debriefings are not intended to be operational critiques, those matters should be dealt with separately. Debriefings are for processing reactions to mission team experiences.

While informed by and indebted to CISM and other resources, the following model is the author's own. He is solely responsible for its content. It was developed out of his mission and crisis intervention experience. The questions are as follows:

1. What was your role today/on this trip?
2. What have been the most meaningful events of today/this trip?
3. What have been the most difficult parts of today/this trip?
4. What spiritual benefits have you gained from this experience?
5. What do you need to pray about?
6. What action steps do you need to take as a result of this experience? (For yourself, for others)

Attendance is mandatory, but participation is voluntary. No one should be forced to speak. Everyone should speak for themselves and not critique others' reactions. This format is easily used by team leaders or their designees. It elicits material that is often common to many in the group, thus normalizing the experience. It also takes the experience through a biblical/spiritual grid. Participants hopefully will gain some sense of eternal perspective regarding their experience.

It is wise to maintain a referral list of competent pastoral and psychological professionals to whom you can refer team members whenever necessary. Be especially aware of warning signs such as: inability to sleep, obsessive focus on an incident, persistent crying, difficulty doing daily tasks, and suicidal thinking. Those individuals are likely in need of professional assistance.

Resources

1. The American Association of Christian Counselors offers training in Critical Incident Stress Management
2. Mission Training International offers training for ministry and mental health professionals who work in missions. It also offers week-long debriefing and renewal sessions for returning missionaries.
3. International Critical Incident Stress Foundation offers training and literature in the internationally recognized standard of care in dealing with critical incidents.
4. Figley, Charles R., and McCubbin, Hamilton I., *Stress and the Family*, (Vols. I and II), Brunner/Mazel, NY, NY, 1983.

Relevant Reading

1. Carr, Karen. *Trauma and posttraumatic stress disorder among missionaries.* Evangelical Missions Quarterly, July 1994, 246–255.
2. Carr, Karen. *Crisis intervention for missionaries.* Evangelical Missions Quarterly, (1997) vol. 33, no. 4.
3. International Critical Incident Stress Foundation, 3290 Pine Orchard Lane, Suite 106, Ellicott City, MD 21042 (offers training and resources).
4. Patterson, Frank and Ericksson, Cynthia. *Missionary Trauma on the Front Lines*, Christian Counseling Today, (2003) vol. 11, no. 3, 18–22.
5. O'Donnell, Kelly, ed. *Doing Member Care Well: Perspectives and Practices from Around the World*, William Carey Library, Pasadena, CA, 2002.
6. O'Donnell, Kelly, ed. *Missionary Care: Counting The Cost For World Evangelization*. Willam Carey Library, Pasadena, CA 1992.
7. Foyle, Marjory. *Overcoming Missionary Stress*, Evangelical Missions Information Service, Wheaton, IL., 1987.

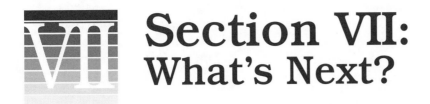

Section VII:
What's Next?

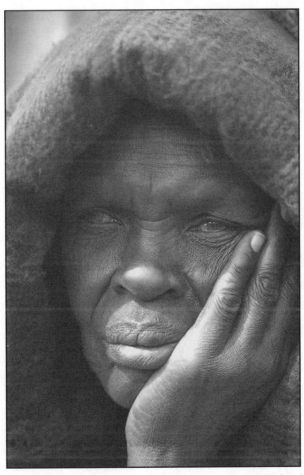

Ted Kuhn/
"What Does the Future Hold?"

Farewell to the Last Spring

W. "Ted" Kuhn

Small droplets of fresh dew glisten on the delicate yellow rose clinging to the white trellis in the morning sun. It's spring in Georgia and the air is full of beauty, hope and new life. The view from my front porch is fresh, colorful, and reviving. Confederate jasmine budding, yet still lacking a few days before releasing its intoxicating fragrance. A mud wasp flies motionless, suspended in time, approaching a crack in a broken shutter. Squirrels scurry gathering acorns. A bird crafts a nest in the fork of an ancient water oak, Spanish moss draped majestically over the limb. The sun on my face is warm and inviting. I am at home, at rest, at peace, and loved.

It is hard to remember that only a few days ago, I walked the colorless hallways of Manila's infectious disease hospital. It now seems more like a thousand years. The malaria ward had been nearly empty owing to the dry season. I noted resting mosquitoes on the walls of the dengue ward, perhaps digesting their latest blood meal. A young woman with the dengue rash lay in bed eating supper with her husband and children. I had purposely walked slowly past the rabies ward. There were black steel bars across the door. Patients locked in, a potential threat to the staff. The newly dead body of an 11-year old boy lay shrouded inside. Steel bars flung open- the child no longer a threat. A pediatric casualty in a microscopic war. More wards, more patients, more hallways. Nurses doing chores. Residents writing on charts. The smell of disinfectant. Chipped paint. Private conversations in hushed tones. Overhanging white signs here and there: meningitis, chicken pox, dengue, measles and cholera.

The tuberculosis ward was isolated from the main hospital. A low, one story structure of nondescript construction. Benches with idle patients lined the hallways. There was a musty smell. Deadly bacilli, too small for the human eye to see filled the air. My physician friend had pulled a handkerchief from his pocket and covered his mouth and nose. Instinctively I held my breath. Past the first ward then around the corner to the next. Unable to hold my breath any longer I decided to take short shallow breaths in a vain attempt to limit my own exposure.

Halfway down the next corridor was the tuberculosis dying room. A large rectangular room, with windows for viewing from the hallway. The designated place for patients with overwhelming infection or drug resistance. Fourteen beds. No nurses or residents running in or out. Isolated, alone. Unlike other patients on other wards, they did not turn to look or stare. No smiles, no greeting. Patients unwilling to be even momentarily distracted from the grave business of the day. Two beds held newly shrouded bodies. Sentinels, neatly wrapped in white, waiting patiently for someone, perhaps anyone who cared. The barely living and the newly dead, side by side. Emaciated bodies, hollow cheeks, blank stares. Despair written in their eyes. Expressions of silent acceptance and hopelessness. Separated by us, for us. The living dead nearing the end of their last journey. One door in, one way out.

I am alone on my front porch in the warm Georgia sun enjoying life's simple pleasures. Content to be here-yet an inconvenient memory hangs over me. My cup of coffee empty, the tasks of the day beckon like an unsolicited intrusion into the quiet. The mud wasp now safely inside the shutter. A honeybee visits the yellow rose. My daughter gets ready for school.

Cars to be driven, meetings to make, and events of the day that will suppress the painful vision of the dying room and the questions I am afraid to ask, and even if asked, dare not attempt to answer. Why me? Why the good fortune of birth and God's special grace? What special merit has placed me on my springtime Georgia porch-and not on the stretchers of the dying room? In the counsel of the Almighty before the foundations of the earth, why was I chosen? And the knowledge that to whom much is given, much is expected.

The beauty of springtime in Georgia -a lifeless rectangular room in Manila. The fragrance of confederate jasmine-the musty smell of antiseptic. A yellow rose-the gray corridors. The green leaves- the white shrouds waiting for someone, anyone. Anticipation for tomorrow- despair sufficient for today. New life, and no life. Many roads to take-only one way out. The task of living, the task of dying. And the bittersweet sorrow of a farewell to the last spring.

42 Principles for Long Term Health Ministry

Brian D. Riedel

"Discernment is not a matter of simply telling the difference between right and wrong; rather, it is telling the difference between right and almost right."
C. H. Spurgeon (1834-1892)

The scope of health ministry in support of the worldwide ministry of the Christian church is very broad indeed, spanning continents, rural to urban settings, formally educated to preliterate societies, and the entire range of economic conditions from exceedingly wealthy to unspeakably poor. No single model of ministry can be expected to apply to such a range of settings.

Nonetheless, the inclusion of this chapter on the topic of models for ministry implies the existence of at least some fundamental principles to guide us in thinking about and implementing long-term health ministry, regardless of the specifics of one's particular local context. It is these guiding principles that this brief chapter seeks to highlight. Fortunately, much has been learned in this regard during the past 150 years of medical experience on the global missions front so that we can learn from those who have gone before us – both their God-given successes and blessed failures – rather than having to reinvent this work

from the ground up.[1] This chapter will attempt to summarize the extensive literature dealing with health and community development among the poor.

Although it's natural for our thoughts to run toward the mechanics of health ministry – the factor of *"what"* we ought to be doing – it is also tremendously important to take the time to reflect upon the ideas of *how* and *by whom* and *for whom* we implement these ministries as having similar, if not greater, influence on the long-term impact of our work.

Learning from History: Dismantling the Traditional Model

Within evangelical Christian circles, the model of traditional "medical missions" in developing nations over the past few decades has focused on a western, curative approach to medicine, typically delivered from fixed mission clinics or hospitals. While this has offered a first-world quality of medical care in the places where it's been developed, this model is intrinsically limited and unsustainable for several important reasons:

- It is extremely expensive, draining missions' budgets.
- It almost always creates *dependency* on the continued presence of highly trained expatriate professional health workers for continuation of the work; conversely, such work frequently collapses within a very short interval after withdrawal of the expatriate presence.
- It may contribute to *perpetuating systemic injustice,* by relieving acute pressure upon

local authorities and governments to address the health of their people.

- Most importantly of all, it communicates *erroneous ideas* regarding the nature and source of health.

The traditional 'medical missions' model mistakenly implies that:

- Health comes from outside of the community—it can and must be "delivered" by experts; the community residents have neither power nor control over their own health.
- Health is a right to be demanded rather than a responsibility to be guarded2.
- Health is found in institutions, in fortresses or islands separated from the daily reality of local residents.
- The North American model of high-tech health care is to be most highly sought after, despite its cost and unsustainability.

Very little in the North American health care professional's training and experience in the U.S. prepares him or her to think in ways outside of this dominant model. As a result, we typically enter uncritically into a new host culture without ever pausing to even consider the appropriate questions regarding whether our approach is well-suited to the context and whether it will truly produce the desired fruit we seek through medical missions.

As a general rule, this results in a top-down, sickness-care model centered on the health professional, which is effective in relieving suffering in the case of acute illness for as long as the expatriate professional remains[3]. While such an approach is often personally gratifying, it sadly does little to actually raise the standard of health over time at the community level. When such externally-driven work withdraws from the community for whatever reason, the population may actually be left in *worse* condition than prior to the effort, as now the people not only have the same unmet health needs but in addition, their expectations of what health care is supposed to look like and from where it should come have been dramatically altered, for good or for ill.

Assumptions

Recognizing this historically dominant model and its limitations, what then should be our response? In light of our goal of extending the Kingdom of God through compassionate health ministry, a series of key questions must be asked to guide our activities:

- From where does health come?
- What makes a community healthy?
- Are we more interested in treating sickness or in promoting health (which, it must be understood, are <u>not</u> the same thing)?
- How may our health ministry reflect the gospel in a truly integrated sense, and not simply as a "carrot" or drawing card to attract people to a church service afterwards?

Our honest answers to these questions reveal much about our preconceptions and cultural biases. This matters because how we define health, sickness and disease will, in large measure, drive our response, whether consciously or unconsciously:

- Poor health defined as merely a lack of curative resources will lead to investment in medicines, doctors and technology.
- Poor health defined as merely a lack of access to services will lead to the building of clinics and hospitals.
- Poor health defined as systemic injustice and oppression of the poor will result in political activism.
- Poor health defined as social inequities (racism, unbiblical views of women, domestic issues, etc.) leads to efforts directed at social reform.
- Poor health defined as a lack of Biblical *shalom* (see below) ought to lead to the broadest approach of all, including many of the above-mentioned elements, but far more comprehensive in its reach. This sweeping approach aimed at pursuing the *shalom* of a community must produce an integrated presentation of gospel in multiple dimensions.

Bryant Myers defines poverty as fundamentally a *spiritual* problem, resulting from the marring of the God-given identity of (or God's image within) the poor, and implying the need for spiritual solutions.[4] By extension, it can be argued that poor health stemming from poverty is similarly a spiritual matter at its root, with the solution necessarily requiring attention to the recovery of God's image, His design, for those afflicted in their physical, relational and spiritual dimensions. It very often has as much to do with a crippling worldview as with a lack of material resources.

Happily, in recent times, we are again rediscovering from our Hebrew roots the concept of *shalom,* variably translated as peace, harmony, wholeness, or wellness, and capturing like no English language equivalent the idea of humankind in the state of complete positive wellness for which it was designed by its Creator.[5,6]

Implicit within this shalom definition, of course, is that a healthy community is not something that can be delivered from without, no matter how well-intentioned the effort. Individuals and the community as a whole must take responsibility for their own health. Outside help may certainly be needed, in the sense of guidance, ideas, advocacy, start-up capital for projects, and even well implemented medical care. However, the fundamental goal is always to seek to raise up local leadership, engender local ownership and transmit a vision for health that is within the grasp of the community, while at the same time stimulating it to look beyond and think more holistically than it had before. In such a model, the outside expert's input is seen more in the form of catalyst, stimulus and collaborative consultant than in up-front, take-charge, imposed design and implementation.

One important caveat of such a grass-roots, community-based approach to health ministry that is sometimes hard for us to accept is the truth that *some communities cannot be helped.* That is to say, whether due to prior exposure to less developmentally-oriented models, lack of vision or whatever other reason, there will be some communities which do not wish to invest in their own health and may choose to continue to wait for someone from the outside to "deliver" health to them. Difficult though it may be to do, in such cases, limited precious resources are best directed toward other communities that demonstrate the ability to learn and grow.

A word is in order here regarding the challenge of cross-cultural communication. Whether we are traditional church-planting missionaries or have a specific focus on health ministry, the success of our efforts hinges on our effectiveness in communicating our message across cultural boundaries. As Paul Hiebert emphasizes, "Communication occurs only when the sender and the receiver have something in common...[Our] communication must be measured not by the messages we send but by the messages the people receive. In other words, *our communication must be receptor-oriented.*"[7] The only way this can possibly occur is if we become students of the culture we are serving.

Principles

Much good has come out of recent emphasis in Christian community outreach circles from recapturing the tight integration between word and deed ministries as more faithful representations of the gospel than mere preaching (word) or social ministries (deed) would ever be alone.[8] Gary Waldecker broadens this idea even further, coming from the starting point of how God reveals Himself to us in history, arguing that this constrains our approach to life and ministry, given that we are citizens of His Kingdom. Waldecker speaks not only of the modalities of word (proclamation) and deed (acts of mercy) as central aspects of God's self-revelation, but also of God's *presence* (or *character*), referring to the truth that some of what we know about God, and by extension some of how we will make Him known through health ministry, can only come through traveling together down the road of life, of shared experience.[9] Only in this way do we come to truly know someone at the deepest level: by the testimony of God's faithful walking with His people through the generations, we know more of His character; by our similar walking through both the joyful and difficult places of life with those we serve with health ministry, we can more completely incarnate the gospel among them. Recalling always that our central focus in health ministry is to make visible the good news of the gospel, it is incumbent upon us to seek to most faithfully communicate the complete, well-rounded character of our God taking advantage of all means available to us.

Building upon this framework of word, deed and presence, and in order to result in a health ministry that promotes real, sustainable increments in the health of a community while at the same time pointing people to Christ as their greatest need for health at the most profound level, many of the following elements are likely to be part of a well-designed program:

Central Focus

- The emphasis is on health ministry and NOT on medical care; it can better be conceived of as a diaconal ministry of the people of God rather than the provision of medical services per se.
- The activities of the ministry reflect the emphasis on health (e.g. education, wellness campaigns, health promotion) and NOT on sickness.

Goals

- The goal is the development and transformation of the community and NOT the construction of a medical clinic.

Integration

- The ministry is seen as a seamless part of the larger gospel witness in the area and NOT as a separate ministry or merely a tool for outreach.

Structure

- The ministry arises organically from the local church with the full support of the leadership and members and NOT as a stand-alone, parachurch activity.

Ownership

- From the earliest stages, community input is actively solicited and respected and NOT merely imposed from without.

- *Local leadership* is encouraged and developed and NOT *marginalized*.
- *Local resources* are identified and mobilized and NOT superseded by importation from *external sources*.
- Individuals are educated that they must *invest in their own health* through small, often symbolic fees for services rendered and NOT that *health is free, of little value and to be dispensed from without at no cost.*

Process

- Value is placed NOT ONLY on *what* is done BUT ALSO on *how* and *by whom* and *for whom.*

Activities and Personnel

Guided by the above-mentioned principles, it becomes easier to see the broad palette of activities and personnel that may comprise such a health ministry. Far beyond traditional medical campaigns, clinics or hospitals, activities may include primary health care, health education, community development, the education of children, and advocacy and justice efforts, in addition to traditional medical care.

Similarly, the types of skills needed to accomplish such wide-ranging activities will come not only from physicians, nurses and other medical professionals, but will also require contributions from educators, nutritionists, community developers, engineers, social workers, administrators and lawyers, among others. Preference is almost always given to national workers, including training them when necessary, recognizing that at the outset the local talent pool may not allow this in all cases.

Thinking along these lines will likely require a significant paradigm shift for the highly educated medical professional who is accustomed to being the focal point of the ministry, to one of truly shared multifunctional team, the medical component of which is one small portion – and not even the central part at that. Difficult though it may be, it still remains a necessary shift in order to move toward the broader goal of health.

Unanswered Questions and Challenges

A fair criticism that could be leveled at this approach to health ministry is that it is impractical or unreachable. It seems far simpler to build a clinic than to truly enter into people's lives over time and pursue deeper changes in habits and worldview. While that may be true, nonetheless it is also true that durable, meaningful increments in the health of a community require such changes to take place.

As with much of human existence, the key lies in pursuing and managing relationships well. In the final analysis, it's generally not primarily a matter of resources that undermines this type of ministry; nor is it even principally a matter of persuading skeptics that the vision is sound, for at some level we can implicitly recognize its validity. Rather, it comes down to a series of key relationships such as:

- Between mission hospitals/clinics and the holistic, community-based health initiative;
- With host governments & established medical systems;
- Relating to conflicting worldviews and culture (the issue of contextualization; views of disease);
- Ability to achieve synergy with national coworkers and leaders.

In large measure, the ability to successfully implement a health ministry of this nature in a given place has very much to do with team commitment to the principles and the ability to generate "buy in" on a larger scale via positive relationships.

A second criticism may be that this approach condemns those in developing nations to a substandard level of care in comparison with the norms in more developed nations, by which the critic means technologically advanced care such as intensive care units or perhaps organ transplantation. The response to that may depend on one's frame of reference regarding the timing or pace of change. Certainly, a nation with lesser demands on its human resources in the form of the lifelong detrimental effects of malnutrition, early death, lost productivity due to the ravages of completely avoidable public health maladies, and the constraints of a limited worldview, is a nation which is bound to prosper and develop in ways that will include increasing access to higher levels of technology-based medicine.

On the other hand, more rapid advancement towards a higher standard of basic levels of medical care in developing nations would require that we examine the sacred cows of market forces and social justice issues on a global scale, as elucidated by Harvard physician Paul Farmer,[10] a risky but ultimately gospel-centered thing to do, especially if we pause to consider the close scriptural linkage between the Hebrew concept of compassion or mercy (*chesed*) with which we typically associate health ministry, and the broader Biblical concepts of justice, righteousness and rectitude *(tsedeqah, mishpat)*.[11]

Conclusion: Measuring Success

Good stewardship and accountability to sponsoring agencies require that we look for ways to measure what we're accomplishing through our health ministries. Fortunately, many of the activities mentioned in such a holistic health ministry readily lend themselves to a quantitative approach to assessment. This may include following trends in traditional public health measures such as infant mortality, rates of malnutrition, access to potable water, etc., along with more distinctly missions-oriented outcome measures such as numbers of churches planted and new converts professing faith.

A word of caution is needed at this point. When the goal is *shalom* health, or the further breaking in of God's Kingdom in a place, it must be emphasized that there are certain intangibles that, though they defy quantification or itemization on spreadsheets, are nonetheless essential and valid markers of the effectiveness of a ministry. In this category we can think of gradually shifting cultural attitudes toward women, marriage, fidelity, alcohol abuse and the nurture of children, among others.

Sylvia Babu speaks in terms of the *narrative* of success[12]—the story of one transformed life that will reach down through future generations of that family and others whom it touches, in the same way our Lord deals with the redemption of His creation one person at a time, even though such a solitary but profoundly important story may never make a blip in a statistical analysis. The point is not that quantifiable results are not impor-tant, only that they're often incomplete in capturing the full impact of what's truly happening in a place.

As we move out into the world seeking to implement holistic ministries of health, it is well to keep the goal in mind, which is the full display of God's splendor through word, deed and presence ministry, while listening for the narrative of success in the midst of the masses clamoring for our attention.

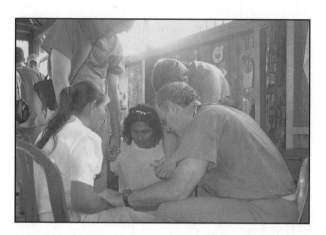

Ted Kuhn/
"Praying with Patient"

References

1. Van Reken DE: *Mission and Ministry. Christian Medical Practice in Today's Changing World Cultures*, Wheaton, Illinois, 1987, Billy Graham Center.
2. Fountain DE: *Health, the Bible and the Church*, Wheaton, IL, 1989, Billy Graham Center.
3. *Ibid.*
4. Myers BL: *Walking with the Poor. Principles and Practices of Transformational Development*, Maryknoll, New York, 1999, Orbis Books.
5. Atkins T: What is Health?, *A New Agenda for Medical Missions*, edited DM Ewert, Brunswick, Georgia, 1990, MAP International.
6. Long WM: *Health, Healing and God's Kingdom. New Pathways to Christian Health Ministry in Africa*, Oxford, 2000, Regnum Books International.
7. Hiebert PG: *Anthropological Insights for Missionaries*, Grand Rapids, 1985, Baker House Books.
8. Keller TJ: *Ministries of Mercy. The Call of the Jericho Road*, 2nd ed., Phillipsburg, New Jersey, 1997, P&R Publishing.
9. Waldecker G: *Toward a Theology of Movement: Missiology from a Christ-centered Kingdom Perspective*, 2002, unpublished manuscript.
10. Farmer P: *Infections and Inequalities. The Modern Plagues*, Berkeley, 1999, University of California Press.
11. Scott W: *Bring Forth Justice*, Grand Rapids, 1980, Wm B. Eerdmans Publishing.
12. Babu S: Redefining Success in Community Health, *Upholding the Vision. Serving the Poor in Training and Beyond*, 2nd ed., edited D Caes, Philadelphia, 1996, Christian Community Health Fellowship.

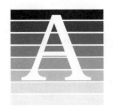

A Resources for the Traveling Medical Professional

Hartmut Gross and W. "Ted" Kuhn

Safe Travel
Travel Clinics
Travel Health Information
International Health Insurance
Physicians Overseas
Emergency Information and Assistance
Medical Supplies
Vaccine Sources
Vaccine Wholesalers
Vaccine and Disease-Specific Advice
Reference Laboratories for Tropical
   and Parasitic Diseases
Women's Health Issues
The Compromised Traveler
Mail Order Camping, Hiking, Climbing
   and Performance Supplies
Wool Clothing and Camo Clothing
Toilet and Water Supplies
Travel Agencies for Overseas Travel
Governmental Organizations
Information Resources
International Multilateral Organizations
Membership Organizations
Non-Governmental Organizations
Job and Field Placement Opportunities

(Listing does not imply endorsement by author or organization and is not intended to be comprehensive but representational of services available)

Safe Travel

Association for Safe International Road Travel. 301-983-5252, Provides traveler with a report on hazardous road conditions in 60 foreign countries.

The Safe Travel Book, a Guide for the International Traveler, Peter Savage (MacMillan Publishing Co. 100 Front Street, Box 500, Riverside, NJ 08075-7500)

RISKNET
305-865-0072
Information services on terrorism, kidnappings, plane hijacking, etc.

State Department Travel Warnings and Consular Information Sheets
http://travel.state.gov/
http://travel.state.gov/travel/warnings_current.html
http://travel.state.gov/travel/warnings_consular.html

US Embassies and Consulates
http://travel.state.gov/visa/questions_embassy.html

US Customs Forms
http://www.customs.gov/xp/cgov/toolbox/forms

Global Weather
http://www.weather.com

Travel Clinics

Travel Medicine, Inc. Listing of more than 700 travel clinics and identifies specialists in travel medicine. Also free download of the *2001 International Travel Health Guide* by Stewart Rose, MD (one chapter at a time in pdf format)
http://www.travmed.com

International Society of Travel Medicine (ISTM). Directory of physicians in the U.S. and overseas who provide travel medicine services.
http://www.istm.org/

American Society of Tropical Medicine and Hygiene (ASTMH) Directory of Travel Clinics and Consulting Physicians. Lists physicians who specialize in travel medicine and tropical diseases,
http://www.astmh.org/publications/clinics.cfm

Travel Health Information

CDC International Fax Information Service (directory sheet). General advice on travel health issues.
888-232-3299 (toll free fax)
404-332-4559

CDC's Travel Information Home Page
http://www.cdc.gov/travel.htm

WHO International Travel and Vaccination Requirements
http://www.who.org

Health Information for International Travel
Superintendent of Documents
U.S. Government Printing Office
Washington, DC 20402
202-783-3238

US Department of State Overseas Citizens Emergency Center Blue Sheet (updates the health information for international travel biweekly).
202-647-5226

Hospital for Tropical Diseases
Healthline–England
(0839) 337-733

Immunization Alert—computerized database

Health Information for International Travel by the CDC. Order from the Public Health Foundation.
1-877-252-1200
http://bookstore.phf.org.

Physicians' Guide to Travel Abroad—Available through the American Medical Association
http://www.ama-assn.org/
800-621-8335

International Association for Medical Assistance to Travelers (IAMAT),
716-754-4883

Travel Health Information Service
5827 W. Washington Blvd.
Milwaukee, WI 53208

Shoreland, Inc.
414-290-1900
800-433-5256
www.shoreland.com
Travax information systems

International Health Insurance

Travel Assistance AIG
800-821-2828

International S.O.S 800-523-8930
http://www.internationalsos.com

Highway to Health, Inc.
1-877-865-5979, or if overseas, call 1-610-254-8772 collect

AirMed Traveler
205-443-4840
800 356-2161
www.airmed.com

Physicians Overseas

International Association for Medical Assistance to Travelers (IAMAT)
716-754-4883 or try 519-836-0102
Lists English speaking physicians and health clinics worldwide.

Emergency Information and Assistance

United States Department of State
Citizens Emergency Center
202-647-5226

Divers Alert Network (DAN)
919-684-9111
800-446-2671
Emergency information of scuba diving
   injuries and accidents

Medical Supplies

MAP International
Contact: Sharron Bullock
912-265-6010
912-265-6170 fax
Will provide medical supplies and medications at minimal cost. They have "travel
   packs" which are boxes of mixed medications sufficiently ready to take on a
   short term medical mission trip. They
   require about 6 weeks notice for any
   order.

International Aid
616-846-7490

Schein Medical
May provide medication at discount for
   missions
Contact: Allison Formal

Janssen Pharmaceuticals
Will provide mebendazole at no cost
   for missions
   http://www.janssen.com/
   800-JANSSEN (526-7736)

Eli Lilly, Lilly Global Cares—Will provide
   a box of antibiotics free for doctors and
   dentists.
   800-545-6962
   11-877-419-8530

Blessings International
   http://www.blessing.org

King Pharmaceutical Benevolent Fund, Inc.
   Contact: Art Yannucciello
      or Jean Collins
   1-800-321-9234 or 540-466-3014

Johnson and Johnson
   Contact: Lisa Crosby
   Manager at Medical Missions Program

Glaxo, Smith, Kline
   Medical Missions Dept.
   Customer Response: 1-888-825-5249

Medshare International
   Contact: A.B. Short / Bob Persons
   770-323-5858

Missionaide
   Contact: Grey Jorges
   423-624-5060

Health Volunteers Overseas
   www.hvousa.org
   1-202-296-0928
   fax 1-202-296-8018

Americares
   Contact: Leonie Gordon
   161 Cherry Street
   fax 203-972-0116
   email—info@americares.org

Worldwide Laboratory Improvement—Will
   provide laboratory supplies at reduced
   cost and technical advice for medical
   missions.
   Contact: Carol and Ed Bos
   269-323-8407
   http://www.wwlab.org
   E-mail: carolbos@wwlab.org

Edmund Scientific—Scientific supplies,
   free catalogue. Microscopes, batteries,
   optical/solar equipment, etc.
   http://www.edsci.com

TECH (Technical Exchange for Christian
   Healthcare)
TECH is an affiliation of ministries which
   are involved with the technical support
   of Christian health organizations in
   the developing world. Some members
   are concerned with the procurement
   and distribution of medical equipment.
   Others receive this equipment for use
   in the field where their organizations
   are active in health care delivery.

Chinook Medical Gear, Inc.— Medical instruments, travel kits, high altitude supplies
Phone: 970-375-1241
Toll Free: 800-766-1365
http://www.chinookmed.com

Ward's Natural Science Establishment Inc.—Science supplies, mainly for teaching.
800-962-2660
http:Medical instruments, travel kits, high altitude supplieswww.wardsci.com

Claude Good—Worm Pill Project
claudeg@mrn.org
albendazole and mebendazole

SonoSite—Portable ultrasound machines.
www.sonosite.com

Vaccine Sources

Wyeth-Ayerst Lab
800-666-7248

Berna Products
800-533-5899

Merck & Company
800-637-2579

Glaxo, Smith, Kline
Customer Response: 888-825-5249

Vaccine Wholesalers

AmeriSource Corporation
800-562-2526

Exotic Tropical Disease Drug Information and Support

Division of Control of Tropical Disease.
World Health Organization
41-22-791-3868

Vaccine and Disease-Specific Advice

CDC International Advice Lines:
* General advice on travel health issues 404-332-4559
* Malaria hotline 404-332-4555
* Rabies Branch 404-639-3095
* Meningitis and special pathogens branch 404-639-3534

Reference Laboratories for Tropical and Parasitic Diseases

Offer serologic tests for anisakiasis, babesiosis, Chagas' disease, crypto-sporidiosis, cystercercosis, echinococcus, E. hystolytica, fascioliasis, filariasis, giardiasis. leishmaniasis, malaria, paragonimiasis, schistosomiasis, strongyloidiasis, toxocariasis toxoplasmosis, trichinosis

Specialty Laboratories
800-421-4449

Microbic Tech Reference Laboratory
800-histodg

Women's Health Issues

Teratogen Information Services (information on medication risk during pregnancy)
http://orpheus.ucsd.edu/otis/
http://www.motherisk.org/

Worldwide Assistance Services Inc. Provides travel health insurance to pregnant women.
800-821-2828

International SOS
800-523-8930

The Compromised Traveler

American Diabetes Association—Provides monographs that are helpful when traveling, especially regarding portable insulin delivery systems, eating out in other cultures, buying supplies over-

seas and time zone changes and insulin dosages.
800-DIABETES (342-2383)
http://www.diabetes.org

The Diabetic Traveler (an ADA bulletin, may be ordered from following address)
P.O. Box 8223 RW
Stamford, CT 06905

Insulin delivery systems for travelers—Novolin dial-a–dose insulin delivery device.
Novo Nordisk Pharmaceuticals Inc,
800-727-6500

International Diabetes Federation Groups
40 Washington Street, B-1050
Brussels, Belguim

Lispro insulin (short acting insulin useful when traveling)
Eli Lilly and Co
http://www.lillydiabetes.com/
product/humalog.jsp?reqNavId=5.1

Sammons Preston (Rehabilitation supplies and durable medical goods)
800-323-5547
E-mail: sp@sammonspreston.com

Mail Order Camping, Hiking, Climbing and Performance Supplies

Campmor
888-226-7667
www.campmor.com
(sells mosquito nets, water purifiers and personal hygiene supplies)

The Sportsman's Guide
800-882-2962 or 888-844-0667
http://www.sportsmansguide.com/

L.L. Bean
800-441-5713
www.llbean.com

Sierra Trading Post
800-713-4534
www.sierratradingpost.com

Sahalie (formerly Early Winters)
877-718-7902
800-458-4438
www.sahalie.com

National Running Center
800-541-1773
www.nationalrunningcenter.com
high performance athletic clothing

REI —Store locations available through the Internet (sells water purifiers and climbing/rescue gear).
800-426-4840
www.rei.com

Norm Thompson
877-718-7899
www.normthompson.com

Adventure Medical Kits—supplier of medical kits for wilderness travel.
510- 632-1442

Medichoice— Kendrick Traction Device
619-258-0105

Mountain Safety Research—High performance stoves and water filters.
206-624-7048

Outdoor Research—Tote bags, medical travel kits for international travel.
800-643-8616

Seaberg Co
503-867-4726
SAM splints

Travel Medicine Inc,
800-872- 8633

Day One Camouflage— Books and supplies for international travel, including insect repellents, clothes, and mosquito nets.
800-347-2979

Wool Clothing and Camo Clothing (Specialized Clothing)

Raven Wear— Fleece cold weather clothing and thermal underwear.
800-387-2836
www.ravenwear.ca

BackCountry—Survival kits, smart wool clothing, emergency equipment, stoves, rain gear.
800-381-5437
www.backcountryinc.com

Schnee's Boots and Shoes
888-922-1510
www.schnees.com

Ice Breaker Boots—Insulated overboots.
800-343-Boot

Muck Boots—Insulated boots.
903-838 0530 www.muckboots.com

Wiggy's Inc.— Cold weather clothing and sleeping bags, Lamalite sweaters.
800 748-1827
www.wiggys.com

HeadSokz—Head and neck covers.
800-946-8824
www.headsokz.com

Northern Outfitters— Extreme cold weather clothing, boots plus clothing for less severe conditions, rain jackets, and pants.
800-944-9276
www.northernoutfitters.com

Bug Shirt Company—Insect protective clothing.
705-729-5620
800-998-9096
www.bugshirt.com

Carol Davis Sportswear— High performance, hydrophobic, anti-microbial body sock (one-piece thermal underwear).
402-991-4447
www.cdsportswear.com

Gransfors Bruks—Ultra soft wool underwear (while it initially looks like they only sell axes, look under "Products").
843-875-0240
www.gransfors.com

OutdoorSafe, Inc
719-593-5852
www.outdoorsafe.com

Fox River Mills— X-Static® socks and liners.
www.foxrivermills.com

Toilet and Water Supplies

U-dig-it®
208-939-8656
U-dig-it@worldnet.att.net.
Palm-sized stainless steel trowel with a folding handle and belt sheath

Four Corners River Sports—The Coyote Bagless Toilet System® (a polyethylene box that has a separate raised toilet seat assembly, weighs nine pounds with a capacity for 55 user-days).
800-426-7637
www.riversports.com

River Bank System—Outdoor portable toilet.
www.riverbankdesign.com/toilets.htm

Partner Steel Company—The Jon-ny Partner® (portable toilet with an aluminum holding tank, automatic pressure release valve and a pressure nozzle attachment for a hose for fresh water flushing).
208-233-2371
www.partnersteel.com

Green River Headquarters—The Bano® toilet (a molded plastic holding tank with aluminum handles, stainless steel fasteners, and a hard plastic seat).
800-684-6323
www.holidayexpeditions.com

Jon Green—The Bano® toilet.
801-355-2830

Restop®—(Disposable bags for liquids that contain polymers which immediately gel liquid waste. Separate bags for solid wastes are available). www.whennaturecalls.com

911 Water—Water purifiers. http://www.911water.com/index.html

Travel Agencies for Overseas Travel

Provide low cost air and land fare to missionaries.

MTS (Missionary Travel Services)
800-444-3004
719-471-4514
fax 719-471-0629
Emergency & after hours:
    800-823-2971

SIAMA (Society for the Interest of Active Missionaries) ($15 per couple to join)
Based in Netherlands
Tel 31-71-5163535
Fax 31-71-5163536
e-mail siama@siama.antenna.nl

IHEC International Medicine Resource Listing[1]

Governmental Organizations

Agency Health Care Policy Research is a major sponsor of research related to clinical practice outcomes and policy. Though primarily concerned with domestic research, some AHCPR work is concerned with international research, comparative studies, and cross-national practice standards. Entering the word "international" in AHCPR's search engine can access studies with international relevance.
    http://www.ahcpr.gov/

Canadian International Development Agency is the agency that directs and manages Canadian development assistance.
    http://www.acdi-cida.gc.ca

Centers for Disease Control, Office of Global Health is CDC's unit responsible for IH activities with information on current projects, global health plans and services; programs; staff roster; OGH capabilities; information resources and country-specific information; information for travelers and consular information sheets; CDC global partners; and links with other organizations. CDC also offers international internships.
    http://www.cdc.gov/ogh

Institute of Medicine (of the National Academies). Wide overview of global health related activities.
    http://www.iom.edu/topic.sp?id=3722

International Development Research Council is Canada's agency for funding development research, including many health-related projects. Much important research has been carried out with IDRC support.
    http://www.idrc.ca

US State Department Travel Warnings and Consular Information Sheets provides country-by-country information relevant to health, safety, visa and entry requirements (this is especially important since travelers may be unable to board planes if they don't have the necessary visa), medical facilities, consular contact information, drug penalties, etc.
    http://travel.state.gov/travel/
        warnings.html

US Agency for International Development provides foreign assistance and humanitarian aid. Listed site provides a wealth of information about population, health and nutrition. — http://www.usaid. gov/ is the home page and for global health, population and nutrition, go to:
    http://www.usaid.gov

US Dept. of Health & Human Services (http://www.hhs.gov) is the principal federal agency concerned with health services and data in the USA.

Information Resources

Centers for Disease Control Travel Information — Sections include: Reference Material (a wealth of information about diseases, locations, specific precautions); Disease Outbreaks; Additional Information; Geographic Health Recommendations.
   http://www.cdc.gov/travel/

CIA Publications and Factbooks includes among its sections: World Factbook [provides a wealth of information on virtually all countries]; CIA Maps and Publications Released to the Public; Handbook of International Economic Statistics (use search tool to find).
   http://www.odci.gov/cia/publications/
      index.html

Eurosurveillance Weekly publishes news of infectious disease incidents and surveillance data as they are released, at least once a week, reporting on outbreaks as they happen.
   http://www.eurosurveillance.org

Ford Foundation is one of the largest U.S. foundations active in national and international health.
   http://www.fordfound.org/

Hardin Meta Directory of Internet Health Sources at the Univ. of Iowa has a comprehensive list of the best health-related sites, organized by disease or system category. There is no specific category for IH or for tropical medical and related conditions.
   http://www.lib.uiowa.edu/hardin/
      md/index.html

Healthy Cities describes the Healthy Cities project, now well established in the US and gaining links overseas. This project seeks a comprehensive approach to the development and maintenance of healthy urban life.
   http://www.healthycommunities.org/

Hesperian Foundation publishes low cost, practical books for use in all aspects of IH practice at the community level.
   http://www.hesperian.org

International Health and Traveler's Medicine [Medical College of Wisconsin/ Milwaukee]
   http://www.intmed.mcw.edu/
      travel.html

Library of Congress Country Studies Detailed information on many of the countries of the world prepared by the Federal Research Division of the Library of Congress. The site has an impressive search engine that can search across the data base for any combination of words, ranks the hits in order of closeness to your search terms, and then provide links to the desired text.
   http://lcweb2.loc.gov/frd/cs/
      cshome.html#toc

Medicine & Global Survival Journal is a publication of the British Medical Journal group and features articles on war and peace issues.
   http://www.ippnw.org/MGS/

Population Reference Bureau [PRB] provides a wealth of information about U.S. and international population trends, and links to numerous population-related websites.
   http://www.prb.org/

Research funding opportunities are listed by the Univ. of Illinois at Urbana-Champaign Researcher Information Service, with links to resource institutions, and includes a search engine for resources by persons based at participating institutions.
   http://www.library.uiuc.edu/iris/

Teaching Aids at Low Cost lists & distributes many health-related teaching aids that are provided in low cost format and often multiple languages for use by health care providers and patients in developing countries.
   http://www.talcuk.org/

Intellicast provides national and international weather forecasts plus lots of more detailed weather-related information.

http://www.intellicast.com

International Multilateral Organizations

International Red Cross provides a country listing of ICRC activities and special sections on topical issues such as civil wars, disasters, land mines, etc.

http://www.icrc.org/

United Nations & Related International organizations can be found at the index page below, with links to all agencies within or related to the United Nations system. Of special relevance to IH are:

http://www.unsystem.org/

UNAIDS

http:http://www.unsystem.org/
www.unaids.org

UN Food & Agriculture Organization

http://www.fao.org

UN Development Programme

http://www.undp.org/

UN Development Fund for Women

http://www.unifem.undp.org/

UNICEF

http://www.unicef.org/

UNICEF Progress of Nations Report

http://www.unicef.org/pon00/

UN Population Fund

http://www.unfpa.org/

World Bank

http://www.worldbank.org

World Health Organization

http://www.who.ch/

Membership Organizations

Am. Public Health Association represents >30,000 health professionals working in public health, including >1500 involved working in IH activities. Student memberships are available and the annual fall meeting provides an excellent opportunity to learn about public health and international health.

http://www.apha.org/

Canadian Society for International Health (CSIH) sponsors many IH activities and provides links with Canadian and international websites.

http://www.csih.org

Global Health Council (formerly the National Council for IH) provides access to the many activities of the largest U.S.-based membership organization concerned with IH, and includes information on IH career opportunities, jobs, advocacy, and links to other IH-related programs.

http://www.globalhealth.org/

Physicians for Human Rights, an organization of health professionals, scientists, and concerned citizens, uses the knowledge and skills of the medical and forensic sciences to investigate and prevent violations of international human rights and humanitarian law.

http://www.phrusa.org/

Non-Governmental Organizations

MacArthur (The John D. and Catherine T.) Foundation is one of the largest U.S. foundations, with a major commitment to national and international health, development, and population issues. The site provides internet links to organizations supported by the Foundation as well as to general resources in the philanthropic community.

http://www.macfdn.org/

Population Institute works to alert policymakers and the public about the key issues relating to population growth and to the need for population stabilization.

http://www.populationinstitute.org/

Robert Wood Johnson Foundation is one of the largest U.S. foundations specifically oriented towards health issues. Though the RWJF does not fund international projects, it may be useful in funding or reporting on projects relevant to IH.

http://www.rwjf.org

Rockefeller Foundation provides information about the Foundation, its programs (many of which are at overseas sites), grant recipients and amounts awarded, and sites where research is being done.

http://www.rockfound.org

Job and Field Placement Opportunities

Africare is a private, non-profit organization, dedicated to improving the quality of life in rural Africa. It provides assistance in five principal areas: agriculture, water resource development, environmental management, health, and emergency humanitarian aid.

http:///www.africare.org/

American Academy of Family Physicians (AAFP) has had a recent expansion of international activities and has now added international activities (http://www.aafp.org/int) onto the academy web site.

http://www.aafp.org/

American Council for Voluntary International Action is a consortium of 150+ non-profit organizations working worldwide in the health, educational, development and other related fields, and is a source of jobs and volunteer resources. The site includes hotlinks to all of its members.

http://www.interaction.org/

American Medical Student Association is an excellent resource for IH activities, advocacy, resources and field placements.

http://www.amsa.org/global/ih/

American Society of Tropical Medicine and Hygiene provides listings of overseas opportunities and much other information. The Am. J. of Tropical Medicine and Hygiene provides an extensive listing of overseas opportunities at approximately three-year intervals.

http://www.astmh.org

See especially information about the Benjamin H. Kean Traveling Fellowship in Tropical Medicine at:

http://www.astmh.org

Belize Rural Elective Program of the Medical College of Wisconsin, Department of Family and Community Medicine, provides a unique rural elective working with Maya Indians in the rainforest of southern Belize. It is designed for family practice residents and faculty in cooperation with the Ministry of Health.

http://www.family.mcw.edu/Belize

Canadian Network for International Surgery promotes the delivery of essential surgical care to the underprivleged. As an educational and research agency, it conducts workshops in essential surgical skills and programs in injury prevention in African countries www.cnis.ca/

Canadian Physicians for Aid and Relief directs and provides emergency relief and support in a wide variety of areas .

www.cpar.ca

Child & Family Health International provides placement opportunities for medical students in years 1-4, and pre-medical students in several locations in Ecuador, Mexico and India. Includes a student handbook with information about the sites, the country, what to expect, and other resources.

http://www.cfhi.org

Christian Connections for International Health lists contacts, placement opportunities, information about how to find a placement, and diverse resources. See especially their "Job Search" section; reference 21 lists 88 organizations providing jobs in IH.

http://www.ccih.org/

Christian Medical and Dental Society (Duke Chapter) lists contacts, placement opportunities, information and diverse resources.

http://www.duke.edu/web/CMDS/

Cuba – Medical Education Cooperation with Cuba (MEDICC), a member of IHMEC. MEDICC medical and public health students four-to-eight week clinical and fieldwork electives in Cuba, with emphasis on community/family medicine. Each elective has a strong component of cross-cultural "Spanish for Health Professionals."

http://www.medicc.org

Doctors Without Borders USA is the famous French-originated organization that sends fully qualified health professionals into some of the most challenging parts of the world.

http://www.doctorswithoutborders.org/

FUNEDESIN (Foundation for Integrated Education and Development) Clinical Rotation Program provides clinical experiences in the Amazon Region of Ecuador. It is open to all levels of students and health professionals in the fields of Medicine and Nursing. Further information can be found on the website http://www.funedesin.org.

The application pack can be requested by e-mailing: clinic@funedesin.org.

Global Service Corps provides short or long-term opportunities to volunteer in health, education and environment projects in Kenya, Costa Rica, and Thailand.

http://www.globalservicecorps.org

International Alliance in Service and Education — IASE offers a Service Learning Program in Tetecala, Mexico (a rural village in the state of Morelos). The program is open to students in health related majors at the undergraduate and graduate level, and offers health and education services to the underserved population of Tetecala and its surrounding hamlets.

http://www.iaseco.org

International Emergency Medicine Rotations Database—Operated by the Boston University School of Medicine, this site provides information about rotations in emergency medicine in all regions of the world.

http://www.ed.bmc.org/iem/search.cfm

International Federation of Medical Students' Association is an independent non-political association of 68 medical stu-

dent associations representing students if 50 countries. It provides information about and facilitates student clinical and research exchanges, and through various standing committees, is involved in medical, public health and other projects.

http://www.ifmsa.org/

International Foundation for Education and Self-Help (IFESH) provides assistance and opportunities for service much in the fashion of the US Peace Corps. The primary focus is sub-Saharan Africa. Through its International Fellows Program (IFP) the Foundation has provided nine-month overseas internships for Americans who are graduate students or recent college and university graduates. Fellows are placed with development-focused organizations working overseas.

http://www.ifesh.org/

International Healthcare Opportunities Clearinghouse provides listings of organizations with internet links, of on-line resources, courses, and books on IH, and information about how to get funding. It has a search engine that can locate organizations according to diverse search criteria and provides links to home pages of organizations where available.

http://library.umassmed.edu/ihoc/

International Health Medical Education Consortium[IHMEC] provides information about courses, curricula, annotated websites, foreign language study courses, and other materials useful for faculty and students interested in international health. See "Resources" section of the IHMEC.

http://www.ihmec.org

International Health Work and Electives Source Book. Arnold Publishers in the UK publishes an excellent 481 pp. book (*The Medic's Guide to Work and Electives Around the World*, by Mark Wilson, 2000) covering IH field experience opportunities in 100 country destinations. The book has a 26 pp. introductory section with suggestions regarding finding a post, getting prepared, and protecting your health and welfare. http://www.hodderheadline.co.uk

Detailed information about the book: www.hoddereducation.co.uk

International Medical Corps is a private, nonsectarian, nonpolitical, humanitarian relief organization established in 1984 by volunteer US physicians and nurses. The home page lists IMC's programs and job openings for doctors, nurses and other health professionals.

http://www.imc-la.org/

International Committee of the Society of Teachers of Family Medicine (STFM) now has online the full text of the Krogh and Pust publication, *International Health: A Manual for Advisers and Students*. This 100+ page downloadable document has abundant information for those interested in IH.

http://www.stfm.org/index_ex.html; Manual for Advisers:
http://www.stfm.org/bookstore/ ItemDetail.cfm?ItemID=135;
.pdf file to download the manual:
http://www.stfm.org/pdfs/ International%20Health.pdf

International Medical Volunteers Assoc. provides much information on why and how to volunteer for IH work.

http://www.imva.org

MAP International is a nonprofit Christian relief and development organization, promoting the total health of people living in the world's poorest communities.

http://www.map.org/

Mission to the World is the mission sending agency of the Presbyterian Church in America. Medical work in multiple countries including long and short term, disaster response ministry, academic ministry and community health and development ministry.

http://www.mtw.org/home/site/ templates/

Network of Community Oriented Educational Institutions for Health Sciences is a global association of institutions for education of health professionals committed to contribute, through education, service and research, to the improvement of health in the communities they serve. The network also has pages for student electives and a student network.

http://www.network.unimaas.nl/

Oxfam is an international organization working to ease poverty and hunger in more than 70 countries.

http://www.oxfam.org.uk/

Swaziland Medical Student Elective is a 4- to 7-week structured service and learning elective for fourth year medical students in the English-speaking African country of Swaziland. This elective, offered through the Dept. of Family Medicine at the Jefferson Medical College, Philadelphia, is open to students in the US and Canada. Priority is given to students whose school is a member of IHMEC and to students whose schools are located in Pennsylvania. The program operates from January through May each year. Applications are accepted from April through October during the year preceding the elective. Full information and links to the readings are provided at the website.

http://home.ptd.net/~nwallace/ index.html

World Organization of Family Doctors (WONCA) is forum for exchanging knowledge and information between member organizations of general practitioners/family physicians concerned with health and medical care throughout the world.

http://www.globalfamilydoctor.com/

References

1. Prepared for the International Health Medical Education Consortium by Thomas L. Hall, Dept. of Epidemiology and Biostatistics, Univ. of California at San Francisco School of Medicine, 500 Parnassus, MU425 West, San Francisco, CA 94143-0560 — Tel: 415/502-7204; Fax: 415/476-6014; E-mail: thall@epi.ucsf.edu. Corrections, suggestions for improvement and additions are welcome. File last updated on 16 April 2002.

Note: The editors of this textbook last verified and corrected all Internet addresses contained in this chapter in July 2006.

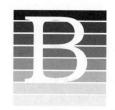

Appendix B:
Emergency Medical Kits
ALS and BLS Supply Bags
Cynthia Urbanowicz

ALS Supply Bag

AIRWAY-large outside top pouch

Intubation Kit:
    Laryngoscope with blades 2.0 Miller,
      3.0 Miller, 3.0 Mac, 4.0 Mac
    2 "C" batteries
    ET-2 each 6.0, 7.0, 8.0
    Stylet (2)
    KY® jelly
    10 cc syringe
    MacGill Forceps (adult)
    ETCO2 detector
    Thomas Tube Holder
    #11 blade
    Curved Kelly
    1 # 16 gauge, #14 gauge angiocatheter
    Heimlich valve
    Chest tube
    Suction device
    Bag/valve/mask with adjustable PEEP
    Space blanket

IV Pouch (Green Pouch)
    1 L Normal Saline
    1 L Lactated Ringers
    IV catheter selection
      2 # 18
      2 # 20
      2 # 16
    2 IV tubing
    IV start kit
    Gloves
    Tape
    Heplock

Yellow Drug Pouch
    1 epinephrine 1:10,000
    1 atropine 1 mg
    2 Solumedrol® 125mg
    1 bicarb 50 Meq
    1 NTG 1/150 tabs or NTG topical
      patches
    2 ASA
    1 epinephrine 1: 1,000
    1 Decadron® 10 mg
    1 Benadryl® 50 mg
    1 succinylcholine (Anectine®) 200 mg
    1 etomidate 40 mg or Versed® 5 mg (2)
    1 vecuronium 10 mg
    1 fentanyl 500 mcg
    1 Ativan® 4 mg
    1 morphine sulphate 10 mg
    2 Lovenox®
    1 Narcan® 4 mg
    HIV post-exposure prophylaxis (PEP)
      kit:
    2 normal saline for injection
    4 Compazine®
    2 ketoralac
    4 Imodium®
    Cipro®
    Levaquin®
    Pepto-bismol®
    Rocephin®
    (For high-altitude: Diamox® 500 mg
      sustained release, Procardia® 10 mg,
      Decadron® 10 mg)

Wound Care
   4x4's
   tape
   saline 250cc bottle
   Kling®
   suture set
   suture selection
   Sam® splint (2)
   Bacitracin®
   sterile drape (1)
   gloves, non-sterile
   gloves sterile
   3 Ace® wrap (2)
   Silvadene® cream
   xylocaine 2 % w/ and w/o epi
   syringe 10cc (3)
   1½" needles 23/25 gauge;
   1½" Steri-strips,® Superglue® or
      Dermabond® or Steri-strips®
   Trauma shears (1)

Nebulizer Pouch
   Bicycle pump with racing valve
      extender
   Nebulizer with tubing and mask (may
      substitute an Omron™ battery
      portable nebulizer for the bicycle
      pump nebulizer)
   Albuterol solution (5)

Side Pouches
   B/P cuff
   Stethoscope
   Pulse oximeter

Survival Pouch
   Caffeine tabs
   Power Bar®
   Venom extractor
   Cigarette lighter
   Iodine tabs for water purification
   Small flashlight
   Rescue rope

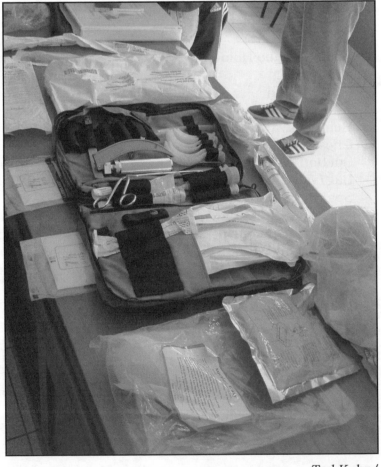

Ted Kuhn/
"Emergency Airway Section of the ALS Bag"

BLS Supply Bag

AIRWAY-large outside top pouch

Oral/Nasal Airways:
    Suction device
    One-way protective barrier mask
      ventilator
    Space blanket

IV Pouch (Green Pouch)
    1 L Normal Saline
    IV catheter selection
      2 # 18
      2 # 20
      2 # 16
      2 # 22
    2 IV tubing
    IV start kit
    gloves
    tape
    heplock

Red Drug Bag
    1 NTG 1/150 tabs or NTG topical
      patches
    2 ASA
    1 epinephrine 1: 1,000
    1 Benadryl® 50 mg inj / Benadryl® PO
    2 Lovenox®
    HIV post-exposure prophylaxis (PEP)
      kit:
    2 saline for injection
    4 Compazine®/Phenergan®
    2 ketoralac
    4 Imodium®
    Cipro® or Levaquin®
    Pepto-Bismol®
    (For high-altitude: Diamox® 500 mg
      sustained release, Procardia® 10 mg,
      Decadron® 10 mg)
    NSAIDS
    BCP's (birth control pills)
    Syringes and needles/ alcohol wipes

Wound Care
    4x4's
    tape
    Kling®
    Steri-strips®
    Sam® splint (2)
    Bacitracin®
    gloves, nonsterile
    gloves sterile
    Silvadene® cream
    saline 250cc bottle
    Superglue® or Dermabond®
    3 Ace® wrap (2)
    Trauma shears (1)
    small Betadine®

Nebulizer Pouch
    Bicycle pump with racing valve
      extender (racing valve extender is
      crucial to operation of nebulizer)
    Nebulizer with tubing and mask
    Albuterol solution (5)

Side Pouches
    B/P cuff
    Stethoscope

Survival Pouch
    Caffeine tabs
    Power Bars®
    Venom extractor
    Lighter
    Iodine tabs for water purification
    Small flashlight
    Rope bag

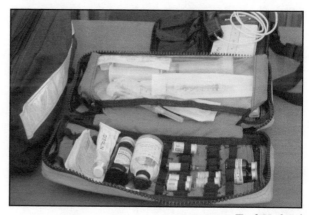

Ted Kuhn/
"IV Medication Pouch"

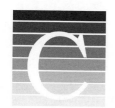

Test and Supply List for Portable Laboratory

W. "Ted" Kuhn and Hartmut Gross

Transport Cases
Sturdy padded trunk for the equipment
  (e.g. Hardigg® case)
    http://www.hardigg.com/hardigg_
      cases/portable_travel_cases.htm
Case for microscope (e.g. Hardigg® case)
Separate waterproof case for stains
  (e.g. Pellikan® case)

Basic Supplies
Customs papers
Microscope slides
Microscope cover slips
Portable timer
Slide rack – wooden
Rack for Sed rate- wooden
Staining rack
Drying rack – Tupperware®
Coplin Jar
Oil for immersion
Forceps
Boundary tape
Battery (e.g. motorcycle) for microscope
Charger for battery
220-110 volt transformer
12 volt battery adapter
Voltmeter (to check battery charge)
Solar panel
Indelible pens – glass markers
Professional business cards
Prescription pads
Information sheets for tests
Tropical medicine textbook
Teaching slides for microscope
Lab results notebook & pens
Table cloths
Specimen containers (for stool, urine,
  sputum)
Duct tape and cellophane tape
Toothpicks and cotton tipped applica-
  tors

Pipettes- small plastic
Ice pack and carry bag for I-STAT®
Wash bottle
Cellophane wrap
Lens paper and filter paper
Scalpel blades
Cigarette lighter/matches
Timer
Paper towels

Phlebotomy Supplies
Blood lancets, 2x2s, 4x4s,
  Syringe and needles, tourniquet
Alcohol wipes
Band-Aids®

Safety
Protective glasses
Gloves
Eyewash
TB mask
Isopropyl gel hand cleaner
Sharps container
Plastic disposal bags

Equipment
Hemacue® and extra batteries
Hemacue® standard cuvette
I-STAT® (bring two)
I-STAT® electronic standard cartridge
Centrifuge and power cord (e.g. Zip-
  Spin®)
Microscope, power cord & extra bulb
Fetal Doppler (e.g. Medasonics®)
Shiotz Tonometer
Capillary glucose monitor
  (e.g. Glucometer®)
Calibrating standard
Ultrasound machine with experienced
  sonographer when available

Micro-hematocrit reader (if not using Hemacue® or I-STAT®)

Stains - (double bagged or in air tight container)
10% potassium hydroxide (KOH)
Saline
Lugol's iodine
Hemaquik 2®
Wright's
    Fixative (Methanol)
    Buffer 6.4 and 7.0
Geimsa
Kinyoun Acid Fast (cold) or Ziehl-Neelson (hot)
    Carbofuschin
    Decolorizer – acid alcohol
    Brilliant green or Methylene blue (counter stain)
Gram's
    Crystal violet
    Gram's iodine
    Decolorizer
    Safranin (counter stain)
    Lab grade sterile water

Immunological Tests
HIV
Hepatitis A or B
Pregnancy (HCG)
Leishmaniasis (in endemic areas)
Malaria (Optimal® or other)

Other Tests and Supplies
Urine Dipsticks (e.g. Uriscan®)
Hemacue® cuvettes
I-STAT® cartridges
    Na, K, Cl, BUN, Glucose, Hct
    Creatinine
    Others available
Capillary glucose test strips
Stool hematest & developer (Beckman Coulter Hemoccult®)
Gastroccult® & developer (Beckman Coulter)
Westergren Sed rate
Centrifuge cuvettes

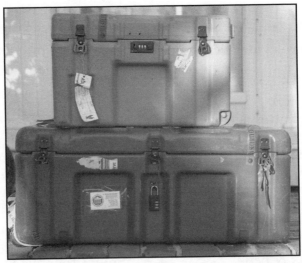

Ted Kuhn/
"Portable Lab"

D Emergency Protocols
Cynthia Urbanowicz

D-1 Evacuation Protocol

Criteria: Illness or injury that will worsen or potentially became fatal if not evacuated

Immediate Evacuation Criteria
1. Animal bite (with possible transmission of Rabies) exposure.
2. Acute Mountain Sickness with or without signs of HAPE (High Altitude Pulmonary Edema) or HACE (High Altitude Cerebral Edema.
3. Abdominal pain with positive pregnancy test.
4. Head injury with decreasing level of consciousness.
5. Chest pain of suspected cardiac origin.
6. Heat stroke.
7. Significant HIV exposure – blood splash to mucous membranes, dirty needle stick (immediately initiate antiviral therapy – see HIV exposure algorithm).
8. Multiple trauma.
9. Psychiatric emergency – disruptive to the team or jeopardizing team safety.
10. Progressive physiologic deteroration with any of the following:
    a. Tachycardia
    b. Bradycardia
    c. Dyspnea
    d. Intractable vomiting and/or diarrhea
    e. Progressive infection\
    f. Bleeding from mouth or rectum if not from obvious superficial source.
11. Near drowning.

12. Hypothermia with drop in core body temperature below 93^0F with altered level of consciousness.

Relative contraindications to Evacuation:
1. Know where you are and where the closest appropriate facility is located, be familiar with the transport method, time and conditions to the facility.
2. Consider the journey – will the journey likely worsen the illness/injury?
3. Consider the facility – will they have personnel/equipment needed to manage the illness/injury.

Evacuation Algorithm
Levels of Evacuation:

Level ONE: Evacuation of critically ill or injured team member, requiring return flight to United States with professional aeromedical assistance.

Level TWO: Evacuation of ill or injured team member to United States with a medical escort via commercial airline.

Level THREE: Evacuation of ill or injured tea member to major medical facility in a developing world country.

Level FOUR: Evacuation of ill or injured team member to local hospital or clinic in developing world country.

Level FIVE: Evacuation of ill or injured team member from local work site to lower altitude, cooler area, warmer area or area more amenable to rest and recovery.

Level ONE Evacuation:
- *Multiple trauma* - Multiple long bone fractures, head injury, chest trauma, abdominal trauma, penetrating wounds to thorax or abdomen.
  - Initially evacuate to major facility for stabilization, contact emergency number to arrange aeromedical transport.
  - Continuously reassess team member status for improvement or deterioration.
- *Illness*-Complicated myocardial infarction or other cardiac event requiring surgical intervention, exacerbation of chronic problem with progressive deterioration; OR,
  Tachycardia, bradycardia, dyspnea, bleeding from mouth or rectum, near drowning with loss of consciousness.
  - Initially evacuate to major facility for stabilization, contact emergency number to arrange aeromedical transport.
  - Continuously reassess team member status for improvement or deterioration.

Level TWO Evacuation:
- Uncomplicated fracture of extremity or extremities (not more than one long bone), dog or other animal bite with possible rabies exposure, exacerbation of chronic health problem without acute respiratory or cardiac complications
  - Initially evacuate to major facility, call emergency number to arrange for medical escort and return travel to USA

Level THREE Evacuation:
- Abdominal pain with suspected surgical need (e.g. positive pregnancy test), head injury with loss of consciousness less than six minutes, no seizure activity, chest pain of suspected cardiac origin, uncomplicated myocardial infarction.
  - Evacuate to closest major medical center.
  - Stop at local facility to stabilize if needed

Level FOUR Evacuation:
- As needed to stabilize for any of the above; OR, dog or other animal bite, psychiatric emergency.
  - Rapidly evaluate personnel/equipment available.

- Don't delay transport to a higher level of care if needed.
- Assess frequently for improvement or deterioration.

Level FIVE Evacuation:
Heat illness without signs or symptoms of heat stroke, acute mountain sickness (AMS), hypothermia
- Evacuate lower altitude, cooler area, warmer area or area more amenable to rest and recovery.
- Reassess frequently for improvement or deterioration.
- Pre-determine and know the altitudes of your escape route.

*Remember even a descent of 2,000 ft in altitude can significantly improve AMS.

Note: When initiating a Level ONE evacuation and calling the emergency number for aeromedical evacuation, it is important to keep the following in mind:
1. Contact the sending agency and let them know about the situation.
2. Contact the medical director for the sending agency. This individual may be able to render assistance in diagnosis of a tropical illness though the use of resources not available in the field (e.g. diagnostic programs and texts, contacting tropical medicine experts around the world).
3. The sending agency and the medical director may be able to assist in the decision of the optimal destination where to fly to the ill patient.
4. Be aware that aeromedical rescue agencies preferentially fly patients to certain designated major hospitals worldwide. These are selected because of available services, as well as logistics arranged for acceptance of patients, landing and transfer arrangements, preprogrammed coordinates, logistics of crossing international borders, etc.
5. Insurance companies that pay for emergency evacuation will pay for only one flight per illness. Once a patient is flown to a selected destination, the terms of the contract are met. The insurance company will not pay for another transfer to a third facility. So select first destination

Appendix D-2   Acute Mountain Sickness

High Altitude Pulmonary Edema (HAPE)
High Altitude Cerebral Edema (HACE)

Criteria:

Known or suspected AMS-rapid ascent in elevation usually over 8,000 ft.

Signs and Symptoms-Acute Mountain Sickness:
- Headache.
- Nausea and vomiting.
- Elevated blood pressure.
- Hypoventilation.
- Periodic breathing.
- Lassitude.
- Dyspnea with exertion.

Guidelines for AMS:
1. Complete AMS worksheet with physical assessment (see appendix—Lake Louise criteria). Include a full set of vital signs.
2. Compazine® 10 mg IM for headache and /or nausea. Compazine® also increases the hypoxic drive.
3. Diamox® 500 mg sustained release (may use lower dose if available). Continue every day for 5 days while at altitude.
4. Increase fluids.
5. Non-steroidal anti-inflammatory medications may also be used for headache relief.
6. Reassess frequently-update AMS worksheet with each assessment.
7. REST
8. Most important *****NO FURTHER ASCENT*****

Signs and Symptoms–HAPE
- May or may not have signs and symptoms AMS.
- Increasing dyspnea-even at rest.
- Central cyanosis.
- Cough, often productive-pink frothy sputum ominous sign.
- Hypoventilation.

Protocol for HAPE:
1. Life threatening emergency. **DESCENT IS MANDATORY.** Do not delay.
   a. Know your current altitude.
   b. Use most rapid evacuation route.
   c. Descent of even 2,000 ft. can produce relief of symptoms
   d. Do not allow patient to walk-if possible
2. Apply oxygen at 4 liters per minute by nasal cannula. Begin AMS worksheet enroute.
3. Procardia® 20 mg SL/ PO, chew and swallow
4. Initiate IV normal saline at 100 cc/hr
5. Compazine® 10 mg (IM/IV) for nausea and vomiting
6. Monitor for signs and symptoms of airway compromise, decreasing level of consciousness. May require intubation.
7. AVOID morphine and Lasix.®

Signs and Symptoms - HACE
- May or may not have sings and symptoms AMS. If signs and symptoms AMS present, may progress to HACE in 12 hours to 5 days.
- Altered level of consciousness
- Ataxia and/or unable to sustain finger tapping test
- Seizure, focal seizure, hemiparesis
- Severe headache, projectile vomiting

Protocol for HACE:
1. **BEGIN DESCENT IMMEDIATELY.**
2. Complete AMS worksheet with initial assessment/ monitor for signs of airway compromise.
3. Apply oxygen, 4 liters per minute via nasal cannula.
4. Initiate IV normal saline at 50cc/hr
5. Decadron® 10 mg IV. May repeat Decadron® 4 mg IV q6h.
6. Compazine® 5-10 mg IV for headache, nausea and/or vomiting.
7. Begin Diamox® 500 mg sustained release PO when tolerated.
8. Ativan® 2mg IV for seizure activity.

Appendix D-3   AMS Worksheet
Based on the Lake Louise AMS Questionnaire

Name_____ Age ____ Sex____ Date _____
Prev Hx AMS/HAPE/HACE?
Meds:

Ascent Profile:
Treatment:

	Time	___	___	___	___	___
	Altitude	___	___	___	___	___

Symptoms:
1.Headache:

No headache 0	___	___	___	___	___
Mild headache 1	___	___	___	___	___
Moderate headache 2	___	___	___	___	___
Severe, incapacitating 3	___	___	___	___	___

2.GI:

No GI symptoms 0	___	___	___	___	___
Poor appetite or nausea 1	___	___	___	___	___
Moderate nausea or vomiting 2	___	___	___	___	___
Severe N&V, incapacitating 3	___	___	___	___	___

3.Fatigue/weak:

Not tired or weak 0	___	___	___	___	___
Mild fatigue/weakness 1	___	___	___	___	___
Moderate fatigue/weakness 2	___	___	___	___	___
Severe F/W, incapacitating 3	___	___	___	___	___

4.Dizzy/lightheaded:

Not dizzy 0	___	___	___	___	___
Mild dizziness 1	___	___	___	___	___
Moderate dizziness 2	___	___	___	___	___
Severe, incapacitating 3	___	___	___	___	___

5.Difficulty sleeping:

Slept well as usual 0	___	___	___	___	___
Did not sleep as well as usual 1	___	___	___	___	___
Woke many times, poor night's sleep 2	___	___	___	___	___
Could not sleep at all 3	___	___	___	___	___

Symptom Score:

___	___	___	___	___

Clinical Assessment:
6.Change in mental status:

No change 0	___	___	___	___	___
Lethargy/lassitude 1	___	___	___	___	___
Disoriented/confused 2	___	___	___	___	___
Stupor/semiconsciousness 3	___	___	___	___	___

7.Ataxia(heel to toe walking):

No ataxia 0	___	___	___	___	___
Maneuvers to maintain balance 1	___	___	___	___	___
Steps off line 2	___	___	___	___	___
Falls down 3	___	___	___	___	___
Can't stand 4	___	___	___	___	___

8.Peripheral edema:

No edema 0	___	___	___	___	___
One location 1	___	___	___	___	___
Two or more locations 2	___	___	___	___	___

Clinical Assessment Score:

___	___	___	___	___

Total Score:

___	___	___	___	___

Using the worksheet.

Patients are assigned a single score for each numbered group. For visual ease, we have designed the worksheet so that this score is entered next to the corresponding symptom severity level.

For example, a person with moderate AMS might get 2 points for moderate headache, 1 point for poor appetite, and 1 point for mild fatigue, for a total symptom score of 4. In addition, this person might get 1 point for facial edema, for a clinical assessment score of 1 and a total AMS score of 5.

Serial evaluations several hours apart give a good measure of whether a patient is responding to treatment or deteriorating.

Resources
1. The Lake Louise Score, International Hypoxia Symposium, Lake Louise, Alberta, Canada, 1991.
2. Dietz, TE, Emergency & Wilderness Medicine. URL: http://www.high-altitude-medicine.com/AMS-worksheet.html Last modified 8-May-2000.

Appendix D-4   Chest Pain & Acute Myocardial Infarction

Criteria: Complaint of chest pain or pain in substernal area, left arm, neck, back or in epigastric area suspicious of ischemia
–and/or–
nausea, vomiting, diaphoresis, dypnea
–and/or–
heart rate 60-130 BPM
–and/or–
systolic b/p > 100 mm/hg

Protocol for chest pain/ AMI (Acute myocardial infarction)

1. Apply cardiac monitor/AED-initiate transport to closest appropriate facility if available and appropriate.
2. Assess airway- consider intubation if:
   a. GCS <8 (Glasgow coma score)
   b. Respiratory rate <10 or >32 breaths/min
   c. Airway obstructed from vomitus/secretions
3. Apply oxygen at 2 liters per minute via nasal cannula if available.
4. Give 2 chewable baby aspirin PO.(160 mg)
5. Rapidly initiate IV.
6. Give NTG 0.4 mg SL or 1 spray SL every 3 minutes until pain is relieved-maintaining   SBP>100 mm/Hg. May give fluid bolus NS 250cc for decrease in SBP<100 mm/Hg.
7. No relief after 3 doses SL NTG and SBP > 100 mm/Hg give morphine sulphate (MS) 2mg IV q5 min until pain is relieved or blood pressure decreases < 100 systolic.
8. Apply NTG paste as follows continuing to maintain SBP >100mm/Hg:
   1" for small person
   1.5" for average person
   2.0" for larger person

9. Reassess for change in chest pain, dyspnea or level of conciousness as needed.
10. If transport is delayed or cardiac catherization is not available, consider anticoagulation therapy.
    a. Give Lovenox® 1mg/kg q 12° **or** heparin 80 units/kg IV as a bolus, then heparin 17units/kg/hr
11. May give Lopressor® (metoprolol) 5mg IV X 2-3 doses **or** Lopressor® 50 mg PO to decrease heart rate to >70 beats per minute.
12. Evaluate evacuation route-
    a. What is the closest appropriate facility?
    b. Is transportation available?
    c. Is the stress of the evacuation greater than the value of the care available?
    d. Uncomplicated MI consider:
       – rest
       – pain control
       – anticoagulation therapy
       – delayed evacuation

Appendix D-5 Heat Illness, Heat Exhaustion and Heat Stroke

Criteria: Exposure to moderate (80° F) or high environmental temperatures and humidity. May occur on the second day of exposure, even if temperatures are lower.

HEAT ILLNESS – may be divided into two categories; heat exhaustion and heat stroke.

Heat exhaustion signs and symptoms:
- Fatigue
- Excessive sweating.
- Nausea and vomiting.
- Dizziness, syncope.
- Rapid heart rate, rapid breathing.
- Muscle cramping.
- Skin may be cool and dry-with "goose bumps" (consider heat stroke).
- Mild confusion (i.e. -forgetting the time).

Heat exhaustion treatment guideline:
1. Remove from the sun to cooler shaded area.
2. Remove excess clothing.
3. If cool water or ice available, sprinkle water on skin and fan to permit evaporative cooling. may immerse in water if no alteration in level of consciousness.
4. Force fluids- give oral rehydration salts or sports drink 1 liter every 2 hours.
5. If unable to tolerate oral fluids, establish IV. Give Lactated Ringers- 1000cc over 2 hours.
6. Obtain oral temperature- if temp is above 104°F, consider heat stroke.
7. REST-may need to rest and increase fluid intake for 24-48 hours.
8. Observe for signs and symptoms of heat stroke- heat exhaustion may rapidly progress to heat stroke.

Heat Stroke signs and symptoms:
Life threatening emergency:
- Altered level of consciousness- (differential to make diagnosis between heat exhaustion and heat stroke) confusion, delirium, and decreasing level of responsiveness or unresponsive.
- Hot dry skin- temp usually >104° F.
- Seizures.

Heat stroke treatment guideline:
1. Remove from sun to cooler shaded area.
2. Assess ABC's—airway, breathing and circulation.
3. Remove excess clothing.
4. Rapidly cool with ice and cool water if available-apply ice packs to axillae, groin and neck if available.
5. If cool water or ice not available, sprinkle water on skin and fan to permit evaporative cooling.
6. Evacuate to closest facility if available and appropriate—see "Evacuation" protocol.
7. May give lorazepam (Ativan®) 2 mg IV for seizure activity.
8. For prolonged seizure activity give sodium bicarbonate 1 meq/ kg IV.

Appendix D-6 Anaphylaxis

Criteria: Known or suspected contact with inhaled, ingested or topical allergen
–and–
Respiratory distress (stridor, wheezing)
–or–
Oropharynx swelling
–or–
Skin signs, flushing
–or–
SBP < 90 mmHg or MAP < 60 mmHg
mean arterial pressure = systolic(Ps) and diastolic (Pd) pressures as follows:
MAP= Pd +1/3(Ps-Pd)

Guideline:

1. Assess airway- high flow O2 if available (consider cricothyrotomy for critical airway)
2. Assess breath sounds-if wheezing or stridor found give albuterol 2.5mg via nebulizer. May repeat as needed.
3. IV resuscitate to maintain SBP >90mmHg or MAP >80 mmHg
   a. Initiate large bore IV (>18 #) with NS at wide open rate.
4. Administer
   a. (1) Epi-pen® or epinephrine 1:1,000 0.3cc SQ
   b. Benadryl® 50 mg IV
   c. Solumedrol® 125 mg IVP
5. Give H2 blocker, such as ranitidine (Zantac®) 75 mg PO, to prevent rebound
6. In extremis:
   a. epinephrine [**1:10,000**]   0.1-0.5 mg slow IVP over 1-2 min
7. If MAP <60mmHg consider epinephrine drip (epi 1mg / NS 250-titrate to MAP> 80mmHg and increase by 1mcg/min q5min)

Surgical Cricothyroidotomy—Open Technique

1. The **most** important step is to correctly identify the cricothryoid membrane. If you are right handed, stand on the victim's right side. Begin by identifying the sternal notch. Lightly run your finger up the tracheal rings until the cricothyroid cartilage is palpated. The cricothyroid membrane is just above the cricothyroid cartilage. If you start from the sternal notch, you are more likely to correctly identify the membrane than if you start from above. Firmly grasp the cricothyroid cartilage with your thumb and middle finger of your left hand. Place the index finger of your left hand on the cricothyroid membrane.

2. Holding a #11 blade in your right hand, make a vertical stab wound through the cricothyroid membrane. Rotate the blade 90°-keeping the blade stationary, use your left hand to insert a curved hemostat. Open the hemostat to dilate the incision. Keep the hemostat stationary in the stab wound. Gently remove the blade.

3. Keeping the hemostat stationary, if needed, extend the incision **downward** (toward the toes), no more than 1". Insert #6.0 endotracheal tube through the opening. Use the curve of the hemostats to guide the tube into place. Gently remove the hemostats. Inflate the cuff of the ETT. Hold securely until the ETT can be sutured in place.

4. Check placement. If the ETT is inserted too deeply, a right (or left) mainstem intubation may occur.

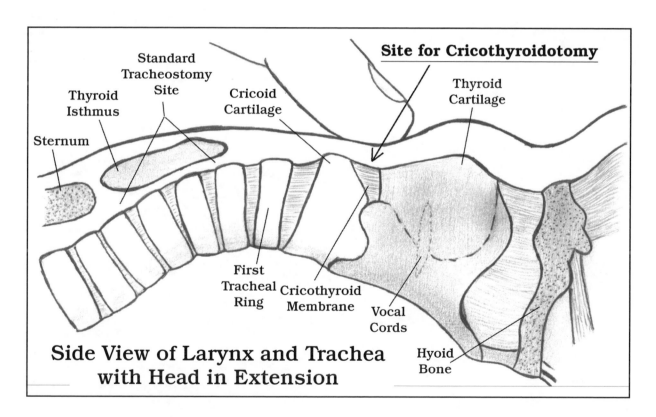

Side View of Larynx and Trachea with Head in Extension

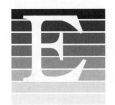 # Team Covenant[1]

Purpose Statement – The purpose of our mission trip is to **serve** the churches and people in and around _____ *(name of country)* through our medical ministry. We will be involved in **evangelistic outreach** to the patients we treat, translators and casuals we work along side of and all others, as opportunities arise, through mercy ministry.

Team Character – We commit to conform to the character of Christ through:

- **Teamwork**:
  We commit ourselves to be a group of individuals who unite as one, striving to accomplish the same goal. The goal is to glorify God in all we do and to help build His church.

- **Communications**:
  We commit ourselves to resolve all team differences and conflicts according to Biblical principles. This involves **prayer** as the first step, **personal confrontation** as the follow-up step, and the **counsel** of a third party (team leaders) as a third and final resort. In all issues we commit ourselves to maintain a humble spirit of confidentiality, while seeking to obey Ephesians 4:29 "Let no evil talk come out of your mouths, but only such as is good for edifying, as fits the occasion, that it may impart grace to those who hear." We also commit to lovingly listen to team leaders.

- **Forgiveness**:
  We commit ourselves to the recognition of sin as our common enemy so that we each may be sensitive to our human shortcomings and forgive each other. We are commanded to forgive just as Christ has forgiven us, and then we forget. In accordance with Hebrews 12:15 "See to it that no one fail to obtain the grace of God; that no "root of bitterness" spring up and cause trouble..." we commit ourselves to resolving any bitterness because we realize that bitterness will drag the whole team down.

- **Spiritual Growth**:
  We commit ourselves to personal worship and fellowship with God through obedience to the Lordship of Jesus Christ and an openness to learn from God's Spirit in all situations. We agree to have the same attitude of Paul the Apostle with respect to failure, Philippians 3:12-14, and with respect to perseverance, I Corinthians 9: 24-27.

How will we work to conform to His character?

1. **We commit** to daily team meetings for devotions, prayer, mutual encouragement, and to share experiences. (Hebrews 10:24-25, Romans 15:4).

2. **We commit** to be as faithful as possible to spend individual time with God at some time during each day as opportunity arises. (Matthew 14:23). We will also pray for other team members and team leaders.

3. **We commit** to praying with one other team member throughout the mission. We commit to affirm one another daily by encouragement through such means as written notes, small acts of service, supportive comments, etc. (Acts - 20:2).

4. **We commit** to manifesting each day the ministry and character of a disciple through being ready to forgive in conflict (confidentially involving the counsel of another only if deemed necessary), to serve as various needs arise, to work to the best of our God-given abilities and to share the Gospel in word, thought and deed as opportunities present themselves at appropriate times (Colossians 3:17 & 23).

How will we evaluate our progress toward fulfilling the Covenant?

1. Are we fulfilling our commitment to daily team meetings, devotionals and prayer (both personal and with our prayer partner)?
2. Are we on time for all team meetings, meals (including breakfast!) and departure times? We're a team, if one is late...we're all late!
3. Are we participating in any conversation that is critical or negative of another?
4. Are we complaining to others or ourselves when things don't go our way?
5. When there is an offense are we following the three-step plan?
    a. Pray
    b. Personal confrontation (go to the individual privately)
    c. Counsel (go to a team leader privately and not to others)
6. Are we exercising forgiveness?
7. When in doubt ask yourself this question, "If Christ were standing next to me (which he is) would He be pleased with the way I am acting, talking, thinking, building, serving, etc.?"
8. Am I doing anything out of selfish ambition? Or, am I esteeming others better than myself? (Philippians 2:3).

I commit myself to the team and team members, serving others before myself. I choose to abide by this covenant to the glory of God.

Signed _____   Date _____

Reference
1. Mission to the World, 2 Week Manual, 1998.

Code of Conduct for Sensitive Countries[1]

I will seek daily to submit my life to the Lord and to the authority of His word. I will ask Him to keep, strengthen, and protect me, for His love to fill me and His Spirit to sanctify me so that in the practical things of life I might be His servant and witness.

I will seek by my lifestyle and attitudes to people and to work to be an example. This includes being modest in dress and neat in appearance. It includes polite speech and behavior and circumspection in my relationships with the opposite sex. I will seek, as far as possible, to identify with my host country friends and colleagues and will avoid overindulgence in things like food and drink. I realize that to drink alcohol could cause offence to national believers and to politely refuse, even when pressed by my hosts, may be a strong unspoken witness for Christ. I will aim to live simply and be content, even if I do not have every modern convenience. I will seek to be a learner and will also willingly share my knowledge and experience with others. I will respect the national culture and customs seeking to understand and appreciate them. I will at all times obey the laws of my host country. I will not engage in political activities or arguments.

I will seek the advice of those in responsibility over me concerning any matter affecting my life and work. I will remember that my life, attitudes, and my performance do reflect on others, on my mission organization, and on the Lord. I wish therefore to be accountable, not merely to "do my own thing." I desire to cooperate with others and be a good "team player."

I will seek to faithfully fulfill my responsibilities to my hosts. I will maintain the highest standards of integrity and professionalism in my work and service. If unforeseen problems arise, I shall seek to resolve them patiently and in a culturally appropriate, as well as Christian way.

As a Christian I have a deep concern for other believers and desire for fellowship with them. However, I realize that it may not always be possible or appropriate for me to meet freely with national believers. My chief concern in this regard should be for their well being. I will remember that. Certain activities acceptable in my home country may not be acceptable in my host country. "Religious activities," such as open distribution of Christian literature or baptizing of people can, if engaged in by foreigners, cause grave misunderstanding or worse. I recognize the importance of one-to-one trusting relationships as a basis of effective sharing. I will seek to humbly and prayerfully be a witness by life and lip but will avoid actions or activities that cause unnecessary offense and which could harm others.

Signature _____ Date _____

Spouse's signature _____ Date _____

Reference
1. Adapted from Tsang, Reginald in msips.org FAQ #9, 2004.

G Medical Team Leaders' Check List

W. "Ted" Kuhn

Carry On

1. Names and addresses of all team members and emergency contact numbers
2. Insurance card and emergency contact numbers including your doctor
3. Names and addresses and contact numbers of contacts on the field
4. Flight information on all team members
5. Team finances and accounting sheets
6. Airport tax (if necessary)
7. Personal money and credit cards
8. Calling card, and phone numbers of organizational office and home phones
9. Passport, immunization records, tickets, health insurance card
10. Extra passport photos, copies of tickets, passport, driver's license and medical license
11. Polar Pure® or equivalent water purification solution for disinfection while traveling
12. Pen and legal pad for notes and ideas
13. Reading material, glasses, Bible and team devotional material
14. Extra clothes- sufficient for 1 night stay, including swimming suit and running clothes
15. Shaving kit
16. Alarm clock and extra batteries
17. Jacket or polar tech pull over
18. Sun glasses
19. Addresses and e-mail addresses of family and friends I want to write or contact
20. Medications- Aspirin, Pepto-bismol,® Claritin,® Afrin nasal spray,® chewing gum, malaria medicines, Chapstick,® cough drops, contact lens solution
21. Surveyor's tape (to identify team's baggage), duct tape and luggage straps
22. Camera and film
23. Cable locks/ zip ties to secure luggage
24. Portable pulse oximeter
25. Battery operated jet nebulizer (Omron™)

Personal Check-Through

1. Personal medical instruments (stethoscope, blood pressure cuff, otoscope, ophthalmoscope, fetal doppler with gel and extra batteries, pulse oximeter, altimeter, thermometer, ear curettes, eye chart.
2. Boots and or sandals and or running shoes
3. Clothes (shirts and socks soaked in permethrin, if necessary)
4. Mosquito net (if necessary with recently applied permethrin)
5. Sports bottle for carrying water
6. Emergency bag for team
7. Insect repellant (30% DEET) and permethrin spray
8. Isopropyl alcohol gel for cleaning hands
9. Water purification filter and coffee filters (assign several team members to bring theirs too) if obtaining pure drinking water will be a problem
10. Kleenex,® toilet paper, dirt trowel (if going rural)
11. Sun block (SPF 15-30)
12. Camping equipment (as necessary)
    a. Candles and candle holder and cigarette lighter
    b. Sleeping bag
    c. Sleeping mat and tarp for ground cloth

d. Flashlight and extra batteries
e. Roll of string (for mosquito net)
f. Towel (rapid dry)
g. Camp soap
h. Tupperware® for silverware and cup
i. Hat
j. Polar Tech® socks, pants, pullover and hat for sleeping if in cold climate
k. Pillow case for making a camp pillow

Medical Supply Check-Through

1. Medicines- see medicine list (divided in bags through out team)
2. Nursing supplies including 4x4's, 2x2's, Kerlex,® tape, scissors, bandages etc.
3. Wound care, suture, instruments, blades, Betadine,® bottle of saline, etc.
4. Syringes, needles, tourniquet, IV solution and administration set ups
5. Plastic garbage bags for used supplies (2 for each day) and sharps containers
6. Envelopes for dispensing medicines and extra pens and tape
7. 5x7 cards and Baggies® for demographic information, vital signs and medical history and physical
8. Tarps for ground cover or for hanging for shade (4 x 8 feet)
9. Reference texts
   a. *Sanford Guide to Antimicrobial Therapy*
   b. *Harriet Lane Handbook*
   c. *Tropical Medicine* text
10. Roll of paper towels

Lab Supplies Check-Through

(see Portable Lab Appendix C)

Suggested Packing List for the 10-14 Day Trip

W. "Ted" Kuhn

Carry On

(Check weight limit ahead of time- may be 10 kg or less)

1. Names and addresses of team members and emergency contact numbers
2. Travel insurance card and emergency contact numbers including medical
3. Names and addresses and contact numbers of contacts on the field
4. Flight information on team members
5. Personal monies and credit cards (clean bills)
6. Calling card, cell phone or satellite phone
7. Passport, immunization records, tickets, health insurance card
8. Extra passport photos, copies of tickets, passport, driver's license and medical license
9. Pen and legal pad for notes and ideas
10. Reading material, glasses, Bible, field educational material
11. Extra clothes- sufficient for 1 night stay
12. Shaving kit/toiletry kit
13. Alarm clock and extra batteries
14. Jacket or Polar® fleece pull over
15. Sun glasses
16. Addresses and e-mail addresses of family and friends you want to write or contact
17. Medications- Aspirin, Pepto-bismol,® Claritin® (or similar non-sedating antihistamine), Afrin nasal spray,® chewing gum, Chapstick,® cough drops, contact lens solution, prescription medicines, Diamox,® (for altitude if applicable)
18. Camera and film (in lead packing if available)
19. Cable locks/ zip ties to secure luggage

Personal Check-Through

(One bag- check weight limit- most international and domestic flights limit check-through to 50 pounds each

1. Personal medical instruments (stethoscope, blood pressure cuff, otoscope, ophthalmoscope)
2. Boots and or hiking shoes
3. Clothes (shirt and pants dipped in permethrin if going into a malaria endemic zone)
4. Sports bottle for carrying water
5. Sun block
6. Insect repellant (30% DEET) and permethrin spray
7. Isopropyl alcohol gel for cleaning hands
8. Kleenex,® toilet paper
9. Camping equipment as necessary
   a. Sleeping bag
   b. Sleeping mat for ground
   c. Flash light and extra batteries
   e. Towel (rapid dry)
   f. Camp soap®
   g. Hat
   h. Pillow case for making a camp pillow
   i. Mosquito net as needed (dipped in permethrin)
   j. Water purification supplies as needed
   k. Cooking supplies as needed
   l. Dirt trowel (if you expect to need a pit latrine)

Team Check-Through

(Check weight limit- probably 50 lbs each bag)

"One bag for you-one bag for the team." (prepare to be asked to carry medical supplies, lab equipment, or educational materials in one of your check-through bags). Make sure you know what is in this bag before check-in at the airport. Airport security will question you about the contents of the bag and whether someone else gave it to you and what it contains. Know before you go.

IMPORTANT NOTE: Don't carry any knives or sharp implements in carry-on, including nail scissors and small pocket knives. They will be removed and confiscated during security check. You can carry in your check-through luggage. Also if you carry medical equipment, e.g stethoscope, otoscope etc. in your carry-on, keep it separate from your personal items and place in container for laptops before going through x-ray. It will keep security from going through your personal belongings.

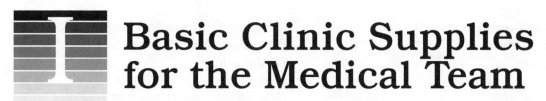

Basic Clinic Supplies for the Medical Team

Sharon C. Kuhn and W. "Ted" Kuhn

General: triage, set-up and patient evaluation
- Charts
- Tarp
- Indelible markers
- Pill bags (small Baggies®)
- Pens
- Labels
- Tongue depressors
- Pill counters
- "Caution" tape or surveyor's tape
- Pill cutters
- Duct tape
- Syringes (3cc, 5cc, 10cc and 60 cc)
- Rope or twine
- Alcohol wipes (a lot)
- Thermometers
- Needles
- B/P cuffs
- Garbage bags
- Broselow tape®
- Rubber bands
- Otoscope /opthalmoscopes
- Scotch® tape
- Pen lights
- Hand sanitizer
- Scissors
- Paper Towels (1-2 rolls)

Wound Care
- Hydrogen peroxide
- Saline for irrigation
- Betadine®
- Gloves
- Sterile gloves
- Gauze: 4x4's, 2x2's (some sterile, some not)
- Steri-strips®
- Kling®
- Non-stick dressings
- Super glue® or Dermabond®
- Ace® wraps 3"
- SAM® splints
- Tape 1", 2"
- Antibiotic ointments, Silvadene®

Instruments for Suturing and Other Needs:
- Suture material, assorted
- Hemostats
- Forceps
- Scissors
- Needle drivers
- Skin stapler
- Xylocaine 1% with & w/o epinephrine
- Scalpels
- Sterile field supplies
- Iodoform packing gauze

IV Supplies
- IV fluids, normal saline or lactated ringers. (Most in liter bags, but consider taking some smaller bags for small children and for giving medicine.)
- IV tubing
- IV catheters and butterflies, in assorted sizes
- IV start kits (tourniquets, alcohol wipes, tape)
- Heplock® caps
- Heparin flush
- Sharps container
- Sterile saline and sterile water for mixing IV/IM medications

Pelvic Exam Equipment
    Speculums
    KY Jelly®
    Gloves
    Flashlight

Limited Lab Supplies
(For full laboratory inventory see "Test and Supply List for Portable Laboratory")
    Urine dipsticks
    Urine pregnancy tests
    Small plastic cups for specimen collection

Hemacue® (hemaglobinometer)
Glucometer® with test strips
Dextrosticks®
Lancets
Hemoccult® w/ developer

Supplies that can be obtained in country:
Buckets and basins for wound care and for cleaning instruments.
Chlorine bleach for cleaning instruments

Suggested Medicine List

Sharon C. Kuhn

Antibiotics

- Include different classes and coverage.
- Liquid and chewable formulations for children.
- IM or IV antibiotics for severe infections.
- You may use 10-20 courses per 100 patients.

Amoxicillin
Augmentin®
Zithromax®or erythromycin or clarithromycin
Fluoroquinolones (Cipro®Levaquin®
Cephalosporins (Keflex,®Rocephin,® a second generation formulation)
TMP-SX (Septra DS®) (Take much more when ministering to HIV/AIDS patients for propylaxis or treatment of PCP pneumonia)
Metronidazole
Doxycycline, tetracycline
H. pylori treatment packs in areas of high prevalence
Antibiotic eyedrops or ointment (10)
Ear drops (5-10 eg. Cortisporin)
Antibiotic skin ointment (10-20 tubes)

Antimalarials

Quinine
Fansidar®
Chloroquine

Antifungals

Creams (20 tubes)
Vaginal creams or tabs (10 courses)
Pills: Nizoral,® Diflucan® (200-300 tablets depending on destination. For treating tinea capitis and severe skin infections, for candidal esophagitis in AIDS patients, for vaginal yeast infections.)

Analgesics

Most frequently prescribed medicines for adults: Allow for at least 10 days of therapy. Much of the pain is chronic. Only a few bottles of liquid or chewable medicines for kids with fever or pain will be needed.
NSAIDS (ibuprofen, naproxen)
Acetaminophen
Also helpful:
Aspirin
Ultram®
Muscle relaxants
Kenalog® for injection
Toradol® injectable
Note: Controlled substances can only be taken into a country in small quantities with proper licensing and documentation.
Migraine: A triptan class medication

Vitamins and Iron

Adult
Children's chewable and liquid
Prenatal (including folic acid and iron)
Iron (ferrous sulfate)
Consider a small amount of IM B12 and thiamine
(Usually give 30 days worth)

Cardiovascular/Antihypertensive

Quantity needed varies depending on destination, e.g. very few needed for the Indians of Peruvian jungle but more helpful in Philippines. Generic medicines that may be available in the country of destination are best.

Beta blockers
ACE Inhibitors (may use in low doses
    where diabetes is also common)
Diuretic
ASA
Furosemide (small amount for urgent
    use)
Nitrates (a few tabs or patches)
Cardura® or terazosin (enough for 2-3
    patients with BPH) if it's available

GI Medicines

H2 Blockers
Proton Pump Inhibitors
(UGI pain is a very common complaint
    in many areas. 5-10 pts per 100
    and many need 30 days of treatment
    if possible)
TUMS® or Maalox®
Promethazine (a few-25-50 tabs for team
    and patients.)
Loperamide (few unless treating AIDS
    patients)
Gatorade® or other rehydration pow-
    der.
IV fluids: normal saline of lactated ring-
    ers are most useful

Diabetic Medicines

Diabetes for some destinations (rare in
    Indians of Peruvian Jungle, common
    in Hispanics)
Glucophage®
Glypizide,® etc.

Respiratory

Inhalers (few, including albuterol)
Singulaire,® etc. or Albuterol® tabs for
    one or 2 pts/100
Antihistamines
Decongestants

Antiparasitic

Metronidazole
Albendazole or Mebendazole for worms
    (10 /100pts)

Psychiatric and Chronic Pain (in small
    amounts)

Antidepressants
Amitriptyline
Trazadone®

Miscellaneous

Epinephrine for allergic rxn
Prednisone (50-100 tabs only for severe
    asthma or allergic rxn.)
Diphenhydramine (IM and PO) or Atarax
    (for itching, allergies, etc.) 100 tabs or
    less
Skin: Steroid creams (tubes 10-20)
Silver sulfadiazine, Silvadene® for
    burns
Scabies medicine, if available (more com-
    mon in cities and street kids.)
Medicine for altitude sickness in helpers
    (Diamox,® nifedipine)

Nursing Supplies: (See "Basic Clinic Supplies" also in this appendix for more complete listing)

IV fluids (normal saline or lactated ring-
    ers): several liters.
May include smaller bags of 250cc or
    500cc for children or giving IV
    meds.

Remember: IV tubing, tourniquets, angio-
caths, butterflies, alcohol swabs, needles
and syringes. Sterile saline and sterile water
for mixing IM/IV meds.

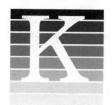

Guidelines for Worm Pill Distribution (Albendazole)

Adapted from Worm Pill Project[1]

Worm pills, mebendazole, Vermox® and albendazole (Albenza®), are a great asset to people suffering from intestinal worms. They act to remove the adult worms from the intestinal area where they formerly fed on the nourishment intended for the human body.

The pills are flavored and chewable so are easily administered. They can be taken before or after eating. Some children may experience some stomach uneasiness as an after affect. Since many people, and especially children, have an aversion to pills it may be wise to ask them to stick out their tongue to be sure they have chewed and swallowed it.

The pills have a shelf life of about three years. They should be stored in the driest area of a building and away from direct sunlight. The dosage of Albendazole® is just ONE 400 mg. pill for anyone above two years of age (World Food Program recommendation). (If you have mebendazole or Vermox® 100 mg instead of Albendazole, you may need to give several doses. You should check with a doctor or pharmacist for the appropriate dosing.)

A few cautions are in order: Administering the pill to a child under two years of age should only be done under the supervision of a doctor. Also, recent research indicates that it is safe for a pregnant woman to take the pill. However, in some countries they are still following former guidelines where it is prohibited to give the pill to any woman of child-bearing age. It is necessary to check with the ministry of health in your particular country to see what the rules are. Otherwise legal problems may arise. Some countries may require the distribution be done under the supervision of a doctor. Even though there is no statistical significance of problems if given in the first trimester of pregnancy it is advisable to tell a pregnant woman to keep the pill and take it after the first trimester (if that country allows pregnant women to be treated).

The large Ascaris can migrate out of the child's nose or mouth. In this case one dose of Piperazine prevents this. Piperazine is inexpensive and widely available.

In general, the pills should be distributed every six months. However, some countries have a policy of dispensing every four months if the infestation is severe. Usually a program should be run for two to three years. During this two or three year period it is highly recommended that steps be taken to improve sanitation such as:

1. Education on washing hands (especially before meals) AND fingernails (one group sent a large number of clippers along to pass out to families).
2. Work toward a safe drinking water supply.
3. Building latrines. Until this is done the Biblical injunction to "...dig a hole and cover up your excrement" (Deuteronomy 23:13) should be followed.

In the washing of hands and fingernails the life cycle of the worm is broken since the worm eggs are picked up in the soil. If not, the eggs (200,000 a day by one adult female) are swallowed and then hatch in the intestinal area. Doing these three steps the worm population can be greatly reduced.

It is also recommended that an entire community be treated within a one week period so as to keep one area from infecting another. If this is not possible the second best is to assure that an entire family be treated at the same time.

Although not directly related to the worm problem, the nutritional deficit is often exacerbated by the introduction of highly refined, empty calorie "foods" into poor communities such as cookies, candies, cakes and sodas. They lure people to spend their very scarce food money on these high-cost items with little or no return in nourishment. One chicken or duck egg costs far less than a soda but provides much needed protein and fat in areas where these are in very short supply.

References
1. Adapted from Claude Good- Worm Pill Project

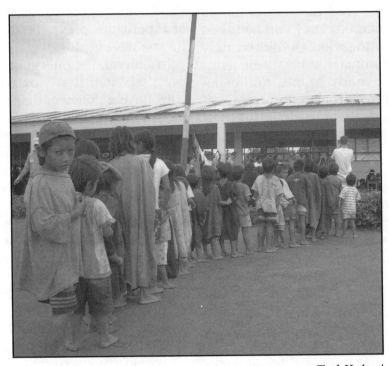

Ted Kuhn/
**"Worm Pill Distribution to School
Children in Amazon"**

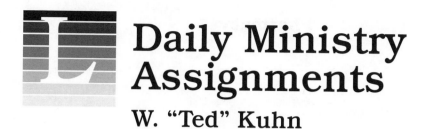

Daily Ministry Assignments

W. "Ted" Kuhn

Daily Ministry Assignments

DAY and DATE:

Village:

Team Leader-

Morning Devotions

1.

Evening Debriefing

1.

Medical Providers

1.

2.

3.

4.

5.

6.

**Students Seeing Patients
with Provider**

1.

2.

3.

4.

5.

6.

Laboratory

1.

2.

Pharmacy

1.

2.

Triage

1.

2.

3.

4.

Evangelism and Prayer

1.

2.

3.

4.

Home Visits

1.

2.

3.

4.

Emergency Bag
(keep bag with team at all times)

1.

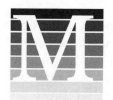

Sample Prayer Requests

Brian Stansfield

1. *"For I long to see you, that I may impart some spiritual gift to strengthen you-that is, that we may be mutually encouraged by each other's faith, both yours and mine."* (Rom 1:11-12) We long to go to encourage the church there and to be encouraged. Pray for us and them that we will continue in our passion for one another now and long after our return. Also that we might all be spiritually refreshed.

2. *"In your goodness, O God, you provided for the needy."* (Psalm 68:10) We are all in need of God to provide. Pray with us that God would provide the necessary money to go to ..... Please pray that God would provide us with facilities to practice medicine. Most important, that He would provide an overflow of his Spirit into each of us and to those that we meet.

3. *"No lion shall be there, nor shall any ravenous beast come up on it; they shall not be found there, but the redeemed shall walk there."* (Isa 35:9) We need God's sovereign and safe hand upon us. We are going into unfamiliar territory with only the Lord at our side and a few churches in our sight. Pray that the Lord will provide safety and open doors for the team and the churches.

4. *"For there the Lord has commanded the blessing, life forevermore."* (Psalm 133) David spoke these words in reference to the unity of brothers. A team that stands together, moves together, and thinks together will find great success. Pray that our team will interact in such a way, that those we meet will yearn for fellowship such as ours. May selfishness be pushed aside and brotherhood be the theme.

5. *"And the Lord will take away from you all sickness..."* (Deut 7:15) In order for us to complete the task set before us, we must be functioning as health care providers. Pray that God would keep us well so that we might complete the mission in its fullness.

6. *"Ascribe to the Lord the glory due his name; bring an offering and come before him! Worship the Lord in the splendor of holiness."* (1 Chron. 16:29) May we wake every morning in praise to God. May we work with diligence as an offering unto Him. May we spend each evening in the splendor of holiness. For only in worship unto God will we find joy in our task.

7. *"But his delight is in the law of the Lord, and on his law he meditates day and night."* (Psalm 1:2) In this time, we desire intense reading and studying of the word of God. Pray that God grants us the discipline and joy that comes from meditating on his holy scriptures.

8. *"And he said to the reapers, 'The Lord be with you!' And they answered, 'The Lord bless you.'* (Ruth 2:4) Pray that we are able to greet one another with a kind word and encourage one another with the word of the Lord.

9. *"I remember the days of old; I meditate on all that you have done; I ponder the work of your hands."* (Psalm 143:5) We look forward to all the great things our Lord will do in ..... May we remind ourselves often of his raised victorious hand and the power of his deeds.

May we see the Lord work in ways that enlarge our vision of Him.

10. *"And let us not grow weary of doing good, for in due season we will reap, if we do not give up."* (Gal 6:9) God has brought us to this place for a special purpose. Please pray that we work with all our hearts in everything we do so that the glory of God might be revealed in its fullness.

11. *"Then Abraham prayed to God, and God healed Abimelech."* (Genesis 20: 17) This verse is full of rich meaning for both of us. For you, the power of prayer is revealed in such a simple way. Thus please pray with faith that God is mighty to do everything that you ask. For us, we may bring health to these people only through God for it is He that heals the sick. May we aid in healing their bodies, but more so, aid in healing their souls.

12. *"And the king granted me what I asked, for the good hand of my God was upon me."* (Nehemiah 2:8b) Only as the good hand of God is upon us, may we accomplish anything that we have set out to do.

This is by far an inexhaustive list of prayers that we need before, during and after our time in... But imagine if only this group of prayers were answered. How awesome and successful would this trip be. But our God is bigger than the heavens and the earth and he can accomplish whatever pleases him. May we be pleasing in His sight.

Please commit to us in prayer. It gives me courage to know that God has brought people along side us to provide the prayers necessary for the salvation of a nation. We **are** ready!

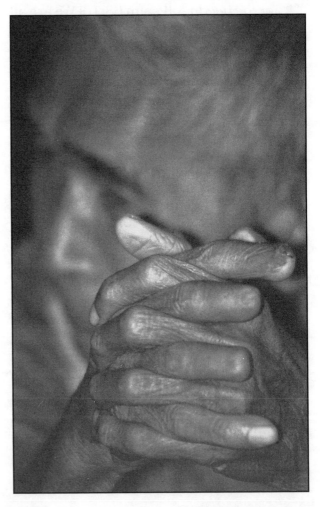

Lydia Kuhn/
"Folded Hands"

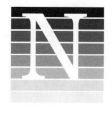 # Non-Denominational Christian Statement of Faith[1]

1. We believe in the one, holy, sovereign, creating and redeeming God, eternally existing in three Persons, Father, Son and Holy Spirit.

2. We believe in the divine inspiration, the inerrancy of the original manuscripts and the entire trustworthiness of the Bible: its infallible teaching and supreme authority in all matters of faith and conduct; and its normative value for all peoples, at all times, in all cultures.

3. We believe that all people without distinction are made in the image of God, but all are now sinners and have incurred both God's holy wrath and their own shame and guilt. All are therefore in utter need of redemption.

4. We believe in Jesus Christ our Lord, the incarnate Son of God, uniquely God-man and the only Savior. We believe in His virgin birth, sinless life, sacrificial death, bodily resurrection and ascension. We believe He has achieved the final defeat of Satan and all evil powers.

5. We believe in the justification of sinners by God's grace, through faith in Christ alone.

6. We believe in the Holy Spirit and in His convicting, regenerating, sanctifying and reviving work. He guides and empowers individuals and churches in their service to God and man.

7. We believe in the unity and priesthood of all believers who together form the one, holy, universal, apostolic church.

8. We believe in the visible, personal return of Jesus Christ in power and great glory to judge both the living and the dead. We believe that the scriptures set out only two destinies for humanity: the joyful prospect of eternal life in the presence of God for those who have received Christ, and the agonizing prospect of eternal separation from God for those who have rejected Him.

Having carefully read this Doctrinal Statement, I declare my acceptance of it as embodying my convictions concerning the Christian faith.

Signed _____   Date _____

Reference
1. Adapted from Tsang, Reginald in msips.org FAQ #7, 2004.

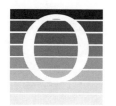 # List of Medicines for Home Visits to AIDS Patients

MTW Medical Department

When making home visits to HIV/AIDS patients, some of whom may be too ill to travel to a clinic or hospital, a simple supply of medicines is helpful to address the medical needs of these patients. These can be easily carried in a small back-pack. The following list is the result of several years experience in visiting the homes of these patients.

Trimethoprim-sulfa (Septra,® Bactrim®) - good for treatment of AIDS patients with wasting
Quinolone (Cipro,® Levaquin®)
Cephalexin - great for Staph or Strep skin infections
Fluconazole (Diflucan®) for thrush
Gentian Violet for thrush
Metronidazole (Flagyl®)
Albendazole (Albenza®) for worms
Anti-scabies cream
Anti-fungal cream
Steroid cream
Topical antibiotic cream
Antibiotic eye drops/ointment
"Magic mouth wash" (viscous lidocaine, Benedryl® liquid, and Maalox®) for use in sore mouth secondary to thrush or HIV related gingivo-stomatitis
Analgesics/antipyretics: acetaminophen (Tylenol®) and NSAIDs (ibuprofen) for fever and pain
Vitamins for adult and children (Do not use preparation with iron for patients with TB)

Iron Supplements
ORS (Oral rehydration solution) or just instruct, 2 small spoons of sugar and 2 pinches of salt in a cup of boiled water that has cooled

Guideline for the Prophylactic Use of Trimethoprim/Sulfa (Bactrim®) in AIDS Patients[1]

Administer one Bactrim DS® or Septra DS® daily for clinical stage 2 or 3 of the WHO staging system for HIV.

Clinical Stage 2:

Weight loss, <10% of body weight
Minor muco-cutaneous manifestations
Herpes Zoster within the last 5 year
Recurrent upper respiratory tract infections, and/or performance scale 2: symptomatic, normal activity

Clinical Stage 3:

Weight loss, > 10% of body weight
Unexplained chronic diarrhea, >1 month
Unexplained prolonged fever (intermittent or constant), > 1 month
Oral candidiasis
Oral leukoplakia
Pulmonary TB, within the past year
Severe bacterial infections and/or performance scale: bed-ridden, > 50% of day during past month

Reference
1. Lancet, May 1, 1999, Vol. 353:1463-1468

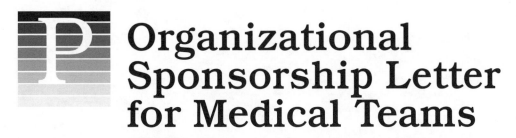

Organizational Sponsorship Letter for Medical Teams

MTW Medical Department

Organizational Letterhead

Certificate of Donation

To Whom It May Concern:

This is to certify that the items appearing on the listing of donations to

_____ **MD**

Dated (**DATE**) are donated at no cost from **Sending Agency** to

Destination Country

and any costs involved are paid for by contributions of **Sending Agency** and various other people and companies in the United States of America outside of

Destination Country
with no Currency of
Destination Country
to be involved in the transaction.

These items are not for resale and are to be used solely for the charitable medical work of:

Sending Agency

Sincerely,

Director of sending agency   Organizational seal   and

Address of sending agency   Notary stamp

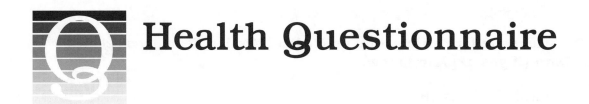

Health Questionnaire

Health Questionnaire for Participation on Medical Mission Team
(Modified from The Outdoor Leadership Handbook, Green P. Tacoma, Washington 1982, Emergency Response Institute)

Medical Team Leader

Trip Coordinator _____

Dates of Trip _____ Location of Trip _____ Difficulty Level _____

Name _____

Address _____

_____

Phone (   ) _____ E-mail _____

Age _____ Height _____ Weight _____

Person to contact in emergency, address, and telephone number

Name _____

Address _____

_____

Phone (   ) _____ E-mail _____

Name of personal physician, address, and phone

Name _____

Address _____

_____

Phone (   ) _____

Name address and contract number of health insurance carrier

Name _____

Address _____

_____

Phone (   ) _____ Group Number_____

Overall Health Status (circle one)   Poor Fair   Good   Excellent

Overall physical condition (circle one)   Poor   Good, but out of shape

Can jog/run 3-5 miles   Excellent aerobic fitness   Fit for extreme conditions

Health Questionnaire for Participation on Medical Mission Team *(page 2)*
Medical Data (if yes explain below)

1. Allergies (drug, food, insects, etc.)
2. Diabetes, thyroid, endocrine
3. Seizures, migraine, stroke, black-out spells
4. Heart problems (heart murmur, coronary artery disease, irregular heart beat)
5. High blood pressure
6. Lung problems (emphysema, asthma, bronchitis, shortness of breath)
7. Kidney problems, frequent infections, kidney stones
8. Injuries or problems with joints (list joints affected) Ankle, knee, hip, fingers/toes, wrist, elbow, shoulder, back/spine, other
9. Anemia or blood disorders, problems with liver
10. Pregnancy, irregular vaginal bleeding, vaginitis
11. Urinary, bladder or prostate problems
12. Visual or hearing problems (glasses prescription)
13. Other (infections, etc.)

Explain all positive answers here or on supplemental sheet.

Immunizations (Circle immunizations that are current)

influenza	measles	mumps	rubella	tetanus
diphtheria	polio	typhoid	hepatitis A	hepatitis B
yellow fever	cholera	varicella	BCG	rabies
meningococcal	pneumococcal			

Are you taking malaria prophylaxis?   yes   no   Which drug?
Are you taking any drug to treat or prevent travelers' diarrhea?   yes   no

Wilderness/ travel history   (circle if you have ever had and explain below)

mountain sickness	hypoxia	nosebleeds
frostbite	pulmonary edema	HIV
sun/snow blindness	heatstroke	hypothermia
envenomation	malaria	cerebral edema
other tropical disease		

List any medical problems, illness, injuries, chronic conditions that you have had in the last 3 years.

List any medications that you are currently taking including dosing (include birth control pills, vitamins, and natural supplements). What medications are you carrying with you?

What are your fears or weaknesses regarding participation on this team/trip?

What personal strengths do you possess that may contribute to the success or safety of this team/trip?

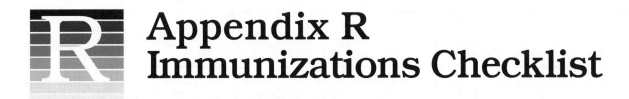
TRAVAX® Traveler Health Report
AMLT
VACCINE INFORMATION

The boxes checked below indicate travel and routine immunizations that have been recommended by your health care provider for your specific itinerary and risk activities. As noted, some vaccines require more than 1 dose to complete the immunization series, so you may need to return for the remaining doses before your trip so that you are properly protected.

Given	Declined	Given at Patient Request	
			Hepatitis A virus causes liver infection with fever and jaundice. Although rarely life-threatening, this illness can be severe and recovery can be prolonged. Infection is passed by consuming contaminated food or water. The initial dose of vaccine protects for a year or more and a second dose (booster) given at least 6 months after the first dose will confer life-long protection. A combined hepatitis A/B vaccine is also available (see below).
			Hepatitis A/B combination vaccine is given in 3 doses (at 0, 1, and 6 months). An accelerated schedule used by many travel medicine practitioners is 3 doses (given on days 0, 7, and 21), which then necessitates a fourth dose at 1 year.
			Hepatitis B virus causes severe liver infection with fever and jaundice. Infection can become chronic and lead to liver failure or cancer. Hepatitis B virus is transmitted by use of nonsterile needles (such as might be found in hospitals in a developing country or used for tattooing or body piercing). The virus also can be transmitted by contaminated blood products and sexual contact. Hepatitis B vaccine is given in 3 doses (at 0, 1, and 6 months) or can be given in an accelerated schedule of 4 doses (at 0, 1, 2, and 12 months) or 3 doses (at 0, 1, and 4 months). An alternate accelerated schedule consists of 4 total doses: 3 doses given on days 0, 7, and 21, followed by a fourth dose 1 year later. This vaccine provides long-term and possibly lifetime protection, once the series is complete. As noted above, a combined hepatitis A/hepatitis B vaccine is also available.
			Typhoid fever is a serious bacterial infection that spreads through the bloodstream, resulting in high fever, belly pain, and either diarrhea or constipation. Infection is acquired by consuming contaminated food or water. One dose of injectable typhoid vaccine protects for 2-3 years. Four doses of the oral vaccine (given on days 0, 2, 4, and 6) provide 5-6 years of protection. Nausea and cramps may occur with the oral vaccine.

Given	Declined	Given at Patient Request	
			Yellow fever is an often life-threatening viral illness spread by mosquitoes in the Amazon basin of South America and sub-Saharan Africa. Yellow fever vaccine may be recommended or required for travel to or from these countries. One dose is given and becomes effective in about 10 days and protects for 10 years or more. Flu-like symptoms might occur 7-14 days after vaccination (occurring in about 2-5% of persons), and rarely, encephalitis can occur. *This vaccine cannot be used by persons allergic to eggs.*
			Japanese encephalitis is a viral infection of the brain that is transmitted by the bite of an infected mosquito incertain rural areas of Asia. Three doses of vaccine (given on days 0, 7, and 30) provide protection for about 3 years. An accelerated schedule of 3 doses given on days 0, 7, and 14 may be used if necessary. Flu-like symptoms may occur after vaccination in about 10% of people. Serious but delayed allergic reactions can occur up to 10 days after vaccination in less than 1/2 of one percent of persons and may be more likely in persons with multiple severe allergies. Neurologic complications are very rare.
			Meningococcal infection is spread by respiratory secretions and causes a severe illness with fever, rash, and (often) meningitis that may lead rapidly to death. Risk is highest during the dry season (December through June) in certain areas of sub-Saharan Africa. A single dose protects for 3 years.
			Rabies is a fatal disease transmitted by animals (most commonly dogs and bats) or other humans; rabies is more common in developing countries. Preexposure vaccination may be advised for prolonged stays, young children, or certain activities in areas where rabies is found. Three doses are given (on days 0, 7, and 21-28). Neurologic reactions can be a concern with some rabies products made abroad. If you are exposed or if there is a potential that you have been exposed to rabies, you must seek medical attention even if you have had the preexposure series.
			Cholera is spread by contaminated food or water and causes diarrhea that can range from mild to very severe. Outbreaks occur mostly after natural and man-made disasters, and the vaccine is indicated mainly for aid or refugee workers. Infection is rare in typical travelers. Vaccination is no longer required for entry into any country. Cholera vaccine is not available in the USA, but oral cholera vaccines are available in Canada and elsewhere and may often be obtained en route. These vaccines provide protection for up to 6 months.
			Diphtheria and Tetanus: Diphtheria is a potentially fatal infection that is common in developing countries. Tetanus (lockjaw) is caused by contamination of cuts or wounds. All travelers should have completed the primary series and receive boosters every 10 years thereafter. More frequent booster doses may be suggested in some cases.

Given	Declined	Given at Patient Request	
			Measles, Mumps, and Rubella: Measles in a potentially serious illness with fever, cough, and rash. Mumps may cause brain infection or infertility in males. Rubella (German measles) usually causes mild fever and rash but can be devastating to a developing fetus. All three diseases are common in developing countries and can be prevented with live MMR vaccine. Persons born before 1957 may be immune already; persons born in or after 1957 may need 1 or 2 doses (given 28 days apart) before travel. Fever and/or rash may occur 5-12 days after vaccination.
			Polio is a viral illness that is spread by contaminated food and water and can result in paralysis or death. Everyone should have a primary series. A one-time adult booster dose is advisable for persons traveling to risk areas. An injectable killed vaccine is used routinely in the United States and Canada.
			Influenza is a viral infection that causes fever, headache, muscle aches, and lung infection and occurs year round in the tropics. All travelers should consider this vaccine, since outbreaks have been linked to travel by plane, train, and cruise ship, in particular. Persons over the age of 50 years or who have a chronic illness or suppressed immune system should be vaccinated regardless of travel plans. Influenza vaccine is available as an injection (inactivated) or a nasal spray (live weakened virus). After the injection, flu-like symptoms might occur for 1-2 days; after the nasal spray immunization, mild symptoms such as runny nose or nasal congestion, cough, headache, sore throat, chills, and a feeling of tiredness or weakness might occur. *Persons with egg allergy should not use this vaccine.* Vaccine only lasts for the current flu season.
			Varicella (chickenpox) is a viral illness spread by respiratory droplets; it causes an itchy blister-like rash. Bacterial infections commonly follow the illness. Adults are at increased risk of severe illness. Adults who are not immune to chickenpox and who plan long-term travel should consider getting this vaccine. Varicella, a live vaccine, is given in 2 doses 4-8 weeks apart and provides prolonged protection. Uncommonly, a blister-like rash might occur after vaccination.

Reference:
1. Travax Traveler Health Report. www.travax.com, Shoreland, Inc., 2004.

Index

2

6

Global Medical Missions - Index

WHO   262
women, attire for   48
women, personal safety   107
women, social customs   51
women, traveling abroad   53
Worldwide Laboratory Improvement   263
World Health Organization (WHO)
        rehydration formula   140
worm pill   303

wound   194–197
Wright's   280

Y
yellow fever   21–22, 24, 26, 28, 87
yellow fever vaccine   24, 26

Z
Zip-Spin®   279

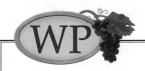

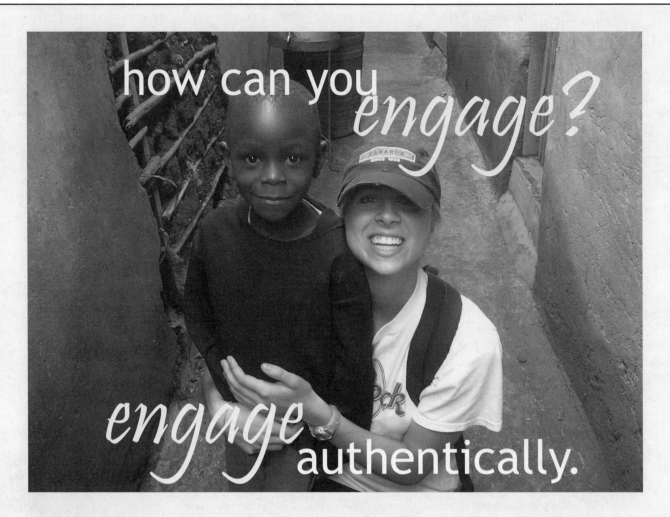

engage. Not simply in medicine, but in heart, touch, authenticity and grace. MTW Global Support Ministries opens the door into medical missions opportunities in more than 20 different countries around the world.

But even with opportunities in more than 20 countries, it may only take one authentic encounter to change your life and the life of another.

go. connect. engage.

MEDICAL MISSIONS
MTW Global Support Ministries
medical@mtw.org

Mission to the World   1600 North Brown Road   Lawrenceville, GA   30043   (678) 823-0004   www.mtw.org